# HEARING DISORDERS IN CHILDREN

# Hearing Disorders in Children

## Pediatric Audiology

EDITED BY

## FREDERICK N. MARTIN

5341 Industrial Oaks Blvd.
Austin, Texas 78735

Printed in the United States of America


**Library of Congress Cataloging-in-Publication Data**

Hearing disorders in children

    Includes bibliographies and index.
    1. Hearing disorders in children.  I. Martin,
Frederick N. [DNLM: 1. Hearing Disorders—in infancy
& childhood. WV 271 H4347]
RF291.5.C45H3183  1987      618.92'0978      86-30594
ISBN 0-89079-144-9

5341 Industrial Oaks Boulevard
Austin, Texas 78735

10  9  8  7  6  5  4  3  2  1     87  88  89  90  91

*To Cathy, David, and Leslie-Anne*

# Contents

# Contributing Authors

**Charles I. Berlin, PhD**
Professor, Physiology and
  Otorhinolaryngology
Director, Kresge Hearing Research
  Laboratory
Louisiana State University Medical
  Center
New Orleans, Louisiana
(Chapter 5)

**Patricia R. Cole, PhD**
Director, Austin Center for Speech,
  Language, and Learning Disorders
Austin, Texas
(Chapter 4)

**Victor P. Garwood, PhD**
Professor, Communication Arts and
  Sciences and Otolaryngology
University of Southern California
Los Angeles, California
(Chapter 13)

**William R. Hodgson, PhD**
Professor, Speech and Hearing
  Sciences
University of Arizona
Tucson, Arizona
(Chapter 6)

**Linda J. Hood, PhD**
Postdoctoral Fellow
Kresge Hearing Research Laboratory
Louisiana State University Medical
  Center
New Orleans, Louisiana
(Chapter 5)

**David M. Luterman, DEd**
Professor, Division of
  Communication Disorders
Emerson College
Boston, Massachusetts
(Chapter 9)

**Frederick N. Martin, PhD**
Lillie Hage Jamail Centennial
  Professor
Department of Speech
  Communication
The University of Texas at Austin
Austin, Texas
(Chapter 8)

**Antonia Brancia Maxon, PhD**
Director, UCONN Mainstream
  Project
Department of Communication
  Sciences
The University of Connecticut
Storrs, Connecticut
(Chapter 11)

**A. Boyd Morgan, MD**
Private Practice in Otolaryngology
Austin, Texas
(Chapter 1)


**Laurie Newton, PhD**
Principal, Deaf-Blind Department
Texas School for the Blind
Austin, Texas
(Chapter 10)


**Polly E. Patrick, MS**
Coordinator, Audiology Clinics
Oklahoma Teaching Hospitals
University of Oklahoma Health
  Sciences Center
Department of Otorhinolaryngology
Oklahoma City, Oklahoma
(Chapter 12)


**Peter V. Paul, PhD**
Associate Professor, Department of
  Human Services Education
The Ohio State University
Columbus, Ohio
(Chapter 2)


**Stephen P. Quigley, PhD**
Professor, Education and Speech and
  Hearing Science

University of Illinois at
  Urbana-Champaign
Urbana, Illinois
(Chapter 2)


**Ross J. Roeser, PhD**
Associate Professor and Chief of
  Audiology
Callier Center for Communication
  Disorders
The University of Texas at Dallas
Dallas, Texas
(Chapter 7)


**Deborah S. Rose, MD**
Psychiatrist in Private Practice
Palo Alto, California
Assistant Clinical Professor
Department of Psychiatry and
  Behavioral Sciences
Stanford University
Palo Alto, California
(Chapter 3)


**Wende Yellin, MS**
Faculty Associate
Department of Otolaryngology
University of Texas Health Science
  Center at Dallas
Dallas, Texas
(Chapter 7)

# *Preface*

*I*n the past decade we have gained many new insights into the language deficits experienced by children with hearing loss. The profession of audiology has experienced quantum leaps in the area of amplification, as seen in the latest forms of wearable hearing aids and other assistive listening devices. The emphasis on early detection of hearing loss is even greater today than ever before, with the talents of teams of experts utilized whenever possible.

The contributing authors bring to this book a great deal of sophistication in dealing with problems of auditory disorders in children. Each has a significant amount of clinical experience with children and is a recognized scholar. For this reason I have asked each of the authors to depart from the traditional third person in their writing and to clearly identify their own philosophies, theories, and even their biases. The reader will thus be aware of differences between the authors' personal opinions and prevailing views of the literature.

The purpose of this book is to provide information for persons who work or plan to work at the professional level with hearing-impaired children and their caretakers. Each author was advised to assume no knowledge on the reader's part beyond the basic audiology course and to take the reader as far as possible in each particular subject within the allotted space. I believe they have done this very well.

Frederick N. Martin

*The child who is normal, and easy to teach,*
  *Will need and deserve our care.*
*But the child with a problem has further to reach,*
  *And should get a more bountiful share.*

                                    *A.J.S.*

# PART I
## Causes and Effects

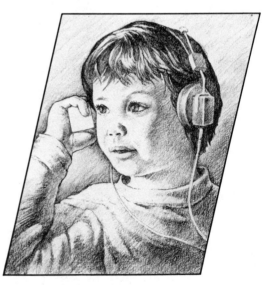

*B*efore remedial work can begin with the hearing-impaired child, the professional worker must understand the causes of hearing impairment, the effects of such impairment on the development of speech and language, the psychological implications of hearing loss, and the ways in which language disorders caused by factors other than hearing loss may make diagnosis and treatment more difficult.

In Chapter 1, Boyd Morgan outlines hearing impairments in children from a practical clinical point of view. The illustrative cases help the clinician to understand these disorders without requiring an in-depth background in otology. Peter Paul and Stephen Quigley, in Chapter 2, bring the reader up to date on the speech and language difficulties experienced by the hearing-impaired child, contrasting the development in normal-hearing children to their acoustically handicapped peers. Deborah Rose brings her experience and training as a clinical psychiatrist to bear in Chapter 3 as she explores the psychological experiences of hearing-impaired children. Her unusual and fascinating approach illustrates some universal individual and family experiences through a case history. Finally, in Chapter 4, Patricia Cole uses her expertise as a seasoned speech-language pathologist to help audiologists recognize children with language disorders.

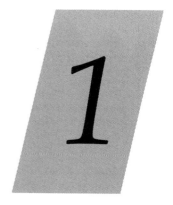

# Causes and Treatment of Hearing Loss in Children

## A. BOYD MORGAN

Caring for sick children is a special privilege and responsibility with benefits beyond the usual satisfactions of practicing medicine. Watching children grow and enjoy the benefits of good health and a normal listening experience is one of the rewards. Children with medical disorders affecting their hearing have always presented a special problem in examination, diagnosis, and treatment. Now new developments in testing and treatment are available and require us to be even more diligent than before.

Over the last decade CT scanning, magnetic resonance imaging, and auditory brainstem response testing have somewhat simplified the difficult task of evaluating infants and young children. In addition, medical advances have improved the care of diseases once untreatable and the detection of illnesses once undetectable. Still, the incidence of hearing loss from unknown causes is unacceptable—approximately 25% (see Table 1.1). As the developmental ramifications of hearing loss become more apparent, detection of hearing loss at an early age has become a priority. Screening of at-risk infants is now the standard. The development of cochlear implants for the profoundly impaired gives new hope to those who care for these children, but the prospect of rehabilitation should not divert us from the primary goal of preventing hearing loss. The most sophisticated methods of hearing augmentation available today are no substitute for normal hearing.

This chapter will review the etiology and pathology of the common medical disorders causing hearing loss in children and will discuss current therapeutic options. The presentation will be from the perspective of a treating physician. The objective is to enhance communication and improve understanding between clinicians in medicine and audiology so

**TABLE 1.1**
**Reported Causes of Deafness, National Census of Deaf Persons 1971**

| Cause | Percentage |
| --- | --- |
| Unknown | 24.6 |
| Congenital | |
| Heredity | 7.6 |
| Maternal Rubella | 5.2 |
| Birth Injury | 2.5 |
| Other | 19.0 |
| | 34.3 |
| Delayed | |
| Meningitis | 9.7 |
| Scarlet Fever | 6.2 |
| Measles | 4.3 |
| Pertussis | 2.6 |
| Fall | 3.1 |
| Other Injury | 2.0 |
| Other Illness | 13.2 |
| | 41.1 |

*Source:* Adapted from Catlin (1978). Data from Schein and Delk (1974).

that they can use their various special skills to work together toward the common goals of detection, treatment, and prevention of hearing loss in children.

# Patient History

The history is the most important part of the initial contact between patient and clinician. This is the period when confidence is built and rapport is established. The parents decide whether they like the clinician and whether they want the clinician to care for their child. The initial interview must be thorough but efficient. The clinician should ask appropriate questions for the child involved. If the problem is chronic otitis media, there is no need to spend a great deal of time picking apart the birth history or the family tree. If the problem is sensorineural hearing loss, however, then of course those aspects of the history should be explored. Efficiency and thoroughness build confidence. It is most helpful when parents fill out a case-history questionnaire before the initial interview, allowing the clinician to concentrate on the most important aspects of the history and saving valuable time in the clinic. The history should begin with a description by the parent of when a problem was first noted, who noted it, and if any immediate causation was apparent. The medical history is of primary importance. Has the child been sick and in the hospital? If so, what for? Has the child ever had meningitis? What kind? What about measles, mumps, chicken pox, pneumonia, encephalitis, flu, or any chronic illness? Does the child have any heart or kidney problem? Has there been a chronic ear infection lasting more than three months or fluid in the ears for that period of time? Have the ears ever drained? What medicine was given for that illness?

The history of the pregnancy is also of great importance. Especially helpful is any information regarding maternal illness during the first three months. Was any rash noted? What about German measles? Was any medication taken? Were any drugs used, including alcohol and tobacco? Were there any problems in pregnancy such as excessive weight gain, bleeding, high blood pressure, or diabetes? Does the mother have a thyroid problem? Is there Rh incompatibility between mother and child? When was the baby delivered—on time, early, or late? How much did it weigh? Was the birth natural or cesarean? Do the parents remember the doctor saying anything about an APGAR score? Did the baby go to the newborn nursery or the neonatal ICU? Was there any jaundice? How long did the baby stay in the hospital?

A joint committee of the American Academy of Pediatrics, American Academy of Otolaryngology—Head and Neck Surgery, American Nurses Association, and American Speech-Language-Hearing Association has developed a list of high-risk prenatal and perinatal conditions (American Speech-Language-Hearing Association, 1982). Any of the conditions listed places the child in the high-risk category for hearing loss and represents a warning signal. These conditions are as follows:

1. Family history of childhood hearing impairment.

2. Congenital or perinatal infection (e.g., cytomegalovirus, rubella, herpes, toxoplasmosis, syphilis).

3. Anatomic malformations involving the head and neck (e.g., dysmorphic appearance including syndromal and nonsyndromal abnormalities, overt or submucus cleft palate, and morphologic abnormalities of the pinna).

4. Birth weight of less than 1,500 grams.

5. Hyperbilirubinemia at a level exceeding indications for exchange transfusion.

6. Bacterial meningitis, especially *Hemophilus influenza*.

7. Severe asphyxia, which may include infants with APGAR scores of 0 to 3 or those who fail to institute spontaneous respiration within 10 minutes and those with hypotonia persisting to 2 hours of age. (An APGAR score is a method of assessing the postnatal adjustment of a newborn baby. On a scale of 0 to 2, it assesses the five vital functions: heart rate, respiratory rate, muscle tone, reflex irritability, and color. The sum of those scores is the APGAR score, the maximum score being 10.

Any of the listed conditions should alert the clinician to the possibility of an increased risk of hearing loss. How much increase in risk, however, is difficult to determine from the studies that have been done to date. Sohmer, Feinmesser, Lev, Bauberger-Tell, and David (1972) reported 0.5% whereas Lubchenco et al. (1972) reported 18%.

Careful attention should be paid to the appearance of the external ear. Is the canal of normal size? Is the auricle malformed? Do the ears look different from each other? Are there any additional appendages, cysts, or sinus tracts? The tympanic membrane is often difficult to visualize due to narrow or angled canals or occluding cerumen, and in the squirming, crying child it is difficult to get a good view. Angulation of the canal will sometimes prevent visual inspection. Pulling the auricle posteriorly and up will usually straighten it so the drum is visible.

The normal tympanic membrane should be translucent, slightly gray, and covered with a plexus of fine blood vessels. The major landmarks of significance are the umbo and the short process of the malleus. Above the short process of the malleus is the pars flaccida, which may be retracted in serous otitis. The cone of light may be visible in normal or diseased ears and seems an unreliable landmark. The best aids to diagnosis are the translucency of the drum, the tympanic capillaries, and the middle ear mucosa. If the drum is dull and the middle ear mucosa and undulations not visible, fluid may be present in the middle ear. An increased number or caliber of blood vessels implies serous fluid or chronic negative middle ear pressure. Serous fluid in the middle ear may contain bubbles, a sign that the eustachian tube is at least partially functioning.

The physical examination of the child with a congenital hearing impairment should include not only the ears but also other organ systems that may have to do with the hearing loss. Examination of the facial bones, jaw, palate, oral structures, and teeth may identify an associated anomaly. The presence of a heart defect, kidney disorder, or ocular or integumentary disorder may indicate a congenital syndrome as the embryologic development of these organs is temporally related to the development of various structures of the ear.

In practice, just holding the child down to perform an ENT exam is an accomplishment, especially if the child is less than 3 years of age. Usually by the age of 3, however, a child responds to gentle reasoning and the examination is easier.

Hearing loss may be caused by damage to the ear before, during, or after birth. The time of presumed injury provides a convenient division into prenatal, perinatal, and postnatal periods. Shimizu reports incidences of hearing loss for each category as 68%, 24%, and 8% respectively. (See Catlin, 1978.) The noxious influence may be due to infectious, toxic, developmental, or hereditary factors and may affect the external or middle ear or may damage the labyrinth, the auditory nerve, or the brainstem. *Congenital* implies only that the condition was present at birth. *Genetic* or *hereditary* implies that a chromosomal mechanism is a factor in causing the abnormality, which may or may not be present at birth.

# Prenatal Hearing Loss

### Developmental Factors of the Inner Ear

Some embryological considerations require discussion. The pars superior, or vestibular labyrinth, consists of the semicircular canals and utricle, and is almost fully developed in the 8- to 9-week embryo. The pars inferior, or cochlea and saccule, develops later, with development continuing into the early part of the second trimester. The embryologic development is thought to reflect phylogenetic age. Thus the pars superior is "older" phylogenetically than the pars inferior. According to conventional wisdom, the older a structure is phylogenetically, the more resistant it is to developmental or acquired disease. This may help to explain the histopathological changes found in common developmental anomalies such as Scheibe's aplasia and maternal rubella, in which the changes are confined to the pars inferior (cochlea and saccule) and the vestibular structures are spared. The saccule and the cochlea are also the primary structures injured in postnatally acquired hearing loss such as that caused by mumps and measles (Paparella & Shumrick, 1980).

Dysplasia of the inner ear may be sporadic, of toxic origin, inherited, or the result of chromosomal abnormalities. The maldevelopment may be of unknown etiology or due to a recognizable syndrome. It is more commonly bilateral but not necessarily equal in degree on each side. Schuknecht (1974) classifies inner ear dysplasias into the Scheibe, Mondini, and trisomy types. He feels that the Bing Siebenmann type (normal bony but underdeveloped membranous labyrinth) and the Alexander type (underdevelopment of the basal turn) are as yet inadequately documented for categorization. Complete inner ear dysplasia, the Michel dysplasia, is rare and of little practical significance (Schuknecht, 1974).

In 1791 Mondini (sometimes Mundini) of Bologna first found the abnormality that bears his name when dissecting the temporal bones of an 8-year-old boy, born deaf. The otherwise healthy boy had died of gangrene after being hit by a horse and cart. The Mondini defect has since been described by other authors and includes a spectrum of inner ear dysplasias. The bony cochlear capsule is flattened with underdevelopment of the apical part of the cochlea and a reduction in the number of cochlear turns. The saccule and endolymphatic duct may be dilated. The degree of structural abnormality in the organ of Corti, stria vascularis, and afferent neural structures determines the degree of hearing loss, which may vary from moderate to profound, however. Cases have been described in which normal hearing was found in the presence of a typical bony Mondini defect. The Mondini dysplasia may lead to cerebrospinal fluid otorrhea from a fistula in the region of the oval window.

The Scheibe dysplasia was first described in 1892. It involves the cochlea and saccule; the utricle and semicircular canals are normal. The stria vascularis of the cochlea is deformed with alternating areas of hyperplasia and aplasia. Reissner's membrane is collapsed on the stria vascularis, and the organ of Corti is rudimentary. The wall of the saccule may be collapsed and the otolithic membrane deformed. The cochlear neurons, however, may be normal (Schuknecht, 1974). The Scheibe type of inner ear dysplasia may account for a large percentage of the inner ear abnormalities found in those with inherited deafness and those with sporadic hearing loss.

The inner ear dysplasias found in the trisomy 13 and 18 syndromes include aplasia of the organ of Corti and stria vascularis, displacement and encapsulation of the tectorial membrane, and a variety of other membranous and bony labyrinthine changes. External ear abnormalities are also found in these dramatic syndromes, including malformations of the pinnae, external canals, and middle ear spaces. Cleft lip and palate, microphthalmia (small eye), micrognathia (small jaw), iris coloboma (a fissure or cleft in the iris), cataracts, glaucoma, and optic nerve aplasia are some of the defects found. Down syndrome (trisomy 21) is the most common of the autosomal aneuploides (an abnormal number of chromosomes), representing 1 out of 600 live births (Schuknecht, 1974). Fortunately, ear anomalies other than partial meatal atresia or stenosis are not a common finding in this syndrome. The sex chromosomal aneuploides such as Turner's and Kleinfelter's syndromes, however, do not present with such dramatic findings, and significant ear abnormalities are not common.

## Case Study

The patient M. J. was 7 years old at the time her hearing loss was detected and quantified. Screening in a sound field had been normal at the age of 3. She is a nonidentical twin of another female with normal hearing. There is no family history of hearing loss. Developmental and other milestones were normal; speech development was normal. There is no history of trauma or toxic drug use. The mother's pregnancy was normal without a history of rash or fever. Delivery was uncomplicated, and there was no hypoxia or jaundice in the perinatal or postnatal period. She has had no significant history of middle ear disease.

The physical examination showed a normally formed pinna and external canal. The tympanic membranes were normally translucent, and the other head, neck, and skeletal structures were normal.

The audiogram is shown in Figure 1.1. Some difficulty in masking was encountered. A CT scan of the temporal bones demonstrated a Mondini defect of the left labyrinth (Figure 1.2). This radiograph demonstrates lack of cochlear turns on the left, with a dilated vestibule on that side. Normal cochlear turns are present on the right. The middle ear and external canal are normal on both sides.

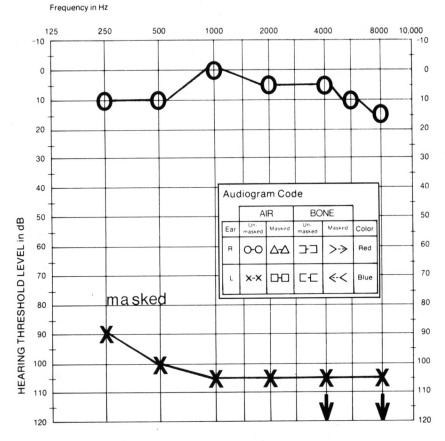

PURE–TONE AUDIOGRAM  **M.J.**

Frequency in Hz

**Figure 1.1.**  Audiogram of patient M. J. showing a profound sensorineural hearing loss in left ear due to a Mondini-type malformation.

## Developmental Factors of the External Ear

The external ear, external auditory canal, middle ear space, and ossicles (except the stapes footplate) are derived from the first and second branchial clefts and arches (embryological folds), as is the lower jaw and related structures. Malformations of these structures result from incomplete or aberrant development of the first two branchial arches. Development of the outer ear is independent from that of the inner ear since the embryo-

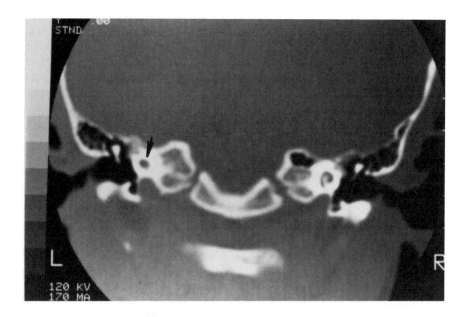

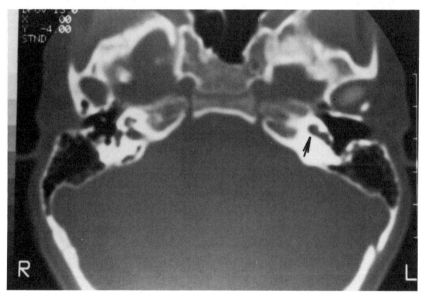

**Figure 1.2.** CT scan showing a dilated cochlea with an underdeveloped bony structure in the left ear characteristic of a Mondini malformation. A, frontal view. B, view from above. Courtesy of David Ray Leake, MD.

logic origins of each are different. The membranous labyrinth is derived from ectodermal otocyst (a cyst of the outer layer of the embryo) and develops independently from the rest of the ear, which is a derivative of the branchial apparatus. The tragus, the head of the malleus, and the short process of the incus are formed by the first branchial (mandibular) arch. The second branchial (hyoid) arch forms the remainder of the malleus, the long process of the incus, and the superstructure of the stapes as well as all of the auricle except the tragus. Improper development of the first and second branchial arches may affect the auricle and result in microtia, anotia, or malposition of the pinna. The ossicles may be malformed, aplastic, or fused. Failure of the first branchial groove to develop may result in partial or complete atresia of the external canal. The jaw may be malformed. All degrees of deformity may be present—from a simple preauricular tag or sinus to a widespread deformity involving hypoplasia of the jaw, temporal bone, orbit, external ear, and base of skull, a condition that might be termed "craniofacial microsomia." The defect is more commonly unilateral than bilateral.

Various schemes of classification have been proposed, based either on the extent of auricular malformation or the surgical approach to be employed in correction. Perhaps the most valuable is Altmann's scheme (quoted in Paparella & Schumrick, 1980, p. 1313):

1. *Group I: Minor external and middle ear malformations.* This group would include preauricular pits and tags, minor alterations in the shape of the pinna, stenosis of the external canal, and malformation, fusion, or absence of the ossicles. In rare instances only a portion of the external and middle ear will be abnormal. A normal tympanic membrane does not necessarily preclude an abnormality in the middle ear space.

2. *Group II: The majority of external ear deformities.* The auricle is rarely normal and is usually represented by a small skin appendage. The external canal is hypoplastic or aplastic. The tympanic bone can be malformed or absent. If it is malformed, it may form an "atresia plate" medial to the normal location of the tympanic membrane, while forming the lateral wall of the middle ear space (Figure 1.3). The cellular development of the mastoid is usually minimal. Normal or near normal pneumatization may imply fairly good differentiation of the middle ear structures. The facial nerve and chorda tympani branch of that nerve may be abnormally oriented or in some cases absent.

3. *Group III: The most extensive forms of malformation.* The auricle is severely malformed or absent (anotia). The external canal is aplastic. The mastoid bone is not pneumatized, and the middle ear space is absent

or represented by a slit. The ossicles are frequently absent. Anomalies of the facial nerve are common, and the inner ear may be malformed, particularly the lateral semicircular canal.

## Case Study

H. D. is now 8 years old. He has a minimally deformed right pinna but a completely atretic right external auditory canal (Figure 1.4). The left ear is normal except for a small preauricular tag. He has had recurrent serous otitis media in the left ear, requiring insertion of ventilating tubes. An audiogram demonstrates normal bone conduction in the right ear (Figure 1.5). Tomograms show bony and soft-tissue atresia of the right external canal, an atresia plate, a small middle ear space, and a malformed ossicular mass. The left side is normal (Figure 1.6).

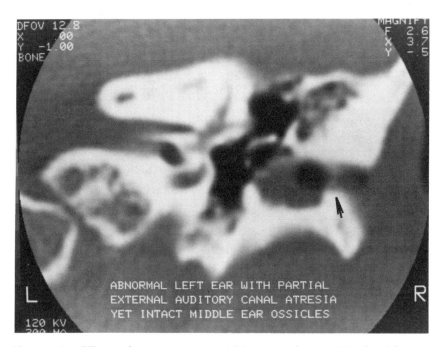

**Figure 1.3.** CT scan demonstrating partial bony canal stenosis in the right ear. Courtesy of Rodney D. Schmidt, MD.

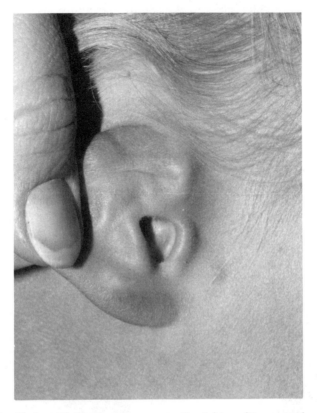

**Figure 1.4.** Patient H. D. showing an atretic right auditory canal with slight deformity of the auricle.

H. D. has had no associated skin, heart, kidney, or neurological disease. Development has been normal. He has five siblings, all of whom have preauricular tags but no canal atresia and no conductive hearing loss. His parents' ears are normal. The pregnancy and birth history are normal.

Because his defect is unilateral, correction will be delayed at least until his mastoid development is complete and he can make his own decision about reconstruction of the atresia.

## Hereditary Factors

Understanding the mechanisms of genetic transmission is fundamental to understanding the disease processes involved. Congenital deafness

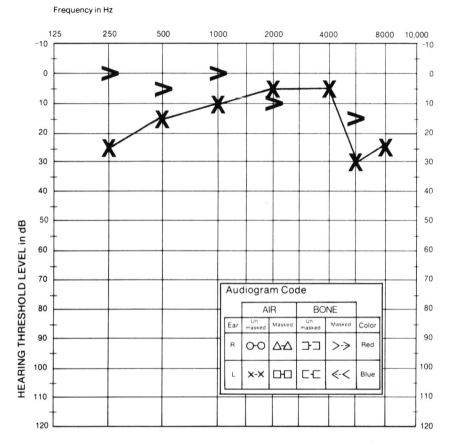

PURE-TONE AUDIOGRAM **H.D.**

Frequency in Hz

**Figure 1.5.** Audiogram of patient H. D. showing normal bone conduction in the atretic right ear.

may be inherited by autosomal dominant, autosomal recessive, or sex-linked genetic mechanisms. Determining whether the deafness is inherited can be a difficult task. Counseling will be even more difficult if the cause is unknown.

Each person's genetic makeup consists of 23 pairs of chromosomes: 22 pairs of autosomes and 1 pair of sex chromosomes. The male pair of sex chromosomes is designated XY, the female pair XX. During fertilization, 22 autosomes and 1 sex chromosome (either X or Y) in the sperm unite with 22 matching autosomes and 1 sex chromosome (X) of the ovum to form the normal chromosomal makeup of the zygote with 46 chromosomes in all. If a trait is autosomal dominant, it will be expressed in the child if the gene for that trait is passed on the autosome from either the father or mother. If a trait is autosomal recessive, the gene for that trait must be present in both the male and female contribution to the zygote in order for that trait to be expressed. If a child possesses a single trait on one chromosome, then the child is heterozygous for the trait. If that trait is autosomal dominant, it will be expressed. If a matching trait is present on the other chromosome, then it will be expressed and the child will be homozygous for it. If it is autosomal recessive, it will not be expressed unless there is a matching trait on the other chromosome of the pair. In other words, autosomal recessive traits are not expressed in the heterozygous state. An autosomal dominant trait is expressed in the homozygous or heterozygous state but may be variably expressed if it is incompletely penetrant. If the trait lies on the sex chromosome, then it is X-linked.

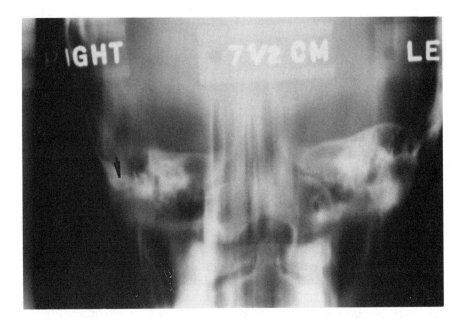

**Figure 1.6.** Tomography of the temporal bones demonstrating atresia of the right external canal. The left external canal is normal. A rudimentary middle ear space is present on the right.

The probability that a trait will be expressed in the child in the case of autosomal dominance is 50% if one of the parents is heterozygous for the trait (Figure 1.7). If both parents possess an autosomal recessive trait, 25% of the progeny will be affected and 50% will be carriers (Figure 1.8).

Thousands of genetic loci are involved in transmitting the information needed to form the auricle, the ossicles, the cochlea, and the other various structures of the ear, so simple concepts of single-gene inheritance do not strictly apply in the transmission of the deafness trait. A trait for sensorineural deafness may be present but, when paired with another recessive trait at a different locus, may not be manifest. Traits may be present as autosomal dominant or homozygous autosomal recessive but variably expressed and thus not apparent.

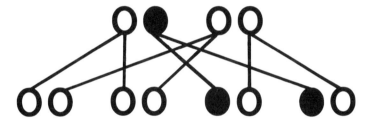

**Figure 1.7.** Autosomal dominant: one parent is affected. Two of four offspring will be affected.

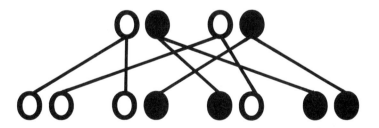

**Figure 1.8.** Autosomal recessive: both parents carry the trait. Of the offspring, one in four is affected, and two in four are carriers.

There is great difficulty in determining the proportion of different types of inheritance involved in hereditary deafness. Studies by Fraser in 1976 (Taylor, 1980) reported 33.2% of patients with autosomal recessive deafness, 15.3% with autosomal dominant deafness, and 1.7% with sex-linked deafness. In other estimates the incidence of autosomal recessive deafness ranges from 30% to 68% (Taylor, 1980). It may be that one third to one half of profound sensorineural loss results from autosomal recessive inheritance. A large proportion of the children with deafness of unknown cause probably would fall into this category.

Various schemes of classifying genetic hearing loss have been employed, including classification by time of onset, by mode of transmission, and by association and nonassociation with various other malformations and organ-system diseases. A certain amount of mental acrobatics is required to assimilate the various schemas and classifications in a useful way and to distill them into a differential diagnosis for a particular patient. Perhaps the most valuable categorization is that provided by Konigsmark and Gorlin (1976), who group genetic and metabolic hearing loss into eight major categories depending on the organ system or metabolic defect involved:

With No Associated Abnormalities
    Dominant Sensorineural Hearing Loss
    Recessive Sensorineural Hearing Loss
    Otosclerosis
    X-Linked Sensorineural Hearing Loss

With External Ear Deformities
    Pre-auricular Pits
    Low-Set Ears
    Anotia

With Associated Eye Disease
    Usher's Syndrome
    Cockayne's Syndrome
    Alstrom's Disease
    Refsum Syndrome
    Cryptopthalmia Syndrome
    Others

With Musculoskeletal Disease
    Treacher Collins Syndrome
    Craniofacial Dysostosis (Crouzon Syndrome)
    Acrocephalosyndactyly (Apert Syndrome)

Otopalataldigital Syndrome
Osteogenesis Imperfecta

With Integumentary System Disease
Waardenburg Syndrome
Others Rare

With Renal Disease
Alport's Syndrome
Potter's Syndrome
Others

With Nervous System Disease
Acoustic Neuromas

With Metabolic and Other Abnormalities
Penred's Syndrome
Mucopolysaccharidoses
Hurler
Scheie
Hunter
Sanfilippo
Morquio
Maroteaux-Lamy
Jerrell-Lange-Nielsen Syndrome

*Genetic Hearing Loss with No Associated Abnormalities.* Genetic hearing loss with no associated abnormality accounts for the largest number of children affected congenitally and includes at least 16 types of hereditary hearing loss, which can be differentiated by severity of loss, shape of audiogram, mode of transmission, and age of onset. Not all genetic hearing loss presents in childhood.

Dominant sensorineural hearing loss may be further categorized as unilateral or bilateral, severe, progressive, or low-, mid-, or high-frequency loss. Although studies differ, these various types of deafness account for about 10% to 15% of those congenitally affected. The majority of patients have a flat audiogram, although any shape of the audiometric curve is possible. The hearing loss is usually bilaterally symmetrical, although this fact should not be used to differentiate congenital from acquired hearing loss (which is usually asymmetrical). The vestibular system is usually not involved, and caloric responses are normal. Studies examining the temporal bones in these patients are lacking, but the extant pathologic studies have shown dysplasia of the organ of Corti and the saccules, a Scheibe type of dysplasia.

A progressive, high-frequency deafness variant has been described by several authors (Konigsmark & Gorlin, 1976). It may be manifest at any age and appears to have complete penetrance in the pedigrees studied. The histopathological changes found have been atrophy of the organ of Corti in the basilar turn and associated degeneration of cochlear neurons.

Otosclerosis, which causes conductive deafness, is rarely found in children under the age of 15. Ninety percent of those affected show onset between the ages of 15 and 60. The mode of transmission is autosomal dominant with about 40% penetrance. The pathological change is otosclerotic fixation of the stapes footplate in the oval window. It is a rare form of hearing loss in children and must be differentiated from congenital malleus fixation and other ossicular malformations.

Hereditary hearing loss of autosomal recessive inheritance is the most important hearing loss of this type since it represents one third to one half of congenital deafness and almost 90% of inherited sensorineural deafness. To produce the defect in progeny, both parents must be carriers of the gene, and if simple Mendelian inheritance patterns apply, 25% of their offspring will be affected. Evidence exists that several different loci carry the deafness trait. For these reasons, a family history is often lacking and studies of pedigrees are infrequently rewarding. The hereditary nature of the deafness may be difficult to establish. It is felt to be more common in consanguinous marriages.

The disease most commonly results in a severe hearing loss early in life, although pedigrees with moderate, nonprogressive loss have been described, and a form termed "early-onset sensorineural deafness" (Konigmark & Gorlin, 1976) exists. The latter variety is manifest by some hearing at an early age with rapid loss to a profound degree by age 5 or 6 (Konigsmark, 1971).

In recessive congenital hearing loss, some retention of low frequencies is often found. This is presumably because the Scheibe type of dysplasia is the most common pathological change and primarily affects the basilar turn of the cochlea. There is associated atrophy of the cochlear afferents.

Considerable genetic hetereogeneity must exist in recessive congenital deafness. Theoretically all of the offspring of two such affected parents should be deaf, but this is not always the case, as demonstrated in numerous pedigrees in which all of the children of such parents are normal. In 1898 Fay examined almost 1,400 children of deaf parents (see Schuknecht, 1974). Among only 14% were all the progeny deaf. Among 79%, the children were normal, and 7% had a combination of normal-hearing and deaf children.

X-linked congenital sensorineural deafness is uncommon, probably accounting for less than 2% to 6% of those congenitally affected. In these families, deaf males will be born of normal mothers who often have deaf brothers. In those affected, the hearing loss is severe. X-linked sensorineural deafness of early-onset type with progression to a moderate hearing loss in adolescence has been described.

*Genetic Hearing Loss with External Ear Abnormalities.* A number of syndromes of genetic hearing loss with associated external ear deformities have been identified. They are well noted and categorized by Konigsmark and Gorlin (1976). The degree of external abnormality varies from preauricular pits to low-set ears to anotia. The hearing loss may be conductive, sensorineural, or mixed, and the type of inheritance either autosomal dominant or recessive. Some of these syndromes are associated with musculoskeletal disease.

*Genetic Hearing Loss Associated with Eye Disease.* Konigsmark and Gorlin (1976) list 25 syndromes of eye abnormalities associated with hearing loss. Of these the most common is Usher's syndrome. A disease of autosomal recessive inheritance, it is characterized by retinitis pigmentosa, moderate to severe sensorineural hearing loss, and vestibulocerebellar ataxia. Mental retardation and/or psychosis may be present. Progressive loss of vision due to retinitis pigmentosa begins in early childhood and is usually suspected because of night blindness and contraction of the field of vision. Visual loss is progressive, and total loss of vision by the age of 50 occurs in over half the subjects. The hearing loss usually begins at birth, is detected between the ages of 1 or 2, and progresses to a profound loss in 85% of those affected. The inheritance is autosomal recessive with 100% penetrance.

Cockayne's syndrome consists of dwarfism, retinal atrophy, and deafness. Affected individuals are normal at birth, but growth retardation becomes obvious between the age of 1 or 2. Most patients have normal hearing at birth, but a sensorineural loss progresses to a moderate or severe range in most. Almost all patients have retinal abnormalities and enopthalmos (the globe is retrodisplaced in the orbit), which progress slowly from the second year of life until the patient becomes blind during the second decade. Mental retardation is common, with development stopping at the 3- to 4-year-old level. Other abnormalities of the neurological, skeletal, and urogenital systems and the skin become obvious as the child ages. Cockayne's syndrome is autosomal recessive in inheritance. The prognosis is poor, with death usually occurring in the second decade of life.

Alstrom's disease consists of early obesity, atypical retinal degeneration with loss of central vision, childhood-onset diabetes mellitus, and progressive sensorineural hearing loss. Nystagmus with progressive loss of vision begins during the first 2 years of life, and slow deterioration of vision due to retinal degeneration progresses to total loss by the second decade. The sensorineural hearing loss is cochlear in nature and progressive, becoming moderately severe in the second and third decades of life. Other findings may be premature baldness, acanthosis nigricans (a skin condition), and chronic renal disease that manifests in the second and third decades. Studies suggest that the inheritance is autosomal recessive.

The 22 additional syndromes that have been described are quite uncommon. Ocular involvement in these additional disorders ranges from myopia to optic atrophy associated with sensorineural hearing loss. The Refsum syndrome is an autosomal recessive disorder with progressive atypical retinitis pigmentosa, night blindness, cerebellar ataxia, and hearing loss. The cryptophthalmia syndrome is characterized by extension of skin of the forehead to cover the eyes, mixed hearing loss, atresia of the external auditory canals, soft-tissue syndactyly of the fingers, and urogenital abnormalities.

***Genetic Hearing Loss Associated with Musculoskeletal Disease.*** The Treacher Collins syndrome was probably initially described by Thomson in 1846, but Berry in 1889 or Treacher Collins in 1900 is usually given credit for its discovery (Konigsmark & Gorlin, 1976). The characteristics include hypoplastic zygomas with resultant antimongoloid palpebral fissures (a reverse slant to the eyes), coloboma of the lower eyelids, mandibular hypoplasia, malformed or crumpled or misplaced pinnae, and malformed external canals and middle ear structures with conductive deafness of autosomal dominant transmission. It must be differentiated from the oculoauriculovertebral syndrome (Goldenhar syndrome or hemifacial microsomia). The characteristic appearance is unforgettable. Reconstructive efforts involve a team approach to correct the external ear and middle ear deformities, mandibular hypoplasia, and malocclusion.

Craniofacial dysostosis (Crouzon syndrome) would occupy this category of genetic hearing loss as well. It is of autosomal dominant inheritance with ocular hypertelorism, exophthalmos, premature craniosynostosis (fusion of the lines of the skull), and occasional bilateral atresia of the external canals, ossicular anomalies, and mixed hearing loss.

Other disorders within this group include the Apert syndrome (acrocephalosyndactyly, Type I), the otopalataldigital syndrome, and osteogenesis imperfecta. The latter is an important syndrome consisting of fragile bones, mild to moderate conductive hearing loss, blue sclerae, and autosomal dominant inheritance with a wide range of expressivity and degree of penetrance. Van der Hoeve and de Kleijn first mentioned hearing loss as part of the disease, and it occasionally bears the name Van der Hoeve's syndrome. Stapedectomy may be of value in restoring the hearing. Konigsmark and Gorlin (1976) should be consulted for a further listing and description of these diverse syndromes.

*Genetic Hearing Loss with Integumentary System Disease.* The Waardenburg syndrome is the most important disease in this diverse group of syndromes of deafness associated with skin disease. The medial canthi (inside corners of the eyes) are laterally displaced with a usually normal interpupillary distance. The appearance is one of hypertelorism, although true hypertelorism is found in only 10% of these cases. A white forelock, vitiligo, and a broad nasal root are common findings. The hearing loss is variable, from mild to severe, with unilateral or bilateral loss in 50% of those affected. Vestibular hypofunction is found in 75%. The inheritance is autosomal dominant, variably expressed.

Other disorders in this group are rare. Hearing loss combined with malformations of teeth, nails, hair, and skin is the rule.

*Genetic Hearing Loss with Renal Disease.* The Alport syndrome is the most prominent syndrome. The combination of progressive sensorineural hearing loss, progressive nephritis with uremia (decreased kidney function), and ocular lens abnormalities is of autosomal dominant inheritance, with males the more affected sex. Renal failure may be remedied by transplantation. Improvement of hearing following this procedure has been described, but the reasons for the improvement are as yet undiscovered. The pathogenesis of the syndrome is unknown, but immunologic and functional similarities of the membranous portions of kidney and ear may imply a common genetic origin of the defects. This disorder accounts for 1% of genetic deafness (Konigsmark & Gorlin, 1974).

About nine other syndromes of associated hearing loss and kidney disease have been described.

*Genetic Hearing Loss with Nervous System Disease.* These diverse syndromes consist of hearing loss associated with neurologic disorders varying from ataxia to epilepsy. The most important syndrome is that of acoustic neuromas and neural deafness. This syndrome of autosomal dominant transmission accounts for about 4% of persons having acoustic neuromas. Differentiation of this disease from von Recklinghausen's disease must be made. The bilateral acoustic neuromas cause hearing loss and vestibular dysfunction, which is progressive in the second and third decades. Males and females are equally affected, and one half of the offspring of an affected person will have the disease.

*Genetic Hearing Loss with Metabolic and Other Abnormalities.* This miscellaneous category contains several important syndromes. The Penred syndrome, goiter, and profound congenital sensorineural hearing loss may account for as much as 10% of congenital hearing loss. The thyroid enlargement is due to an inborn error in thyroxine synthesis. The hearing loss is bilateral in the moderate to profound range. The Mondini cochlear abnormality has been described in a number of cases; some bony or membranous changes are found in all. The inheritance is autosomal recessive. Treatment is with exogenous thyroid hormone, which may stop the growth of the goiter but does not improve the hearing.

The mucopolysaccharidoses are inherited disorders of mucopolysaccharide (carbohydrate) metabolism. Failure of degradation of these substances leads to increased intracellular storage and excretion of specific mucopolysaccharides. The syndromes of Hurler, Scheie, Hunter, Sanfilippo, Morquio, and Maroteaux-Lamy exhibit these metabolic defects as well as skeletal changes and sensorineural, conductive, or mixed hearing loss. They are autosomal recessive in inheritance, except for the X-linked Hunter syndrome. Mental retardation is a common feature.

The Jervell-Lange-Nielsen syndrome consists of prolonged electrocardiographic QT intervals, recurrent Stokes-Adams attacks (fainting due to cardiac arrythmia) beginning in early childhood, sudden death in some cases, and congenital severe sensorineural deafness. Its inheritance is autosomal recessive. In one half the cases described the patient has died by the age of 15 years.

## Prenatal Infectious Factors

*Cytomegalovirus Infection.* Cytomegalovirus (CMV) is a herpes type of virus that may cause infections of great importance in humans. It is an endemic rather than epidemic disease, always present in the population and characterized by lifelong infection with intermittent reactivation, as with other types of herpes virus infections. The manifestations of this disease may be as minimal as a rash and fever or as severe as microcephaly, mental retardation, and profound sensorineural hearing loss. The infection may be asymptomatic, or death may be the result.

Transmission results from contact with infected body fluids: saliva, blood, urine, cervical secretions, or milk. Infection usually takes place silently in the child. The exposure may be *in utero*, in the perinatal period, or in childhood. A South African study has shown 60% to 100% of mothers may be infected, with the rate of infection directly related to socioeconomic status. The poorer the family, the greater the risk of infection. Probably 0.5% to 2.2% (average 1%) of infants are infected *in utero*. Another 8% to 60% become infected in the first 6 months of life (Pass, Hutto, Reynolds, & Polhill, 1984). Of the approximately 1% who are infected, 90% to 95% are free of disease. From 5% to 17% of infected but asymptomatic children may develop late sequelae such as hearing loss, dental abnormalities, mental retardation, or other neurological deficits. Clinical disease at birth is therefore rare. When present, it is manifested as the well-known CMV syndrome of rash, hepatosplenomegaly, jaundice, microcephaly, low birth weight for gestational age, and intracranial calcifications. It is rare as a cause of lethal disease in the newborn and an unlikely cause of recurrent abortion.

Congenital infection of the fetus may occur after a primary infection in pregnancy but is thought to be more common as a result of maternal secondary reactivation. The latter type of maternal infection is felt to result in more severe, long-term sequelae than the primary type (Stagno et al., 1977). The mode of infection is via placental transfer. Maternal infection, however, does not definitely mean fetal infection. It has been demonstrated that one child in a twin pregnancy might be infected, the other not (Hanshaw & Dudgeon, 1978). Unlike other congenital infections, which are more severe in the first trimester, there is no current evidence to suggest that the time of fetal infection is important.

Sensorineural hearing loss is the most common single-organ, late sequela of congenital infection. Since positive CMV titers are a common finding, its etiologic role in hearing loss of unknown cause is easily assumed but not easily proven. According to some studies (MacDonald & Tobin, 1978), 6% to 17% of congenitally infected infants had hearing loss. That hearing loss may be unilateral but is more commonly bilateral and may progress (Williamson et al., 1982). When congenital infection has taken place in the first 2 weeks and viral shedding in urine is documented, then the sensorineural hearing loss that is detected may be attributable to CMV with confidence. A more difficult question is the older child who is found to have a sensorineural loss and is excreting the virus. Is the presence of CMV causal or coincidental? Paired serologic studies may be helpful in this situation but are rarely available because the congenital infection is usually asymptomatic and unsuspected in the newborn period.

Perinatal infection of the infant may result from shedding of the virus from the cervix during parturition, or via maternal excretion of the virus in milk or saliva. Infection acquired in this period of time is thought to cause fewer late sequelae than when acquired in utero.

Cytomegalic inclusions (characteristic intracellular aggregations) may be found in the cochlea, saccule, and utricle and in the semicircular canals (Schuknecht, 1974). They have been described on the endolymphatic side of Reissner's membrane in the region of the stria vascularis and in the spiral ligament. Infected cells have deeply staining central nuclear inclusions and are three to four times the normal size. A clear halo surrounds the inclusion and extends to the nuclear membrane, forming a characteristic "owl's eye" appearance.

Of recent concern in the epidemiology of CMV disease is the finding of an increased frequency of CMV infection in children in group day-care centers (Pass et al., 1984). Group day care was found to be likely to result in early acquisition of CMV. It was suspected that this exposure might then result in increased rates of infection among parents of children in those centers. Subsequent studies have borne out that suspicion (Pass, Hutto, Ricks, & Cloud, 1986). It was found that children often transmit CMV to parents and can be an important source of maternal CMV infection in pregnancy.

Interpretation of positive CMV serologic tests is difficult, considering that it is often a ubiquitous but undiagnosed illness that may silently reactivate without causing overt disease. A variety of tests are available, including culture of the virus from urine or secretions, complement fixation tests, electron microscopy, and enzyme immunoassays (ELISA) for IgG or IgM immunoglobulins. The presence of IgM is felt to indicate infection within the last several months. The presence of IgG antibody in the serum implies a prior infection but does not identify when that infection took place (Cohen & Corey, 1985).

Despite the common nature of the organism and the frequency of infection, prevention is difficult. Experimental vaccines of attenuated virus are available, but they are not approved for general use because of inexperience with them and hesitation about the use of a potentially oncogenic herpes virus.

*Rubella.* Congenital rubella and its associated multiple congenital defects were first described by Gregg in 1941. Congenital cataracts, retinal pigmentation, and microphthalmia were noted. Swan, Tostevin, Moore, Mayo, and Black (1943) described sensorineural hearing loss in the syndrome. The incidence of rubella follows a definite pattern and is subject to seasonal variation. Usually maternal rubella peaks in the spring and early summer. Consequently, 80% of the children with congenital rubella are born between September and February, with the peak between October and December.

The rate of fetal infection is about 90% after maternal infection, but the fetus is not necessarily damaged if infected. The infection is acquired transplacentally due to maternal viremia. The risk of fetal damage is 15% to 35%, with the first trimester being the period of greatest danger. There is less risk from the 12th to 16th week and slight risk from 16 weeks on. Still births are possible.

The congenital defects are well known: sensorineural hearing loss, cataracts, microphthalmia, patent ductus arteriosus, ventricular septal defects, pulmonic stenosis, cerebral palsy, mental retardation, thrombocytopenic purpura, rash, hepatosplenomegaly, osteopathy, and learning disorders (Dudgeon, 1972). Sensorineural hearing loss is the most common defect resulting from intrauterine infection; it is usually bilateral but can be unilateral. The histopathologic changes include degenerative and inflammatory changes affecting the organ of Corti, stria vascularis, Reissner's membrane, and the tectorial membrane (Alford, 1968).

Although the manifestations of the illness may be protean, a significant number of children—40% in one study (Taylor, 1980)—have a single-organ defect: sensorineural hearing loss. A sure sign of infection, retinopathy may be present and detectable but may not impair visual acuity.

Maternal infection is manifested by a macular rash, cervical lymphadenopathy, and arthralgias, but often symptoms are minimal. Other viruses may cause the same symptoms, and a significant number of cases (about 24%) may be subclinical. Paired serologic studies to document an increase in specific IgM immunoglobulin levels are required to document recent primary rubella infection. Immunoglobulin M is the largest of the five types of antibodies produced by the lymphocytes of our immune system. Specific IgM may be elevated for 6 to 8 weeks and has been detected in the serum for one year. A congenital infection is diagnosed by serologic tests; attempts at isolation of the virus are not rewarding. Demonstration of specific IgM in fetal blood from cord samples documents fetal infection since maternal IgM does not cross the placental barrier. Radioimmunoassays and enzyme immunoassays (ELISA) are sensitive and are employed to detect IgM antibodies. IgG may be present in serum as well. Detection in a child of specific IgG in the absence of specific IgM indicates a less recent infection with rubella.

The hope for prevention of congenital rubella lies in immunization of susceptible populations with the currently available vaccines.

*Syphilis.* Syphilis is no longer a major cause of sensorineural hearing loss in the Western world and in other developed countries, but it remains a significant factor in less developed countries.

Congenital syphilis occurs from intrauterine transmission of acquired maternal syphilis, with loss of hearing and vestibular function occurring in 25% to 38% of children affected (Karmody & Schuknecht, 1966). The incidence may be higher, since those affected may not manifest the disease until later in life. Two forms exist—early (infantile) and late (tardive), the early form being associated with severe systemic manifestations. The tardive form may present as sudden severe loss in childhood with progression of the loss in most individuals. Loss of vestibular function may occur as well, and the presentation may be like that of Meniere's disease. In fact, the otitic pathology in these patients includes endolymphatic hydrops and progressive deterioration of the membranous labyrinth, changes which are also present in Meniere's disease. Other pathologic findings may be osteitis with round-cell infiltration, multinucleated giant cells, and varying degrees of destruction of the bony labyrinth (Schuknecht, 1974). Both Meniere's disease and hearing loss due to congenital syphilis may present with the clinical findings and symptoms of episodic vertigo as well as symmetrical and fluctuating sensorineural hearing loss, predominating at the low frequencies initially and becoming flat and more severe as the disease progresses. The Tullio phenomenon (vertigo with loud sounds) and Hennebert's phenomenon (a positive fistula test in the absence of middle ear disease) may also be present. Other sites of involvement may be the cartilage and bony framework of the nose (snuffles), periostitis of the cranial bones (bossing of the skull), periostitis of the tibia (sabre shins), injury to the teeth (Hutchinson's teeth), and interstitial keratitis (cloudy cornea) (Schuknecht, 1974). Suspicion of congenital syphilis on a clinical basis should lead to serological studies that will allow diagnosis. Treatment with adequate doses of penicillin and occasionally systemic steroids should be curative and, in some cases, improve the hearing.

# Perinatal Factors

Certain perinatal factors have long been known to have a high probability of causing sensorineural hearing loss. Whether a particular child's loss can be traced to perinatal events, however, depends on the exclusion of prenatal and postnatal etiologies. Lack of appropriate studies to exclude those causes makes the diagnosis uncertain. Not only are multiple factors to be considered, but the time between traumatic birth or toxic event and the diagnosis of hearing loss is often long, sometimes several years. Because of the multiple factors surrounding a child's birth, often the diagnosis is one of exclusion, reached by eliminating intrauterine events and postnatal etiologies. Hypoxia, traumatic birth, hyperbilirubinemia, prematurity, and otoxic drugs are the most frequent suspect etiologies. Other contributing factors are recurrent apnea, sepsis, acidosis, and low birth weight.

## Prematurity

Prematurity, in the absence of other problems at birth, is associated with an increased risk of hearing loss. The incidence of such loss may range from 3.3% to 10% (Catlin, 1978). In addition, premature infants are subject to a variety of perinatal events that increase the risk of central nervous system complications. Any child born weighing less than 1,500 grams should be considered at risk.

## Hypoxia

Hypoxia due to asphyxia during the birth process may lead to hearing loss. The central auditory pathways and cochlea are quite sensitive to oxygen deprivation, more so in the child with low birth weight or premature child. Nintey-one percent of ischemia cerebral lesions are due to antepartum and intrapartum asphyxia (Brown, Purvis, Fortar, & Cockburn, 1974). Three patterns of damage to central pathways have been described by Wigglesworth and Pape (1978): cerebral edema and necrosis, infection of boundary zone areas, and necrosis of nuclei in the brainstem and thalamic regions. They have also suggested that damage to the brain as the result of asphyxia may be determined by the extent to which vasodilatation from hypoxia and hypercapnia may maintain cerebral blood flow. The site and severity of the hypoxic lesion may depend on the infant's stage of development. Periventricular leukomalacia may be the lesion found in preterm infants, whereas term infants may show necrosis of neurons. Hemorrhage into the cochlea may occur as a result of asphyxia (Hall, 1964), although this type of lesion has also been linked to trauma during delivery (Buch, 1966).

The preterm infant is more susceptible to the effects of hypoxia than the term infant. Lack of surfactant in lung tissue may lead to the development of hyaline membrane disease and the respiratory distress syndrome. In addition, the proportion of fetal hemoglobin, with its high affinity for oxygen, is advantageous in fetal life but can lead to tissue hypoxia in the newborn.

Other than birth asphyxia, recurrent apnea in the newborn may result in hypoxia. These events are more common in preterm infants. The association of frequent, recurrent apnea attacks and low-birth-weight babies having a hearing loss has been reported (Anagnostakis, Petmezakis, Papazissis, Messaritakis, & Matsoniotis, 1982). Animal experiments indicate that repeated hypoxic episodes may have a cumulative effect (Newton, 1985), but studies in humans are lacking.

## Kernicterus

Hyperbilirubinemia in the perinatal period with resulting kernicterus has been widely reported as a cause of sensorineural hearing loss. Bilirubin is a toxic, lipophilic (fat soluble) agent that may alter cellular metabolism by affecting mitochondrial function in the cochlear nuclei and basal ganglia. Increased levels may arise from overproduction of bilirubin combined with decreased clearance of that product of metabolism. In addition, decreased conjugation of bilirubin due to hepatic immaturity may lead to increased levels of the relatively fat-soluble (and thus able to penetrate the CNS), unconjugated bilirubin. Deafness as a result of kernicterus associated with hemolytic disease of the newborn has been described (Fisch & Osborn, 1954).

Bilirubin is transported in the bloodstream bound to albumin, a combination felt to be nontoxic. The high affinity of albumin for bilirubin assumes that little unconjugated bilirubin is free to diffuse into other tissues. A low albumin concentration in the low-birth-weight neonate would result in more bilirubin precipitate in that newborn. Acidosis may predispose to kernicterus since uptake of bilirubin by the mitochondria increases as pH decreases (Brodersen, 1977). Sepsis may result in significant increases in bilirubin concentration by one of several mechanisms and lead to an increased risk of kernicterus. Increased bilirubin levels have been reported in bacteremic infants (Rooney, Hill, & Danks, 1971). It has been shown that hypothermia may decrease binding of albumin and bilirubin and lead to increased levels of free bilirubin, thus compounding the effects of acidosis and sepsis (Schiff, Stern, & Leduc, 1966). The association and dissociation of bilirubin and albumin may occur rapidly, so detection and measurement of free bilirubin in the newborn may be difficult. Thus, the etiology of kernicterus as the cause of hearing loss may be difficult to prove. However, the neonate of low birth weight with associated hypoxia, acidosis, and sepsis is at increased risk for the toxic effects of hyperbilirubinemia (Newton, 1985).

### Temporal Bone Trauma

Trauma to the temporal bone may be a complication of traumatic delivery. Hemorrhage into the inner ear or brainstem or cochlear concussion may occur. Buch (1966) studied the temporal bones of 73 newborn infants and concluded that trauma played a major in causing hemorrhage in the inner ear. The incidence of this complication and its clinical importance remains difficult to estimate, however, since documentation depends on autopsy.

### Incubator Noise

The ambient noise in neonatal intensive care units and in incubators in particular has raised a great deal of speculation about whether the noise level is sufficient to cause hearing impairment, especially when combined with other factors such as ototoxic drugs. The level of noise has been variably measured from 56 dBA to 77 dBA (Northern & Downs, 1984), with transient elevations above that level in some instances. Most authors, including Abramovich, Gregory, Slemich, and Stewart (1979), have now concluded that ambient noise from the incubator is not a factor in the hearing loss of infants in intensive care units. Most incubators maintain levels in the range of 60 dB or below.

A single entity leading to sensorineural hearing loss is often difficult to determine, since sick, premature, or low-birth-weight babies may be exposed to multiple toxic and traumatic factors. In some infants a single etiology can be recognized; yet others exposed to the same insult escape injury. The perinatal causes of sensorineural hearing loss in the neonate may be more often obscure and multifactorial rather than obviously due to a single cause.

# Postnatal Hearing Loss

Hearing loss acquired in the postnatal period may be due to a variety of causes, including otitis media, serous otitis media, chronic suppurative otitis media, and chronic otitis media with cholesteatoma as well as meningitis, injury, and ototoxic agents. Depending on the pathology involved, the hearing loss will be sensorineural, conductive, or mixed. In some cases the acquired loss may be profound, as is often the case with hearing loss following meningitis.

## Otitis Media

Otitis media implies the presence of bacteria-laden fluid in the middle ear space. It is more common in those children who have had persistent middle ear effusion. The symptoms are pain, fever, irritability, and sleeplessness. In a very small child the symptoms may be vague and the problem not obvious to the parent.

Examination will reveal a red tympanic membrane, usually but not always bulging. Engorgement of the vessels on the drum will be obvious, and the ear will be difficult to examine because of its tenderness. The infection usually occurs with or follows an upper respiratory tract infection. The otitis is more often bilateral in infants than in older children. Blisters or "bullae" may be present on the eardrum, and occasionally the ear will be draining a clear or yellowish fluid. When the ear begins to drain, the pain usually subsides promptly.

Otitis media is commonly due to one of three types of bacteria: *Hemophilus influenza* type b (having nothing to do with "the flu"), *streptococcus pneumonia* (pneumococcus), and *beta-hemolytic streptococcus.* Occasionally an unusual type of bacteria, mycoplasma pneumonia, will cause an infection, usually of the bullous type and frequently after a respiratory infection. This type may require treatment with erythromycin.

Treatment is usually straightforward. The appropriate antibiotic is given, usually for 10 days. Myringotomy and drainage of the ear may or may not be needed, depending on the severity of the child's illness and its response to antibiotics. Prompt resolution of the infection is common, although persistent infections requiring multiple changes of antibiotics are not uncommon.

The complications of otitis media include chronic suppurative otitis media with mastoiditis, meningitis, brain abscess and otitic hydrocephalous (enlargement of the ventricular spaces in the brain), and sigmoid sinus thrombosis (an infected blood clot in the mastoid bone). Sensorineural hearing loss may occur, presumably due to the effect of bacterial toxins on the cochlea. The loss may be in the high frequencies because of the vulnerability of the basilar turn of the cochlea. Persistent infection of the middle ear space may affect the tissues of the eustachian tube, and sufficient swelling or scarring may prevent adequate drainage. Artificial ventilation may then be required for complete resolution of the problem. This may include either myringotomy alone or insertion of a ventilating tube. Adenoidectomy or occasionally tonsillectomy and adenoidectomy may be required for resolution of chronic, recurrent otitis media.

If recurrent, chronic ear infections may progress to perforation and chronic suppurative otitis media with mastoiditis. This condition implies a chronic infection of the middle ear and mastoid air cells with chronic or recurrent drainage through a perforation of the drum. Occasionally the mastoiditis will be so extensive that drainage through the tip of the mastoid bone and skin behind the ear will occur, a so-called Bezold's abscess. In the worst cases acute otitis media will extend through the thin plate of bone separating the ear from the brain and cause a brain abscess.

## Serous Otitis

Serous otitis media or seromucinous otitis media is a common disorder of childhood. It is the most frequent childhood illness seen in the otolaryngologist's office, and the frequency of diagnosis is increasing, no doubt a result of improved and more readily available diagnostic equipment, more screening programs, and increased clinician and parental awareness. Some have implied that the incidence of the disorder itself is increasing because of the growing number of day-care centers, where large groups of children gather at an early age. True or not, this assertion is difficult to prove. Serous otitis media and its attendant complications have been described at least since the time of Hippocrates (Black, 1984). Some authors claim its existence was unjustly denied in the early part of the twentieth century, resurfacing as a new and popular disease for medical discussions in the 1940s and 1950s. Perhaps it was overlooked, and improved methods of testing and visualization of the middle ear space have made the diagnosis easier. Certainly the treatment of serous otitis media has improved a great deal over the last two decades, with the widespread use of tympanostomy tubes.

The disorder is characterized by the accumulation of fluid, either serous (thin) or mucinous (thick) fluid behind the tympanic membrane and in the air spaces of the mastoid bone. In some cases the fluid may be almost gluelike (glue ear). Experimental evidence (Silverstein, Miller, & Lindeman, 1966) and clinical observation suggest that the disorder is associated with dysfunction of the eustachian tube. This obstruction may be caused by mucosal or lymphoid swelling resulting from allergy or infection. In some cases the eustachian tube is underdeveloped or shortened, or a muscular abnormality of the palate impedes its opening. Children with midface deformity, cleft palate, submucous cleft palate, and other facial deformities have a greatly increased incidence.

In this disorder the eardrum appears dull, and the mucosal surfaces of the middle ear cannot be seen. An air-fluid level or bubbles will occasionally be evident. The frequently mentioned "cone of light" is an unreliable sign, as is the use of pressure otoscopy while visualizing the movement, or lack of movement, of the eardrum. The most helpful signs are the appearance or projection of the short process of the malleus, the relative concavity of the drum, the presence of enlarged tympanic vessels, and the inability to see the convoluted musosal surface of the middle ear. Experience in examining tympanic membranes is the best teacher.

The disorder of serous otitis media includes a spectrum of ear disease ranging from those with persistent negative pressures to those that become glue ear. Over a period of time, clinical experience shows that tympanic membranes exposed to chronic negative pressure or fluid accumulation will eventually weaken and retract. Occasionally the retraction will be so severe that the tympanic membrane drapes itself over the ossicles, most commonly the incus and stapes. If the membrane adheres to these structures, the bones may be deprived of their blood supply and dissolve. Chronic retraction may lead to formation of a squamous tissue-lined pocket in a recess of the tympanic cavity, attic, or antrum. A so-called "cholestatoma" may develop. Clinical experience and more recent experimental evidence suggest that the presence of serous fluid in the middle ear space increases the risk of acute otitis media. Adequate ventilation of these spaces either through the eustachian tube or a tympanostomy tube removes the fluid and decreases that risk.

Serous otitis media is properly treated through the restoration of normal middle ear ventilation. Occasionally the eustachian tube dysfunction will disappear over time, and once the upper respiratory tract infection has cleared or the allergic stimulus is gone, the fluid subsides. The period of resolution usually takes at least several weeks. The persistence of fluid should not be a concern until several weeks have passed. Usually 3 to 4 months of observation are warranted before contemplating surgical ventilation of the middle ear spaces. However, if a worrisome change in the appearance of the drum takes place during this period, such as atalectasis and adherence of the drum to the incus, then ventilating tubes may be inserted earlier to preserve the integrity of the tympanic membrane.

The surgical treatment of serous otitis media almost always includes insertion of ventilating tubes. These are usually made of Teflon, although they may be made of a variety of materials such as silicone, stainless steel, titanium, and gold. They have a small (usually 0.04 inch) opening in a grommet-shaped tube and are placed in the eardrum through an incision. This is done under general anesthesia since proper placement of the tube cannot be easily accomplished if the child is awake and squirming. The tubes usually stay in position about 6 months, after which time they come out on their own. Depending on the type of tube used, however, they may stay in place for 12 to 24 months. Whenever prolonged ventilation of the middle ear space is required, a permanent type of tube is inserted. Myringotomy without tube insertion may be beneficial in a limited number of cases. The problems encountered with ventilating tubes are few, and the benefits usually greatly outweigh the risks. Complications from tubes include perforation of the eardrum and tube-induced cholesteatoma. The latter is rare, and, in fact, perforation of the drum is uncommon with the currently available tubes.

Treatment in the past has included insufflation of the middle ear through the eustachian tube, adenotonsillectomy, and even irradiation of nasopharyngeal lymphoid tissue. Although adenoidectomy may still be useful in the case of persistent or recurring serous otitis media, the other older methods are not currently in vogue.

## Chronic Suppurative Otitis Media

Chronic suppurative otitis media will usually be manifested by a perforation of the drum and drainage of purulent material. Continued drainage and infection can lead to the secondary problems of ossicular fixation or destruction of the ossicular chain. A fistula may occur if the otic capsule is eroded.

Perforations are characterized according to their location, extent, and relationship to the annulus. For instance, a 30% anterior, inferior, marginal perforation of the pars tensa would mean that the hole in the tympanic membrane is in the front lower portion of the eardrum, involves about 30% of its surface area, and lies adjacent to the bony annulus. The distinction between marginal perforations and central perforations is important. Marginal perforations may allow the ingrowth of squamous epithelium and lead to the formation of cholesteatoma. Central perforations seem more resistant to this complication.

The long-term complications of chronic otitis media include hearing loss due to perforation alone or due to perforation and fixation or dissolution of a portion of the ossicular chain. The maximum conductive loss will be about 60 dB if discontinuity exists; any lesser degree of loss may depend on the amount of fixation and the location of the perforation. Another long-term complication of chronic suppurative otitis media is an infection of the bone, an osteitis that may be exceptionally difficult to cure.

If left untreated, this infection may lead to dissolution of the otic capsule, fistulization of the labyrinth, and eventually destruction of the inner ear and complete loss of hearing in the affected ear.

The treatment of chronic suppurative otitis media may include surgical removal of infected bone and tissue and closure of the membranous space behind the eardrum. Closure of the eardrum is termed *tympanoplasty* and may be one of several types (designated types I–V), depending on the amount of reconstruction of the ossicular chain that is required. A type I tympanoplasty is the simplest, involving only closure of the perforated eardrum without ossicular reconstruction. Tympanoplasty combined with mastoidectomy may be required if the mastoid bone is chronically infected or if keratoma has involved the mastoid cavity or middle ear space. Mastoidectomy may involve extensive removal of bone and middle ear mucosa and ossicles (a so-called radical mastoidectomy), or it may involve a removal of involved bone and air cell system with preservation of the middle ear space and any remaining ossicles (a modified radical mastoidectomy). Depending on the surgical technique involved, the posterior bony external auditory canal may or may not be preserved. The current surgical trend in tympanoplasty and mastoidectomy is to keep the external canal wall intact because its preservation improves the hearing and lessens the required postoperative care.

Chronic suppurative otitis media seems to be decreasing in frequency. The use of ventilating tubes and the frequent use of antibiotics over the last several decades are probably responsible for this decrease. Mastoiditis with its attendant complications is now quite uncommon except in populations that lack access to proper medical care.

Surgical closure of the eardrum and middle ear cavity is reserved for those children who can demonstrate adequate ventilation of the middle ear through a functioning eustachian tube. Repair of the drum will do no good if a poorly functioning eustachian tube causes immediate recurrence of the problem. Usually the age of 7 or 8 is a good time to contemplate tympanoplasty if the opposite ear is used as an indicator of eustachian tube function and that ear remains disease-free. Preferably the ear to be operated on should be without drainage or infection for a period of 5 to 6 months prior to surgery.

## Keratoma

Keratoma is uncommon in the pediatric age group. It has been commonly termed *cholesteatoma*, but *keratoma* is a more proper term since the disease process is one of invasion of the normally mucosal-lined spaces of the middle ear and mastoid with keratin-producing epithelium. The keratoma may be either primary or secondary and may be congenital or acquired. A secondary acquired cholesteatoma, for example, would be one arising from ingrowth of squamous epithelium through a marginal perforation. A congenital cholesteatoma implies one that arises from a "rest" of epithelial cells behind an intact tympanic membrane. Congenital cholesteatomas are quite rare.

The pressure of a skin-lined tract behind the tympanic membrane may lead to continued ingrowth of the sac and destruction of middle ear structures, dissolution of bone, and invasion and fistulization of the otic capsule or the facial canal. The destruction of bone is the result of resorption, which may be due to pressure from the keratoma or to enzymatic activity at the bone and skin interface. The resulting hearing loss may be conductive or mixed, depending on the structures destroyed. The most common area for formation of a keratoma is in the area of the pars flaccida, where it will appear as a small perforation with extrusion of whitish keratin material.

A well-known clinical phenomenon is the aggressiveness and destructiveness of keratomas found in children compared with those found in adults. The reasons for this difference are not entirely clear but may be due to the less well developed mastoid air cell systems in adults who have had longstanding ear problems with resultant decreased pneumatization of the temporal bone (Derlacki, Harrison, & Clemis, 1968). Infection of the keratoma greatly speeds its destructive growth.

## Meningitis

Bacterial meningitis is the most common cause of postnatal, profound, sensorineural hearing loss in children, accounting for 9.7% of all causes of deafness (Schein & Delk, 1974). The incidence of hearing loss following meningeal infection has decreased by a factor of only 2 since 1920 (from 18% to 9.7%), a fact probably accounted for by an increased rate of survival from the disease compared to the preantibiotic era (Catlin, 1985). Survivors of meningitis exhibit a hearing loss in 2.4% to 29% of cases. The risk of profound loss is quite dependent on the bacteria responsible. Kaplan and others found 7% of children with meningitis developed hearing loss. In that study, pneumococcal meningitis caused a loss in 33%, *Hemophilus influenza* type b in 9%, and meningococcal meningitis in 5% (Kaplan, Catlin, Weaver, & Feigin, 1984). *Hemophilus influenza* type b (Hib) is the causative agent in most cases in childhood meningitis, with an incidence of 3 to 59 per 100,000 children. It is a common cause of systemic disease in children under 2 years of age (Kaplan, Catlin, & Weaver, 1984).

Other types of *H. influenza* are not as virulent and are rare as a cause of meningitis.

*Hemophilus* b polysaccharide vaccine is now available for prophylaxsis against systemic Hib disease. Its routine use should decrease the incidence of meningitis due to *Hemophilus*. Unfortunately, its use is limited to children 24 months of age or older. In high-risk individuals it may be used as early as 18 months of age, although the antibody response is not as great as that in older children. The vaccine's age restriction limits its usefulness as a preventative agent in Hib diseases.

*Hemophilus influenza* type b is a difficult organism to treat since a high percentage of the organisms have developed a resistance to ampicillin. Treatment is possible with some of the newer cephalosporin antibiotics and with chloramphenicol. When meningitis occurs, the hearing loss is usually severe to profound, presents early in the course of the disease, and is bilateral and flat in most cases.

Meningitis is caused by invasion of the subarachnoid space with bacteria, usually via the bloodstream, upper respiratory tract, or ear. The hearing loss is probably a result of suppurative labryrinthitis, although bacterial toxins may also be a factor. The rare case of improvement in a postmeningitis hearing loss may be due to resolution of a toxic labyrinthitis.

The most common bacteria are *H. influenza*, pneumococcus, and meningococcus. Other less common microorganisms such as fungi and mycobacteria may be responsible in the rare case. Treatment is with an appropriate antibiotic that crosses the blood/brain barrier. Prompt treatment increases survival rates, but since hearing loss occurs early in the disease process, it may not prevent the occurrence of hearing loss.

## Measles

Measles (rubeola) may be a cause of sensorineural hearing impairment. The National Census of Deaf Persons (NCDP) found a 4.3% incidence of hearing loss due to this disease (Catlin, 1985). The mechanism may be encephalitis with resultant injury to cochlear structures. The involvement is bilateral with moderate to severe permanent loss of auditory and sometimes vestibular function (Schuknecht, 1974). Pathologically the changes include degeneration of the organ of Corti, spiral ganglion, and vestibular organs. Cochlear neurons may be lost. No specific treatment is available, and prevention of the disease through adequate vaccination programs is the key to decreasing the risk of hearing loss.

## Pertussis

Pertussis (whooping cough) is recognized as a cause of sensorineural hearing loss. It is much less common now than in the past. Immunization programs have been effective in reducing the incidence of the disease, although recent concerns about postvaccination complications threaten this success. Recent studies have shown, however, that the risk of serious postimmunization complications is much less than the risk of fatality from pertussis infection.

## Mumps

Hearing loss due to mumps is most commonly unilateral and may vary from a mild high-frequency loss to profound impairment. The cochlea is usually the site of involvement, and vestibular function is rarely affected. Because it is frequently one-sided, the loss may go undetected until the child is of school age or older. Early immunization has greatly decreased the incidence of mumps.

## Scarlet Fever

The National Census of Deaf Persons lists scarlet fever as the cause of 6.2% of hearing loss in a 1971 survey (Schein & Delk, 1974). This disease is due to beta-hemolytic streptococci, which are quite sensitive to most commonly used antibiotics. Its importance as a cause of hearing loss, although difficult to estimate now, is certainly less than in the preantibiotic era.

## Ototoxicity

Ototoxicity may occur from a variety of drugs—from antibiotics to antineoplastic drugs. The most important drugs to consider are the aminoglycoside antibiotics, which may be cochleotoxic and/or vestibulotoxic in some situations. These antibiotics are used to treat life-threatening infections and prolonged exposure to high levels, especially in the presence of decreased kidney function, may result in hearing loss. There is some speculation that a combination of noise and aminoglycoside administration may increase the risk of sustaining hair cell damage in the cochlea (Catlin, 1985). Antiinflammatory drugs and diuretics such as furosemide (Lasix) may also be ototoxic, usually in a reversible way.

## Noise Exposure

Excessive noise exposure, being more common in older individuals, is often overlooked as a cause of hearing loss in children. Insidious exposure to excessive noise levels occurs at rock concerts or from hi-fi equipment. In addition, there may be exposure to shooting noises while hunting or to firecrackers during the holiday seasons. The loss is characteristic, usually bilateral with high-frequency notching at 4000 Hz to 6000 Hz.

# Diagnostic Evaluation of Hearing Loss

There is an average delay of 2.5 years between birth and the detection of sensorineural hearing loss (Pappas & Mundy, 1981). For the one child in 1,000 born with the handicap of a sensorineural loss, this delay may unfortunately extend well into the early years of speech development. A large proportion of children with varying degrees of sensorineural impairment will appear normal at birth. They are born without the obvious risk factors of familial hearing loss, viral exposure, ear deformity, hyperbilirubinemia, or low APGAR score. Many will not be small at birth or premature. For these children, screening at birth or in the first 6 months of life may provide the only chance to diagnose their hearing loss definitively and help them at an early age. Identification of a hearing loss early in life usually generates an intensive search for the cause. This search can be very expensive and lead to an extensive battery of screening tests from CT scans to karyotypes. Clearly a rational approach is needed.

The following outline presents a sequence of evaluation steps that can be useful in diagnosing hearing loss:

If hearing loss is suspected:
    Detailed physical examination
    Family history
    Assessment of high-risk factors
    Auditory screening, ABR

If screening tests are abnormal or questionable:
    Complete blood count (CBC)
    Urinalysis
    Urine for mucopolysaccharidoses
    EKG

Polytomography of the temporal bones
Urine for CMV
Repeat screening in 6 weeks

If screening tests are abnormal after the age of 3, and the cause is not obvious:

EKG
Thyroid function studies
Urinalysis
Ophthalmologic examination
SMA screen
Polytomography
Viral studies—not helpful

Cytomegalovirus is the most common infectious cause of hearing loss, and examination of a urine specimen for CMV within the first week of life is the most sensitive method of detection of intrauterine infection. Urine or serum samples obtained in the later months of life will not definitively document a CMV infection. For children 0 to 3 years of age with objective documentation of hearing loss, evaluation should include a urine or serum test for CMV. In addition, a detailed physical examination not only of the ears, nose, and throat but of the skin and skeletal system should be done. Thyroid size should be noted, but thyroid function studies are not needed at this age. Polytomography of the cochlea may indicate a structural abnormality, and an electrocardiogram may document characteristic changes of the Jervell-Lange-Nielsen syndrome or associated cardiac abnormality. Pappas recommends a routine battery of polytomography, EKG, complete blood count (CBC), urinalysis, and a urine test for mucopolysaccharidoses in addition to a urine specimen for CMV and a careful physical examination. In this age group, testing for retinitis pigmentosa is not fruitful, and thyroid function tests are nonrevealing since the hormonal manifestations of Penred's syndrome are not apparent until after the age of 3. A CBC will provide information of the child's general health, and a urinalysis may document hematuria associated with Alport's syndrome (Pappas & Mundy, 1981).

After age 3, the manifestations of the mucopolysaccharidoses will become more apparent, and opthalmologic examination for the changes of Usher's syndrome will be more revealing. An SMA screen (multiple metabolic studies) including blood-urea-nitrogen (BUN) and creatinine tests to screen for renal abnormalities will be valuable in the 3- to 6-year-old age group. Neurologic studies such as brain scans and EEGs are generally superfluous since most neurologic syndromes do not become apparent until later and brain damage by this age is usually readily apparent. A karyotype to screen for a genetic syndrome is usually not indicated and its routine use an expensive waste.

The most valuable studies are still objective audiometry (BSER), polytomography, CBC, urinalysis, and viral studies of urine or serum within the first week of life (Pappas, 1981). Other studies should be ordered based on objective, clinical evidence.

# Prevention

Emphasis in the past has been on alleviating the condition of deafness once it has been identified. Great progress has been made in the last decade, particularly in the early diagnosis of sensorineural impairment, and opportunities now exist to reduce significantly the number of children born deaf. These opportunities include diverse new technologies from genetic manipulation to advances in immunization against viral and bacterial illness.

Early diagnosis is important. Identification of the profoundly deaf child in the first few months of life combined with parental guidance and genetic counseling may decrease the number of subsequent children born with the same defect to the same family. Perhaps sensorineural hearing loss should be a reportable condition. This policy would focus public and professional attention to the problem and perhaps unify efforts of study and prevention. A uniform screening program would be beneficial.

Maintenance of immunization programs for rubella and development of new vaccines for CMV would greatly decrease the prenatal acquisition of hearing loss of infectious origin. Early detection of CMV infection is mandatory, since detection later in life obscures the diagnosis of prenatally acquired hearing loss. Hearing loss due to meningitis, particularly *Hemophilus influenza* type b, remains a problem. Perhaps utilization of *Hemophilus influenza* type b vaccine and development of a vaccine that can be used with children younger than 24 months of age would decrease the number of children affected with meningitis.

The emphasis should be on early detection, unified study, standardization of screening procedures, genetic counseling, and elimination of viral and bacterial risk factors.

# Summary

Hearing loss in children can be conveniently divided by time of onset into prenatal, postnatal, and perinatal groups. Although not always absolute, these groups provide a convenient basis for discussion. The majority of children acquire their hearing loss in the prenatal period, usually due to maternal viral infection or more commonly due to genetic factors. Of the latter group, bilateral sensorineural hearing loss acquired by autosomal recessive inheritance is most common. Since detection of the carrier state of the deafness trait is not yet possible, we are not now able to decrease the frequency of this devastating problem. Research in this area remains one of the great challenges of the next several decades.

Meningitis remains the most common cause of postnatally acquired sensorineural hearing loss. Efforts at early diagnosis and prompt treatment as well as prevention with newly developed vaccines offer the most hope, especially for those affected by *Hemophilus influenza*. The appropriate use of antibiotics and ventilating tubes offer the most hope for those with postnatally acquired hearing loss due to chronic otitis media and serous otitis.

Perinatally acquired sensorineural hearing loss remains a vexing problem since the cause is usually obscure. Hypoxia and prematurity probably account for the majority of cases. These circumstances are most often beyond the control of those in attendance.

Early detection through screening programs and proper diagnosis through prompt utilization of available diagnostic tests will allow coordination of efforts to eventually decrease the incidence of sensorineural hearing loss.

# References

Abramovich, S. J., Gregory, S., Slemich, M., & Stewart, A. (1979). Hearing loss in very low birthweight infants treated with neonatal intensive care. *Archives of Disease in Childhood, 54*, 421–426.

Alford, B. R. (1968). Rubella—*La bete noire de la medicine. Laryngoscope, 78*, 1623–1659.

American Speech-Language-Hearing Association (1982). Joint Committee on Infant Hearing: Position statement. *Asha, 24*, 1017–1018.

Anagnostakis, D., Petmezakis, J., Papazissis, G., Messaritakis, J., & Matsoniotis, N. (1982). Hearing loss in low-birth-weight infants. *American Journal of Diseases in Children, 136*, 602–604.

Black, N. A. (1984). Is glue ear a modern phenomenon? A historical review of the medical literature. *Clinical Otolaryngology and Allied Sciences, 9,* 155–163.

Brodersen, R. (1977). Review article: Prevention of kernicterus based on recent progress in bilirubin chemistry. *Acta Paediatrica Scandinavia, 66* (5), 625–634.

Brown, J. K., Purvis, R. J., Fortar, J. D., & Cockburn, F. (1974). Neurological aspects of perinatal asphyxia. *Developmental Medicine and Child Neurology, 16* (5), 567–580.

Buch, N. H. (1966). Purulent labyrinthitis in a newborn infant. *Journal of Laryngology and Otolaryngology, 80* (9), 875–884.

Catlin, F. I. (1978). Etiology and pathology of hearing loss in children. In F. N. Martin (Ed.), *Pediatric Audiology* (pp. 3–34). Englewood Cliffs, NJ: Prentice-Hall.

Catlin, F. I. (1985). Prevention of hearing impairment from infection and ototoxic drugs. *Archives of Otolaryngology, 111* (6), 377–384.

Cohen, J. I., & Corey, G. R. (1985). Cytomegalovirus infection in the normal host. *Medicine, 64* (2), 100–114.

Derlacki, E., & Clemis, J. (1965). Congenital cholesteatoma of the middle ear and mastoid. *Annals of Otology, Rhinology, and Laryngology, 74,* 706.

Derlacki, E., Harrison, W., & Clemis, J. (1968). Congenital cholesteatoma of the middle ear and mastoid: A second report presenting seven additional cases. *Laryngoscope, 78* (6), 1050–1078.

Dudgeon, J. A. (1972). Congenital rubella: A preventable disease. *Postgraduate Medical Journal, 48* (Suppl. 3), 7–11.

Fisch, L., & Osborn, D. A. (1984). Congenital deafness and hemolytic disease of the newborn. *Archives of Disease in Childhood, 29,* 309–316.

Hall, J. G. (1964). The cochlea and cochlear nuclei in neonatal asphyxia. *Acta Otolaryngologica* (Suppl.), *194,* 1–93.

Hanshaw, J. B., & Dudgeon, J. A. (1978). Viral disease of the fetus and newborn. In *Major problems in clinical pediatrics* (pp. 1–9). Philadelphia: W. B. Saunders.

Kaplan, S. L., Catlin, F. I., Weaver, T., & Feigin, R. D. (1984). Onset of hearing loss in children with bacterial meningitis. *Pediatrics, 73* (5), 575–578.

Karmody, C., & Schuknecht, H. (1966). Deafness in congenital syphilis. *Archives of Otolaryngology, 83* (1), 18–27.

Konigsmark, B. (1971). Hereditary congenital severe deafness syndrome. *Annals of Otology, Rhinology, and Laryngology, 80,* 269–276.

Konigsmark, B. W., & Gorlin, R. J. (1976). *Genetic and metabolic deafness.* Philadelphia: W. B. Saunders.

Lubchenco, L. O., Delivoria-Papadopoulos, M., Butterfield, L. J., Metcalf, D., Hix, I. E., Danick, J., Dodds, J., Downs, M., & Freeland, E. (1972). Long-term follow-up studies of prematurely born infants: I. Relationship of handicaps to nursery routines. *Journal of Pediatrics, 80* (3), 501–508.

MacDonald, H., & Tobin, J. O. H. (1978). Congenital cytomegalovirus infection: A collaborative study of epidemiological, clinical, and laboratory findings. *Developmental Medicine and Child Neurology, 20* (4), 471–482.

Newton, V. E. (1985). Aetiology of bilateral sensorineural hearing loss in young children. *Journal of Laryngology and Otology* (Suppl.), 10, 1–57.

Northern, J. L., & Downs, M. P. (1984). *Hearing in children* (3rd ed.). Baltimore: Williams and Wilkins.

Paparella, M. M., & Shumrick, D. A. (1980). *Otolaryngology: II. The Ear* (2nd ed.). Philadelphia: W. B. Saunders.

Pappas, D. G., & Mundy, M. R. (1981). Sensorineural hearing loss in young children: A systematic approach to evaluation. *Southern Medical Journal, 74,* 965–967.

Pass, R. F., Hutto, S. C., Reynolds, D. W., Polhill, R. B. (1984). Increased frequency of cytomegalovirus infection in children in group day care. *Pediatrics,* 74 (1), 121–126.

Pass, R. F., Hutto, C., Ricks, R., Cloud, G. A. (1986). Increased rate of cytomegalovirus infection among parents of children attending day-care centers. *New England Journal of Medicine, 314* (22), 1414–1418.

Rooney, J. C., Hill, D. J., & Danks, D. M. (1971). Jaundice associated with bacterial infection in the newborn. *American Journal of Diseases of Children, 122,* 39–43.

Schein, J. D., & Delk, M. T., Jr. (1974). *The deaf population of the United States.* Silver Springs, MD.: National Association of the Deaf.

Schiff, D., Stern, L., & Leduc, J. (1966). Chemical thermogenesis in newborn infants: Catecholamine excretion and the plasma non-esterified fatty acid response to cold exposure. *Pediatrics, 37* (4), 577–582.

Schuknecht, H. F. (1974). *Pathology of the ear.* Cambridge, MA: Harvard University Press.

Silverstein, H., Miller, G. F., Jr., & Lindeman, R. (1966). Eustachian tube dysfunction as a cause for chronic secretory otitis in children (correction by pressure-equalization). *Laryngoscope, 76* (2), 259–273.

Sohmer, H., Feinmesser, M., Lev, A., Bauberger-Tell, L., & David, S. (1972). Routine use of cochlear audiometry in infants with uncertain diagnosis. *Annals of Otology, Rhinology, and Laryngology, 81* (1), 72–75.

Stagno, S., Reynolds, D. W., Amos, C. S., Dahle, A. J., McCollister, F. P., Mohindra, I., Ermocilla, R., & Alford, C. A. (1977). Auditory and visual defects resulting from symptomatic and subclinical congenital cytomegalovirus and toxoplasma infections. *Pediatrics, 59* (5), 669–678.

Swan, C., Tostevin, A. L., Moore, B., Mayo, H., & Black, G. H. B. (1943). Congenital defects in infants following infectious diseases during pregnancy with special reference to the relationship between German measles and cataract, deaf-mutism, heart disease, and microcephaly and to the period of pregnancy in which the occurrence of rubella is followed by congenital abnormalities. *Medical Journal of Australia, 2,* 201–210.

Taylor, I. G. (1980). The prevention of sensori-neural deafness. *Journal of Laryngology and Otology, 94* (12), 1327–1343.

Wigglesworth, J. S., & Pape, K. E. (1978). An integrated model for haemorrhagic and ischaemic lesions in the newborn brain. *Early Human Development, 2* (2), 179–199.

Williamson, W. D., Desmond, M. M., LaFevers, N., Taber, L. H., Catlin, F. I., & Weaver, T. G. (1982). Symptomatic congenital cytomegalovirus: Disorders of language, learning, and hearing. *American Journal of Diseases in Children, 136* (10), 902–905.

# *e Effects of Early*
# *ing Impairment*
# *glish Language*
# *⌄pment*

## PETER V. PAUL
## STEPHEN P. QUIGLEY

$I$n the education of hearing-impaired children and youths, considerable attention and research have focused on the development of language comprehension skills. These are important if one of the goals is literacy—that is, the ability to read and write standard English at a mature, sophisticated level (Quigley & Kretschmer, 1982). Despite the concerted efforts of numerous professionals, it is well documented in the research literature that most hearing-impaired students fail to acquire English language skills commensurate with their hearing counterparts (King & Quigley, 1985; Quigley & Paul, 1984a).

The development of English is a formidable task that demands, in the least, the cooperation of teachers, speech pathologists, audiologists, and researchers. Progress may be possible with access to a wider view of the problem, which is often obscured by the details of daily practices. Specifically, the personnel concerned with the welfare of hearing-impaired students should be cognizant of theories and research relating to the development of English language and reading skills. Equally as important is an understanding of the interrelationships of several descriptive variables affecting language development that are uniquely attributable to hearing-impaired students.

There are several objectives of this chapter. First, theories and research regarding normal English language development are briefly discussed. Second, some studies regarding the effects of early hearing impairment on acquisition of the primary (i.e., signs and speech) and secondary (i.e., reading and writing) forms of English are presented, and some tentative conclusions are inferred from the available evidence. Finally, areas in need of further research are discussed. It should be emphasized that the studies selected here are meant to be representative of the issues rather than an exhaustive treatment.

# Definition of Hearing Impairment

To delineate the impact of hearing impairment on English language development, it is necessary to discuss some definitions. There are certain descriptive variables that should be considered: for example, degree and type of hearing impairment; age at onset; etiology; presence of additional handicaps; type of education program; and hearing status, level of involvement, and communication mode of the parents. It is important to define hearing impairment in relation to these variables to avoid the generalization of findings to dissimilar populations (Quigley & Kretschmer, 1982). Unfortunately, it is difficult to find studies that provide complete descriptions of the subjects. In addition, it is also possible that some of this information is not available to the researcher. While these factors should be considered simultaneously, the degree of impairment has assumed the most weight in determining the educational placement of hearing-impaired children (Karchmer, Milone, & Wolk, 1979).

In audiological terms, the degree of an individual's hearing impairment (i.e., hearing threshold level) is represented as a pure-tone average in decibels (dB) across what is known as the speech frequencies (500, 1000, and 2000 Hz) for the better unaided ear. Hearing impairment is a generic term that may be qualified in relation to one of five categories as described in Table 2.1. Students within the first three categories are referred to as hard of hearing whereas those in the last one are labeled deaf. The students in the severe-impairment category are referred to as either hard of hearing or deaf, depending on the use of their residual hearing. Excluding the profound range, the relationships between degrees of hearing impairment and educational achievements have not been investigated extensively. Consequently, there has been little impact on instructional methodologies and materials.

This chapter presents research findings in relation to two broad categories, hard of hearing (up to 89 dB) and deaf (90 dB or greater), which contains the bulk of the evidence. As will be observed, this is not always possible since some studies of deaf students also contain severely hearing-impaired students. These exceptions, however, are noted. Nevertheless, on the audiological continuum, there is a point at which the hearing-impaired individual's primary mode for receiving language and for communication is through vision rather than audition, even with the use of

## TABLE 2.1
### Categories of Hearing Impairment

| Degree of Impairment[a] (ISO)[b] | Label |
|---|---|
| *Slight*<br>27 to 40 decibels | Hard of Hearing |
| *Mild*<br>41 to 54 decibels | Hard of Hearing |
| *Moderate*<br>55 to 69 decibels | Hard of Hearing |
| *Severe*<br>70 to 89 decibels | Hard of Hearing or Deaf |
| *Profound*<br>90 decibels and greater | Deaf |

[a] Refers to better unaided ear averaged across the speech frequencies of 500, 1000, and 2000 Hz.

[b] International Standards Organization.

*Source:* Adapted from Moores (1982) and Quigley and Paul (1984a).

amplification. There is evidence to suggest that this occurs at approximately 90 dB (ISO) (Quigley & Kretschmer, 1982; Quigley & Paul, 1984a; Stark, 1974). Thus, for most profoundly hearing-impaired students, there is little doubt that the use of residual hearing serves as a secondary and supplemental channel. Even the differences in academic achievement observed among these students may be due, in part, to the effective exploitation of residual hearing (Ross & Calvert, 1984). It is likely that hard-of-hearing children have received more exposure than deaf (profoundly hearing-impaired) children to normal aural/oral interactions, which provide the foundation for an auditorially based, internalized linguistic system. According to the findings of the Gallaudet Research Institute's 1982–83 Annual Survey of Hearing-Impaired Children and Youth, the profoundly impaired students comprised approximately 44% of the hearing-impaired student population whereas the severely impaired students make up 21%, and those with lesser impairments, about 34% (Gallaudet Research Institute, 1985).

When degree of hearing impairment is considered in conjunction with the other previously mentioned descriptive variables, research has shown a significant effect on the development of spoken and written English skills (King & Quigley, 1985; Quigley & Paul, 1984a). For example, children who become severely to profoundly hearing-impaired at 6 years of age may have the same degrees of impairment as those who suffered hearing losses at birth; however, their language and communication skills may be very different (Goetzinger & Rousey, 1959; Pintner & Paterson, 1916, 1917; Quigley & Kretschmer, 1982). The importance of investigators providing complete descriptions of the populations under study cannot be overemphasized. This would certainly aid in the interpretation of the results and, consequently, have a greater impact on educational practices. Finally, it should be remarked that those variables of importance in describing the normally hearing student population—for example, intelligence (IQ) and socioeconomic status (SES)—are also applicable to the hearing-impaired student population.

# Acquisition of English: Hearing Students

### Primary Language Development

Typically, primary language development is manifested by the development of speech skills within the conceptual framework of established linguistic components such as syntax and semantics. For most hearing students the comprehension and production of spoken English is a seemingly effortless task. Their ability to understand is limited primarily by the extent of their linguistic and cognitive development (de Villiers & de Villiers, 1978; Schlesinger, 1982).

A theory on the acquisition and use of a language is heavily influenced by the nature (i.e., grammar) of a language (Chomsky, 1957, 1965; Slobin, 1979). In general, theories of language can be grouped into four categories: behavioral, transformational generative grammar, cognitive, and sociocultural (Cruttenden, 1979; Menyuk, 1977; Schlesinger, 1982). While there is debate as to which theory achieves explanatory adequacy or, rather, best fits the data, few recent linguistic studies have been conducted within the behavioristic framework. Behavioristic theories specifically fail to consider the notion of meaning and to account for the productivity of language. The aspect of productivity resulted from the influence of the thinking of Noam Chomsky. Consequently, the major thrust of current linguistic and psycholinguistic analyses of child language has been to describe or explain grammatical errors in relation to a system of rules rather than simply listing or cataloging the errors. This perspective may contain more potential for resolving some of the language problems of language-impaired populations (e.g., learning disabled, educable mentally retarded, and hearing-impaired students).

One of the most astonishing yet debatable issues has been the rate at which most hearing children learn a spoken language. It is generally considered that some important milestones are the one-word, two-word, and three-word stages, which correspond roughly to 1, 2, and 3 years of age respectively. Beyond the three-word stage, children produce and comprehend linguistic forms and functions of a more complex nature, such as major transformations (Bloom & Lahey, 1978; de Villiers & de Villiers, 1978; Schlesinger, 1982). With the emergence of adolescence, most hearing children have reached linguistic maturity in that they have mastered most, if not all, of the finite set of native-speaking adult rules regarding the form, content, and function of their language.

## Secondary Language Development

A preponderant amount of theoretically based and empirical research has been accumulated on the development of secondary language skills—that is, reading and writing (Anderson, 1981; Pearson, 1985; Tierney & Leys, 1984). It appears that secondary language processing is essentially similar to that of primary language: children play an active role by discovering regularities and formulating hypotheses regarding the application of rules.

Current theories of reading can be grouped into three categories: bottom-up, top-down, and interactive. There is increasing evidence to suggest that reading is an interactive process between the linguistic and cognitive structures of the readers and the linguistic aspects of the text (Anderson, 1981; Pearson, 1985). In this view, reading is considered to be driven by higher-order mental processes in which readers construct meaning from the text and interpret it in terms of their background knowledge or schemata. Consequently, instruction in reading should entail the development of decoding and comprehension skills as well as the enrichment of the background or world knowledge of the readers.

It is becoming clear that reading and writing are interrelated (Tierney & Leys, 1984). While the nature of this relationship is disputable, it appears to depend upon the types of measures employed to evaluate these secondary language processes. Tierney and Leys (1984) have argued that the two processes are confounded: "When an individual writes he also reads, and when an individual reads he often writes" (p. 7). Eckhoff (1983) observed that the style of writing is affected by the content of reading materials. For example, if readers understand only language that is stilted in format, then their writing is also likely to be stilted. In light of the continuing research, it is safe to remark that reading and writing have parallels; however, they are not identical.

For most hearing children, reading and writing are secondary language forms superimposed on their internalized, auditory-based primary language forms. While the abilities to read and write require more than just a knowledge of language structures, they are still part of the overall language comprehension process. Thus, it appears that a primary, internalized language needs to be established before secondary language skills can be taught successfully. This view is espoused by Pearson and Johnson (1978): ". . . linguistic competence is an absolute prerequisite for reading comprehension. Such an assertion is almost tautological, since language is the medium of comprehension" (p. 19). As with the acquisition of a primary language form, most hearing students learn to read and write at a sophisticated mature level.

## Language and Communication Systems

Most of the knowledge regarding hearing-impaired students' understanding of English has been derived from their performances on secondary language measures, mainly in the format of achievement and diagnostic tests. These findings should be considered in relation to the nature and extent of the primary communication and language input to which hearing-impaired children are exposed in infancy and early childhood. It has been argued that there are two aspects of this controversial issue: the type of language and the form of communication mode employed (Quigley & Kretschmer, 1982). Two forms, oral and manual, can be combined in a number of ways to produce a variety of pedagogical approaches. The broad categories described here are representative of most of the commonly used approaches: oral English (OE), manually coded English (MCE), and American Sign Language (ASL) (Quigley & Paul, 1984a). Due to the nature of these categories, describing the English language development of hearing-impaired students is a very complicated matter. A brief description of these approaches is provided in the ensuing paragraphs. A more detailed analysis can be found elsewhere (Quigley & Kretschmer, 1982; Quigley & Paul, 1984a).

## Oral English

In the oral English category, three approaches and their variations may be found: acoupedics, aural-oral, and cued speech (Cornett, 1967, 1984; Ling, 1984; Moores, 1982). Traditionally the use of spoken English in the oral form has been the major thrust of these approaches. Cued speech can be placed in this category since its primary function is to enable the hearing-impaired child to disambiguate aspects of the spoken signal. It should be remarked that these approaches have been typically employed with hearing-impaired students in the severe and profound categories as well as with most of those with lesser impairments who are integrated in regular education programs and are thus exposed to the oral English of regular education instructors. A few of the integrated students in the severely to profoundly impaired category, however, may also require the services of oral interpreters (Ross, Brackett, & Maxon, 1982).

*Aural-Oral.*   Since acoupedics (or unisensory) methods are on the decline (Moores, 1982), only the aural-oral approach is discussed here. The major emphasis is on the development of the auditory *and* visual senses of the hearing-impaired child (Ling, 1976, 1984; Ling & Ling, 1978). To exploit the use of residual hearing, some aural-oral approaches have incorporated the acoupedics techniques of early amplification and auditory training. Others (e.g., auditory-visual-oral) have placed equal emphasis on the development of speech reading (lipreading) skills (Ling, 1984; Sanders,

1982). One of the goals of *all* aural-oral programs is the development of intelligible speech. As is discussed later, only a few select profoundly hearing-impaired students can perform well academically with the exclusive use of aural-oral approaches.

*Cued Speech.* In cued speech, eight contrived handshapes are utilized in four positions on or near the face to supplement the spoken signal. Each handshape represents a set of consonantal phonemes (e.g., /m/, /f/, /t/) that are distinguishable to a certain extent by speech reading. Each of the four positions represents a set of vocalic phonemes. The use of these manual cues without accompanying speech is essentially meaningless. When produced in conjunction with speech, they are supposed to provide a message that can be visually perceived by the hearing-impaired child. Despite the tenets of cued speech, very little research has been conducted to assess its effects on the development of English.

## Manually Coded English

In recent years a number of educational signed systems have been developed to represent the structure of written standard English in a manual manner. In general, these systems are considered to be morphologically based; however, they differ in their rules for representing the morphological structures of English (Raffin, 1976; Wilbur, 1979). Within the philosophy of total communication, educators and other practitioners are expected to execute the manual aspects of the systems and spoken English simultaneously (Moores, 1982). The more commonly used systems are briefly discussed here.

*Seeing Essential English (SEE I).* Of the various contrived systems, it is safe to conclude that, in theory, Seeing Essential English (SEE I) provides the closest morphological representation of standard English (Quigley & Paul, 1984a). The selection of signs or sign markers to represent a word and/or its parts is based on a two-out-of-three rule in relation to three criteria: sound, spelling, and meaning. For English words that have several meanings (see the review in Paul, 1984), two of these three criteria are typically similar (i.e., sound and spelling), so the same sign or sign marker is employed for each of the meanings (Anthony, 1966; Raffin, 1976).

*Signing Exact English (SEE II).* A few educators and researchers who found it difficult to accept some of the major principles of SEE I constructed a signed system labeled Signing Exact English (SEE II) (Gustason, Pfetzing, & Zawolkow, 1980). Since SEE II is derived from SEE I, there is some overlap in the use of signs and sign markers (e.g., affixes). Both systems adhere to the two-out-of-three rule described previously; however, they differ in their definitions of a root word or, in linguistic terms, a free morpheme. For example, in SEE II, the English word *butterfly* is represented by one sign. SEE I, however, treats this word as two root words requiring two signs, one for *butter* and another for *fly*. Due to this difference in definition, SEE II contains fewer sign markers for affixes (e.g., *-ing*, *-s*) than SEE I.

***Signed English (SE).***  Signed English (SE) is the result of the work of Bornstein and his associates (Bornstein, 1973; Bornstein & Saulnier, 1981; Bornstein, Saulnier, & Hamilton, 1980). The system was created to provide a language environment for hearing-impaired children similar to that for young hearing children. SE contains signs that represent the most commonly used inflections and words of preschool and lower elementary students. The relationship between a sign and an English word and its meaning(s) is determined by the status of the word in a dictionary of standard English. Each sign corresponds to the meaning(s) of one lexical entry. If a word has two lexical entries and, consequently, two meanings, then each entry would be represented by a different SE sign. Finger spelling may be employed for English words for which there are no sign equivalents.

***Pidgin Sign English.***  Typically, a pidgin is spoken by two speakers who are not competent in the other's language. As a rule, a pidgin contains vocabulary from both languages and adheres to the morphosyntactical structure of the majority language. There are wide variations due to the competence of the speakers and the nature of the communication tasks (Cokely, 1983). A pidgin is a communication system; yet it can become a bonafide language for a second generation of users.

Pidgin sign English (PSE) integrates the signs of American Sign Language (ASL) with the syntax of spoken English (Wilbur, 1979; Woodward, 1973). Like spoken pidgins, there are wide variations among the users of PSE. In one instance ASL-like signs may be executed in an English word order without nonmanual cues (e.g., raised eyebrows) and with the accompaniment of speech. In another instance more grammatical features of ASL may be employed without the accompaniment of spoken English. While PSE is not a contrived signed system like the others previously discussed, it may still be employed as a means of communication in educational environments. Other terms used to describe this communication system are American Sign English (Ameslish), sign English (Siglish), signed English, manual English, and even simultaneous communication (Bragg, 1973; Wilbur, 1979).

## American Sign Language

American Sign Language (ASL) differs from English in grammar and form (i.e., signs versus speech). It also differs from the contrived codes designed to represent the structure of English (Stokoe, 1975; Wilbur, 1979). The use of ASL-like signs in English word order does not reflect the grammar of ASL, just as the use of Spanish words in English word order is not Spanish (Lane & Grosjean, 1980). Since the English-based codes are executed simultaneously with speech, it is not possible to utilize a number of nonmanual cues of ASL (e.g., puffed cheeks, pursed lips) that convey important linguistic information. More important, the signs of the contrived codes do not retain their original syntactical (e.g., directional) and semantic (meaning) properties as present in the context of ASL. It can be inferred that English is a second language for deaf (profoundly hearing-impaired) students who received exposure to ASL in infancy and early childhood from their parents or caretakers.

# Acquisition of English by Hearing-Impaired Students

## Oral English

This section focuses on the language comprehension skills of hearing-impaired students exposed to special oral English methods and/or to the spoken English of regular classroom teachers. Not surprisingly, the students who typically receive special oral methods are those with severe to profound hearing impairments (Moores, 1982; Ross, Brackett, & Maxon, 1982). Of interest here are those who are exposed to aural-oral methods in good, comprehensive oral programs, such as that of the Central Institute for the Deaf (CID) in St. Louis, Missouri. The students with less than severe impairments (i.e., less than 70 dB) who are integrated into regular classrooms constitute the bulk of the hard-of-hearing student population as defined earlier. In theory this group is said to be the most numerous of all handicapped students and the most difficult to identify (Blair, Peterson, & Viehweg, 1985; Davis, 1977). Ross, Brackett, and Maxon (1982) have surmised that students with hearing losses in the better unaided ear up to 70 dB comprised about 1.6% of the general school population or approximately 16 per 1,000 students. It should be remembered that very few profoundly hearing-impaired students are academically integrated, either partly or fully, in regular education settings (Allen & Osborn, 1984; Wolk, Karchmer, & Schildroth, 1982).

*Hard-of-Hearing Students.* Presently it is taken as axiomatic that academic achievement is negatively affected by the degree of hearing impairment. This is not always obvious to some teachers who work with children with slight to mild hearing impairments (Ross, Brackett, & Maxon, 1982). This conspicuous fact can be gleaned, however, from studies conducted nearly 45 years earlier (e.g., Pintner, Eisenson, & Stanton, 1946; Pintner & Lev, 1939). It has also been corroborated by more recent investigations. According to group data, the major conclusion is that even a relatively slight hearing impairment can negatively affect academic performance.

Quigley and Thomure (1968) evaluated the academic performance of students in relation to their degree of hearing impairment. They found an inverse relationship between hearing impairment and academic achievement. For example, hearing-impaired students in the slight category (0–26 dB) demonstrated a resultant lag of a little more than 1 year on educational achievement tests whereas those with moderate impairments (40–55 dB) exhibited about a 3-year retardation when compared with hearing age norms.

Quantitative delays in language comprehension abilities have been substantiated by more recent investigations. Pressnell (1973) and Wilcox and Tobin (1974) examined the ability of students with moderate or greater hearing impairments to understand aspects of the verb system of English. Analyzing spontaneous language samples and the results of the *Northwestern Syntax Screening Test*, Pressnell (1973) found that the performance of her students were similar in manner but different in rate when compared to hearing norms. Using a sentence repetition task, Wilcox and Tobin (1974) reported similar findings. They also found a wide range of performances among their hearing-impaired students when compared to hearing counterparts. Nevertheless, their results lend support to the hypothesis of delay rather than deviance.

More support for this hypothesis can be found in a study of syntactic ability by Davis and Blasdell (1975). Their students ranged in age from 6 to 9 years and in degree of hearing impairment from 35 to 75 dB. The researchers explored the ability of the students to comprehend sentences containing medially embedded relative clauses (e.g., "The man who chased the sheep cut the grass"). As in previous studies, the hearing-impaired students produced more errors than their hearing peers, yet their errors were similar in kind. These quantitatively reduced yet qualitatively similar patterns have also been observed for students with profound hearing impairments in a national longitudinal investigation (Quigley, Wilbur, Power, Montanelli, & Steinkamp, 1976).

Using the *Boehm Test of Basic Concepts*, Davis (1974) documented the vocabulary deficiency of students ranging in age from 6 to 8 years and in degree of hearing impairment from 35 to 70 dB. As expected, the hearing-impaired group performed worse than their hearing counterparts. Interestingly, the discrepancy in scores between the two groups widened with an increase in age.

In a recent study Blair, Peterson, and Viehweg (1985) compared the academic performance of students with hearing impairments ranging from 20 to 45 dB with their hearing grade peers in grades 1 to 4. Analyzing the scores on the *Iowa Test of Basic Concepts,* they found superior perform-ances in favor of the hearing students at each grade level tested for subtests on reading comprehension, vocabulary, math concepts, and arithmetic problem-solving skills. The academic lag reported for these hearing-impaired students was not as great as that reported in earlier investigations for those with similar losses (e.g., Quigley & Thomure, 1968). In fact, the mean grade scores obtained at the end of fourth grade were very impressive and not different from the norms (4.2 to 4.5). Never-theless, since the mean grade scores of the hearing students in fourth grade in the same school district were higher (5.3 to 6.3), the researchers reiterated the finding that general academic performance is negatively affected by a hearing impairment, even in the mild range. They also found some support for the assertion that the discrepancy between hearing and hearing-impaired students increases with age.

The studies reported thus far revealed that the academic performance of most hard-of-hearing students (i.e., up to about 89 dB) is quantitatively reduced yet qualitatively similar when compared either with the hearing norms of the assessment or with the performance of hearing peers in the same school district. There have been a few investigations supporting both quantitative and qualitative similarities. Analyzing the performances of students with moderate and severe hearing impairments, McClure (1977), for example, found that their scores on the reading, spelling, and mathematics subtests of the *Wide Range Achievement Test* fell in the low-average to average grade ranges of hearing norms. In another study, Reich, Hambleton, & Houldin (1977) examined the progress of students with impairments ranging from mild to profound and reported similar results on the language and reading subtests of the *California Achievement Test*. In a more recent study Davis, Shepard, Stelmachowicz, and Gorga (1981) reported that students with mild to moderate hearing impairments performed as well as their hearing peers (norms) on the reading, math, and spelling subtests of a standardized achievement test; however, they exhibited a delay of approximately 1 year or more on assessments of English language development.

The researchers in these investigations attributed the good academic performances of most hearing-impaired students to one or more of the following factors: (1) early diagnosis and use of amplification, (2) intense involvement and education levels of parents, and (3) highly developed oral communication skills. Even in the study by Blair et al. (1985), performances of the students were affected by the length of time associated with the use of hearing aids. (Only 4 of the 24 students, however, wore hearing aids.) These factors enhanced the development of primary, verbal language skills, which form the base for the acquisition of secondary or literary skills in English. This assertion is also true for students with profound hearing impairments.

*Deaf Students.* There are very few investigations that assess the effects of oral English methods on English language skills in profoundly hearing-impaired students (see the reviews in King and Quigley, 1985; and Quigley and Paul, 1984a). Those discussed here employed deaf students exposed *only* to oral approaches either in a good intensive oral program (for example, CID's) or in regular education settings. It has been shown that these few deaf students exhibit select characteristics, such as high IQs and well-developed oral communication skills, which contributed to their educational and vocational successes (e.g., Ogden, 1979).

Lane and Baker (1974) reported the reading comprehension scores of former CID students and compared them with those in other studies. These former students ranged in age from 10 to 16 years and in degree of hearing impairment from 70 dB to the limits of the audiometer. Approximately 90%, however, had a profound hearing impairment. The researchers found that the reading achievement level of the CID group improved 2.5 grades during a 4-year period. This is much greater than the improvement noted in national surveys conducted by the Center of Assessment and Demographic Studies (CADS), formerly the Office of Demographic Studies (DiFrancesca, 1972; Gallaudet Research Institute, 1985; Trybus & Karchmer, 1977). More important, the researchers stated that there was no evidence of asymptote—that is, there was a continuous upward trend in reading growth. It should be noted that mean IQ of the former CID students in the Lane and Baker study was 115. This is considerably higher than the national average of 96.6 for hearing-impaired students (Jensema, 1977) and must be considered a major factor contributing to reading achievement.

In another study Doehring, Bonnycastle, and Ling (1978) investigated the language comprehension abilities of CID students ranging in age from 6 to 13 years and in degree of hearing impairment from severe to profound. These students were integrated in regular education environments and were administered language- and reading-related tasks. The students performed at or above the grade level of hearing peers only on the reading-related tasks. The researchers argued that this was influenced by the fact that the students' auditory-oral training had resulted in well-developed oral skills that, in turn, affect academic achievement.

Even the more recent studies (Messerly & Aram, 1980; Moog, Geers, & Calvert, 1981; Ogden, 1979) support the assertion that deaf students in incontestably good oral programs (some of whom have been integrated in regular education programs) develop significantly better language comprehension skills than deaf students in any other education program. A large number of these students perform on grade level when compared with hearing age norms or peers. In addition to those factors discussed previously, some researchers have argued that another factor which may account for the differences in academic achievement between special oral deaf students and those in other programs is the effective use of residual hearing (Geers, Moog, & Schick, 1984; Ling, 1984; Ross & Calvert, 1984). Indeed, training deaf students to exploit their residual hearing enhances their oral communication skills, resulting in the improvement of speech and speech-reading abilities (Boothroyd, 1984; Hack & Erber, 1982), and subsequently these abilities facilitate the acquisition of secondary English language skills.

*Cued Speech.*  Cued speech (CS) has not been studied extensively. Most of its "successes" have been documented in anecdotal reports in newsletters and other nonrefereed publications. A few research investigations have been conducted and have assessed mainly the reception of CS by severely to profoundly hearing-impaired students. CS has not been compared with other types of instructional approaches.

Ling and Clarke (1975) and Clarke and Ling (1976) examined the effects of cued speech on the receptive abilities of Canadian hearing-impaired students exposed to the system for approximately 2 years. The subjects were required to write their responses, which were then analyzed. The results revealed an order of difficulty for the cued stimuli ranging from easiest to most difficult: words, phrases, and, finally, sentences. It was also reported that most of the subjects experienced great difficulty in proceeding beyond the cued word level. On the positive side, the researchers were able to detect a pattern of phonemic errors during the second year. The discovery of error patterns is important in that it permits the establishment of a systematic remedial program.

More recently Nicholls and Ling (1982) reported on the speech reception abilities of Australian hearing-impaired students exposed to cued speech for 4 years. The subjects were presented stimuli under seven experimental conditions that resulted from all possible permutations of three variables: audition, cues, and lipreading. Superior scores were obtained for lipreading plus cues and for audition, cues, and lipreading. The scores for these two conditions were significantly higher than those for all others. The researchers also asserted that the use of cues did not negatively affect the students' lipreading abilities. Thus, they concluded that CS may be an option for those severely to profoundly hearing-impaired students who are experiencing difficulty in conventional aural-oral programs.

Only one study was found that assessed the effects of CS on English language development. Mohay (1983) studied three children—two profoundly impaired and one severely impaired—who transferred from an oral program to CS. While the two-word combinations of the children increased after exposure to CS, Mohay suggested that factors other than CS may have been responsible, such as the growth of cognitive ability.

## Manually Coded English

During the 1970s, the philosophy of total communication (TC) became dominant in the education of deaf students (Moores, 1982). One of the major tenets of TC has been the use of signs in the classroom, often simultaneously with speech. It has been reported that educational programs use signs with approximately 80% of profoundly hearing-impaired students, 75% of severely hearing-impaired students, and 30% of students with less severe impairments (Gallaudet Research Institute, 1985).

The TC philosophy has also spawned several sign systems that, as discussed previously, are based on the morphosyntactical aspects of written standard English and are supposed to be employed simultaneously with speech. Most have been in use for approximately 15 years; however, very little research data exist regarding their effectiveness. This may be attributable, in part, to the difficulty of using the contrived systems in a consistent manner (Marmor & Pettito, 1979; Mitchell, 1982). More likely, however, it may be that the expectation of developing English literacy skills has not been fulfilled (Quigley & Paul, 1984a, 1984b). The merits of the contrived sign systems are discussed in relation to their placement on a continuum from most representative to least representative of the morphosyntactical structure of English, as shown in Figure 2.1.

*Seeing Essential English (SEE I).*  The use of Seeing Essential English (SEE I) has been investigated by Schlesinger and Meadow (1972) and, more intensively, by Raffin and his associates (Gilman, Davis, & Raffin, 1980; Raffin, 1976; Raffin, Davis, & Gilman, 1978). These investigations documented the use of SEE I markers, especially those representing some of the most common English morphemes, such as those for past tense (*-ed*) and the third-person singular present indicative (*-s*). The results of morphemic acquisition were compared to those of hearing children reported by Brown (1973).

Generally, the findings indicated that the order of acquisition for severely to profoundly hearing-impaired students was qualitatively similar to that of younger, normally hearing children. The rate of development of the hearing-impaired students, however, was slower. In addition, it was asserted that one of the most important factors influencing the acquisition and use of the SEE I markers was exposure to a teacher executing the system in a consistent fashion. It was concluded that if hearing-impaired students are exposed consistently to a morpheme-based sign code, they will internalize the rules of English morphology. This will, in turn, enable them to produce the structures and make judgments of grammaticality. It should be remembered that, despite these assertions, the results indicated a 2- to 6-year delay in hearing-impaired students' acquisition of the morphemes when compared to hearing peers. Finally, the effects of SEE I on the development of English literacy skills like reading and writing have not been explored.

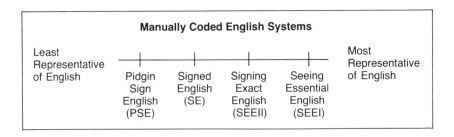

**Figure 2.1.**  Relationship of manually coded English systems to the morphosyntactic structure of standard English. Adapted from Quigley and Paul (1984a).

*Signing Exact English (SEE II).*   Signing Exact English (SEE II) has been reported to be one of the most widely used sign systems in the education of deaf students (Jordan, Gustason, & Rosen, 1979) and has been heavily promoted by its developers (Gustason, 1983; Gustason, Pfetzing, & Zawolkow, 1980). Only one study, however, was found that assessed the effectiveness of this system on the development of English. Babb (1979) studied deaf students who had been exposed to SEE II for approximately 10 years. Half of the students received exposure in the home and school environments and half only in the school environment. The academic achievement, knowledge of syntax, and written language abilities of these two groups were compared to each other, to the groups in a study by Brasel and Quigley (1977), and to a national survey of achievement scores of hearing-impaired students (DiFrancesca, 1972).

As expected, the results showed that the group exposed to SEE II in the home and at school performed significantly better than that exposed to SEE II in school only. The former group also performed as well as the best group in the Brasel and Quigley study (pidgin sign English) and significantly better than the national sample of hearing-impaired students (DiFrancesca, 1972). The median grade achievement of this group on language and reading measures was approximately the seventh-grade level. The importance of the home environment was evident in this study; however, due to limited data, more research is needed in evaluating the effectiveness of SEE II.

*Signed English (SE).*   The effects of signed English (SE) on the development of English has been assessed by Bornstein and his associates and, in a more recent study, by Gardner and Zorfass (1983). Bornstein, Saulnier, and Hamilton (1980) and Bornstein and Saulnier (1981) reported the results of a 5-year longitudinal study of 18 severely to profoundly hearing-impaired students enrolled in residential and day school programs. In general the findings indicated that the receptive vocabulary and syntactic development of the students was qualitatively similar to that of young hearing children, and, as expected, the rate of development was quantitatively slower. Analyzing the productions of the SE sign markers, Bornstein and his collaborators found that very few students were using the markers consistently and systematically. This later finding was substantiated in the 1981 investigation, which revealed that the 10-year-old students were executing only half of the 14 inflectional SE markers after at least 5 years of exposure.

On the contrary, Gardner and Zorfass (1983) reported that the oral language development of their 3-year-old, severely to profoundly hearing-impaired subject was comparable to hearing peers. This student was exposed to SE in a total communication environment from the age of 13 months. Interestingly, as the oral development of this subject *increased*, the production of signs and markers *decreased*. While these results are impressive, a closer inspection of the characteristics of this subject reveals an audiometric configuration resembling a flat contour from 250 to 8000 Hz. As expected, this subject benefited from amplification, which established audition as the primary mode of receiving communication and language, rather than vision, which is the case for most students with severe to profound hearing impairments.

*Pidgin Sign English (PSE).*   It has been suggested that most of the signing that occurs in the classroom resembles some form of pidgin sign English (PSE), owing mainly to the difficulty of executing the various contrived sign systems in a consistent manner (Kluwin, 1981; Marmor & Pettito, 1979; Mitchell, 1982). Descriptions of PSE vary according to the competency of the practitioners being investigated. At any rate, PSE is an amorphous term used to describe the method of signing that combines some grammatical elements of ASL with those of the contrived systems and executes this combination within the framework of standard English syntax.

Within this descriptive view, several studies have depicted the effects of PSE on hearing-impaired students' acquisition of primary and secondary English language skills. Development of vocabulary (Griswold & Cummings, 1974), morphosyntactic structures (Crandall, 1978), and semantic relations (Layton, Holmes, & Bradley, 1979) have been documented. As discussed previously, the growth in these areas was reported to be similar in manner, albeit slower in degree, to that of normally hearing peers. It has even been argued that deaf students can comprehend written stories despite an inability to produce certain morphosyntactic structures (Maxwell, 1983). This seems to support a top-down theory of reading; however, the findings may be contaminated owing to the relatively easy, familiar content of the stories (see King & Quigley, 1985).

A more intensive illustration of the effects of PSE on secondary English language development has been delineated by Brasel and Quigley (1977). These investigators provided insights regarding the merits of *form* of communication (i.e., oral and manual), type of language (ASL and English), and the intensity of linguistic input. Four groups of deaf students were studied: those exposed to manual English (i.e., PSE), ASL (labeled Average Manual in this study), intensive oral English (IO), and average oral English (AO). The parents of the PSE and ASL groups were deaf whereas those of the oral groups were hearing.

The PSE group performed significantly better than all other groups. The ASL and IO groups were about equal, and the AO group had significantly inferior scores in all language and reading areas. Finally, the mean reading grade level of the PSE group was reported to be a little above the seventh-grade level.

The findings of this study corroborated those presented previously regarding the importance of parental influence. In addition, the findings suggest that the *form* of manual communication is essential for secondary English language development. While it is clear that the form should represent English in some fashion, the nature of this representation is still equivocal. This can be seen by recalling that the mean reading grade level of the best group in the Brasel and Quigley study was similar to that of the SEE II group in the Babb (1979) study. These results should be considered in view of the assumption that SEE II is purportedly more representative of English structure than PSE is (see Figure 2.1).

A more recent study by Delaney, Stuckless, and Walter (1984) reported that the achievement levels of some profoundly hearing-impaired students in a TC program were significantly higher than those of students who had been exposed to aural-oral methods in the earlier years of the school prior to its switch to TC. The TC students also had higher achievement levels than students in the transitional period—that is, those exposed to both aural-oral methods and total communication. In addition, the language comprehension abilities of the TC students were equal to the best group in the Brasel and Quigley (1977) and the Babb (1979) studies. More important, the researchers asserted that the achievement of the TC students may not be attributable only to exposure to a total communication program. They proffered other factors for the students' success, some of which have been delineated previously: involvement of parents and school personnel, improvements in curricula, and, interestingly, the presence of *some* oral communication skills.

## American Sign Language

It is now well accepted that ASL is a bona fide language with its own grammar, which is influenced by but not derived from English (Lane & Grosjean, 1980; Wilbur, 1979). While most deaf children are exposed to some form of English in the home (Quigley & Kretschmer, 1982; Quigley & Paul, 1984a), some are exposed to ASL in infancy and early childhood (Lane & Grosjean, 1980). For the latter group, English should probably be taught as a second language in a bilingual or second-language educational program (Quigley & Paul, 1984b).

It is difficult to evaluate the effects of knowing ASL as a first language on the acquisition of English as a second language (ESL). At present, few education programs use (or have used) ASL as an instructional tool in a bilingual or ESL environment (Luetke-Stahlman, 1983; Quigley & Paul, 1984b). The preponderant amount of research data on bilingualism and second-language learning in hearing children, however, can be employed analogously to argue for the use of ASL in teaching English as a second language for those deaf students for whom ASL is the native or home language. The very few studies that examine this issue have been conducted within the conceptual framework of a contrastive analysis approach (Crutchfield, 1972; Jones, 1979). In general, this approach focuses on the manner in which the native language influences the development of the target or second language. Future investigations should consider other approaches—namely, error or noncontrastive analyses that describe the developmental strategies and stages of the second-language learner. The limited data in this area suggest that many educators are not sensitive to the native language (i.e., ASL) of some deaf students. Consequently, this attitude may be somewhat detrimental to the academic development of these students, as has been the case with many minority hearing students in regular education programs.

From another perspective several researchers (e.g., Balow & Brill, 1975; Meadow, 1968) examined the development of English in deaf children of deaf parents (dcdp) in order to shed light on the ASL and ESL situation. They assumed that only dcdp were exposed to manual communication and, in retrospect, that this communication was in the form of ASL. These assumptions, however, are unwarranted. Some dcdp are exposed to a form of PSE (Brasel & Quigley, 1977; Collins-Ahlgren, 1974) and some to spoken English (Corson, 1973). Furthermore, interpreting the *form* of manual communication as ASL must be done with caution since a grammar of ASL has only recently been written (Lane & Grosjean, 1980; Wilbur, 1979).

Despite these caveats, early investigators have compared the performances of dcdp with deaf children of hearing parents (dchp). Most of the findings indicated superior performances on language and reading measures in favor of dcdp (e.g., Quigley & Frisina, 1961; Stuckless & Birch, 1966). The differences between the two groups are attributable to manual communication and parental acceptance, which was supposedly higher in dcdp. As previously discussed, it has been demonstrated that the form of manual communication is important, especially when it conforms to the structure of English (Brasel & Quigley, 1977). In addition, it has been shown that a high level of parental acceptance is not confined to deaf parents who sign to their deaf children; it may be found in deaf parents who *speak* (Corson, 1973). Finally, as emphasized by Delaney et al. (1984) and others, the development of English skills should not be attributable to one all-encompassing factor such as manual communication (*in any form*).

# Factors Related to English Literacy

It is well documented that most hearing-impaired students do not read or write as well as their hearing peers (Blair et al., 1985; Gallaudet Research Institute, 1985). The extremely low literacy levels of most severely and profoundly hearing-impaired students have been reported in national surveys conducted by the Center for Assessment and Demographic Studies. Specific correlates of inadequate English language skills for students at all levels of hearing impairment, however, have been revealed by investigators employing diagnostic measures (e.g., Quigley et al., 1976). In this view, the literacy difficulties may be due to deficits in experiential (background or world knowledge), linguistic (e.g., syntax), and cognitive (e.g., memory) aspects. It should be emphasized that the poor reading and writing levels of some normally hearing students are also attributed to deficits in these areas. A more detailed treatment of these variables may be found elsewhere (King & Quigley, 1985; Quigley & Paul, 1984a). Discussed here are a few of the linguistic and cognitive variables.

## Linguistic Variables

Several linguistic factors suspected of affecting literacy have been reported, including knowledge of vocabulary, syntax, and figurative language. In relation to vocabulary, several researchers have reported that most hearing-impaired students acquire word meanings at a rate slower than that of their hearing counterparts (Rosenstein & MacGinitie, 1969; Schulze, 1965). More recently it has been shown that the rate of acquisition is influenced in part by the frequency and variety of meanings of words (Paul, 1984; Walter, 1978). These aspects contribute to the difficulty of a word, and this, in turn, may affect the ability to read and write.

Like the investigators of students with lesser degrees of impairment, Quigley and his collaborators have demonstrated that most profoundly (and some severely) hearing-impaired students acquire the major syntactic structures in a manner similar to, albeit slower than, that of their normally hearing counterparts (Quigley et al., 1976). This longitudinal project described the extent of knowledge of specific syntactic structures for a national sample of profoundly hearing-impaired students from 10 to 19 years of age. It was also shown that a huge discrepancy existed between the students' understanding of the structures and the frequency of their occurrences in the most popularly used reading series (see Quigley & Paul, 1984a). The discrepancy was of such magnitude that the construction of a reading series specifically designed for profoundly hearing-impaired students was deemed necessary (Quigley & King, 1981–1984). It is possible that this series, controlled for vocabulary and syntax, may be useful for other language-impaired populations (e.g., learning-disabled and ESL learners) who have been shown to have similar language and reading comprehension problems (see Paul, 1985).

In relation to written language, Quigley et al. (1976) and others (e.g., Myklebust, 1964; Powers & Wilgus, 1983; Taylor, 1969) have reported that many hearing-impaired students also have not mastered rules pertaining to the morphosyntactical structures of English. In addition, most severely and profoundly hearing-impaired students have been shown to use strategies (e.g., subject-verb-object interpretation) similar to those used by younger normally hearing children. This has caused difficulty with comprehending and producing the more complex transformations (e.g., relative clauses), which require a hierarchical rather than linear interpretation. Most of the work in this area has lent support to the delay hypothesis discussed previously. Thus, it is concluded that hearing-impaired students with poor writing skills, like young hearing children, operate under a rule-ordered system.

Another linguistic area suspected of affecting English literacy, particularly reading development, is figurative language. The reader may encounter many of these expressions in commonly used reading materials (Dixon, Pearson, & Ortony, 1980). It has been estimated that two thirds of English contains figurative elements such as figures of speech and idioms (Boatner & Gates, 1969). Most of the limited data available suggest that many severely and profoundly hearing-impaired students have difficulty with figurative language (Conley, 1976; Giorcelli, 1982; Payne, 1982). Some investigators have shown that some of these students can understand metaphorical expressions, especially if vocabulary and syntax are controlled (Iran-Nejad, Ortony, & Rittenhouse, 1981). There may be a limit to their understanding, however, since some expressions require a specific set of vocabulary and syntactic items. Additionally it has been reported that mastery of some figurative expressions is correlated with level of reading achievement (Fruchter, Wilbur, & Fraser, 1984), and, as previously discussed, the ability to read is partly influenced by knowledge of words and syntactic structures. More research is needed in this area, especially for students with less severe hearing impairments. Furthermore, the effects of figurative expressions on written language need to be studied.

## Cognitive Variables

The present writers espouse a cognitive-based theory of language acquisition, which essentially argues that the growth of cognitive structures is a requisite for grammatical and lexical development and, subsequently, for the development of literacy skills (Anderson, 1981; Pearson, 1985). The relationship between literacy, particularly reading, and cognition can be seen in the investigations of the internal coding strategies of severely and profoundly hearing-impaired students.

Most normally hearing children develop an internal representation of speech that is used for certain cognitive activities—namely, memory and inferencing tasks. This is true also for most hard-of-hearing and some profoundly hearing-impaired students (see Conrad, 1979; Lichtenstein, 1984). This internal representation of speech or, in other words, a speech-based recoding strategy may be important for processing hierarchical, temporal-sequential items as in reading (Lake, 1980; Lichtenstein, 1984).

This importance has been revealed by investigations of various aspects of information processing and memory, specifically working memory capacity. Based on analyses of errors, a variety of mediating strategies have been discovered: dactylic (finger spelling), phonological (speech-based), sign, and visual (graphemic) (Blanton, Nunnally, & Odom, 1967; Conrad, 1979; Locke, 1978; Odom, Blanton, & McIntyre, 1970). The data suggest that some profoundly hearing-impaired students do use a speech-based mediating code, although most of them employ nonspeech-based strategies when reading.

There is increasing evidence to suggest that a speech-based working memory capacity is essential for reading comprehension. Ehri and Wilce (1985) reported that hearing children shift from visual to phonological processing when beginning to read. Conrad (1979) and Hirsh-Pasek and Treiman (1982) found that good profoundly hearing-impaired readers used a predominantly phonological-based code in mediating print. Lichtenstein (1984) emphasized that speech recoders are better readers than nonspeech recoders owing to a more efficient representation of complex, nonlinear English structures (e.g., relative clauses) in their working memory capacity.

The research on cognition and reading has supported the assertion that a strong relationship exists between primary and secondary language developments. It is a truism to state that reading and writing skills are superimposed upon those of primary language, which are essentially speech-based in nature. This relationship provides some insights into the relatively good literacy levels of most hard-of-hearing and some profoundly hearing-impaired students who have developed adequate speech-based or oral communication skills. It should be remembered, however, that most severely to profoundly hearing-impaired students used non-speech recoding strategies, and, consequently, other means of teaching literacy may need to be developed (King & Quigley, 1985; Quigley & Paul, 1984a).

# Summary

The purpose of this chapter is to describe some effects of early hearing impairment on the development of English literacy skills. It is proposed that such a description is best served when presented in relation to the nature and extent of the language and communication modes to which hearing-impaired students are exposed in infancy and early childhood: oral English, manually coded English, and American Sign Language. To shed additional light on this topic, a brief discussion of the development of English in normally hearing children is also included.

It is probably useful to present the findings in relation to two broad categories based on degree of hearing impairment: hard of hearing and deaf. In general, the hard-of-hearing group represents a range of hearing impairment up to 89 dB (ISO) in the better unaided ear across the speech frequencies of the audiogram. The label deaf is usually reserved for those students with profound hearing impairments, that is, 90 dB and greater. This level is purported to represent the dividing line between a primary dependency on audition and one on vision for the purposes of language and communication. There are, of course, exceptions. For example, some hard-of-hearing students may rely heavily on vision whereas some deaf students may be able to utilize their residual hearing (audition) in a very effective manner.

Regardless of the degree, it is now axiomatic to assert that early hearing impairment has marked effects on all aspects of English language development, for example, morphosyntactic and semantic. The research on hard-of-hearing students has suggested that the development of

English in this group is quantitatively less than, albeit qualitatively similar to, that of normally hearing peers. This pattern is not even affected by type of education program—that is, special or integrated. It should be clear that the support services of the audiologist and speech pathologist are necessary for students with slight to mild impairments of hearing.

Hard-of-hearing students are receiving increasing attention from researchers and educators; yet there is still a need to identify and study more members of this group, especially those in integrated classrooms. Difficulty with the identification process can only mean that these students are not receiving adequate support services. Researchers should also examine the writing skills of hard-of-hearing students as well as develop more diagnostic assessments in light of recent linguistic and reading theories.

The situation is quite different for students with profound degrees of impairment. Although fewer in number, the English language development of this group has been thoroughly investigated and presented in relation to three general communication modes: oral English, manually coded English, and American Sign Language. Regardless of the communication mode, the evidence indicates that language acquisition proceeds at a slower rate than, but in a similar manner to, that of normally hearing peers and of most hard-of-hearing students.

To state that most deaf students acquire English literacy skills at a slower rate than hearing students is quite an understatement. The data presented in this chapter indicate that the average 17- to 18-year-old deaf student performs at a level similar to that of the average 9- or 10-year-old hearing student. Higher achievement is often observed in deaf students with advantageous personal and demographic characteristics like high socioeconomic status and adequate oral language skills. These students can be found in incontestably good oral *or* total communication programs. It should be remembered that factors other than mode of communication have been reported to be important, such as involvement of parents and school personnel along with well-developed curricula.

The most pressing need for hearing-impaired students in the profound category is for researchers and educators to document the effects of the various MCE codes and ASL on the development of English. For more than 15 years, the majority of education programs have used one or more of the various contrived approaches, yet very little data exist on their relative merits. There is little doubt that American Sign Language is the native language for some deaf students; however, very few programs have employed ASL in a bilingual or ESL manner. It appears that most deaf readers, exposed to signing in any form, mediate primarily with a nonspeech code to access meaning from print. Given that secondary language skills are superimposed on primary language ones, it is no surprise that a speech-based code is important for developing literacy skills as demonstrated here. Further research on the MCE codes and ASL is necessary for understanding how spoken secondary language forms (i.e., reading and writing English) can be superimposed on nonspeech-based primary language forms.

# References

Allen, T., & Osborn, T. (1984). Academic integration of hearing-impaired students: Demographic, handicapping, and achievement factors. *American Annals of the Deaf, 129,* 100–113.

Anderson, R. (1981). *A proposal to continue a center for the study of reading* (Tech. Rep. Vols. 1–4). Champaign: University of Illinois, Center for the Study of Reading.

Anthony, D. (1966). *Seeing Essential English.* Unpublished master's thesis, Eastern Michigan University, Ypsilanti, MI.

Babb, R. (1979). *A study of the academic achievement and language acquisition levels of deaf children of hearing parents in an educational environment using Signing Exact English as the primary mode of manual communication.* Unpublished doctoral dissertation, University of Illinois, Urbana-Champaign, IL.

Balow, I., & Brill, R. (1975). An evaluation of reading and academic achievement levels of 16 graduating classes of the California School for the Deaf, Riverside. *Volta Review, 77,* 255–266.

Blair, J., Peterson, M., & Viehweg, S. (1985). The effects of mild hearing loss on academic performance of young school-age children. *Volta Review, 87,* 87–93.

Blanton, R., Nunnally, J., & Odom, P. (1967). Graphic, phonetic, and associative factors in the verbal behavior of deaf and hearing subjects. *Journal of Speech and Hearing Research, 10,* 225–231.

Bloom, L., & Lahey, M. (1978). *Language development and language disorders.* New York: Wiley.

Boatner, M., & Gates, J. (1969). *A dictionary of idioms for the deaf.* Washington, DC: National Association of the Deaf.

Boothroyd, A. (1984). Auditory perception of speech contrasts by subjects with sensorineural hearing loss. *Journal of Speech and Hearing Research, 27,* 134–144.

Bornstein, H. (1973). A description of some current sign systems designed to represent English. *American Annals of the Deaf, 118,* 454–463.

Bornstein, H., & Saulnier, K. (1981). Signed English: A brief follow-up to the first evaluation. *American Annals of the Deaf, 126,* 69–72.

Bornstein, H., Saulnier, K., & Hamilton, L. (1980). Signed English: A first evaluation. *American Annals of the Deaf, 125,* 467–481.

Bragg, B. (1973). Ameslish—our American heritage: A testimony. *American Annals of the Deaf, 118,* 672–674.

Brasel, K., & Quigley, S. (1977). The influence of certain language and communication environments in early childhood on the development of language in deaf individuals. *Journal of Speech and Hearing Research, 20,* 95–107.

Brown, R. (1973). *A first language: The early stages.* Cambridge, MA: Harvard University Press.

Chomsky, N. (1957). *Syntactic Structures.* The Hague: Mouton.

Chomsky, N. (1965). *Aspects of the theory of syntax.* Cambridge, MA: MIT Press.

Clarke, B., & Ling, D. (1976). The effects of using Cued Speech: A follow-up study. *Volta Review, 78,* 23–34.

Cokely, D. (1983). When is a pidgin not a pidgin? An alternate analysis of the ASL-English contact situation. *Sign Language Studies, 38,* 1–24.

Collins-Ahlgren, M. (1974). Teaching English as a second language to young deaf children: A case study. *Journal of Speech and Hearing Disorders, 39,* 486–500.

Conley, J. (1976). The role of idiomatic expressions in the reading of deaf children. *American Annals of the Deaf, 121,* 381–385.

Conrad, R. (1979). *The deaf school child: Language and cognitive function.* London: Harper and Row.

Cornett, R. O. (1967). Cued speech. *American Annals of the Deaf, 112,* 3–13.

Cornett, R. O. (1984). Book review: Language and deafness. *Cued Speech News, 17*(3), 5.

Corson, H. (1973). *Comparing deaf children of oral deaf parents and deaf parents using manual communication with deaf children of hearing parents on academic, social, and communication functioning.* Unpublished doctoral dissertation, University of Cincinnati, Cincinnati, OH.

Crandall, K. (1978). Inflectional morphemes in the manual English of young hearing-impaired children and their mothers. *Journal of Speech and Hearing Research, 21,* 372–386.

Crutchfield, P. (1972). Prospects for teaching English Det + N structures to deaf students. *Sign Language Studies, 1,* 8–14.

Cruttenden, A. (1979). *Language in infancy and childhood: A linguistic introduction to language acquisition.* New York: St. Martin's Press.

Davis, J. (1974). Performance of young hearing-impaired children on a test of basic concepts. *Journal of Speech and Hearing Research, 17,* 342–351.

Davis, J. (Ed.). (1977). *Our forgotten children: Hard-of-hearing pupils in the schools.* Minneapolis: Audio Visual Library Service.

Davis, J., & Blasdell, R. (1975). Perceptual strategies employed by normal-hearing and hearing-impaired children in the comprehension of sentences containing relative clauses. *Journal of Speech and Hearing Research, 18,* 281–295.

Davis, J., Shepard, N., Stelmachowicz, P., & Gorga, M. (1981). Characteristics of hearing-impaired children in the public schools: Part II—psychoeducational data. *Journal of Speech and Hearing Disorders, 46,* 130–137.

Delaney, M., Stuckless, E. R., & Walter, G. (1984). Total Communication effects—a longitudinal study of a school for the deaf in transition. *American Annals of the Deaf, 129,* 481–486.

de Villiers, J., & de Villiers, P. (1978). *Language acquisition.* Cambridge, MA: Harvard University Press.

DiFrancesca, S. (1972). *Academic achievement test results of a national testing program for hearing-impaired students* (Series D, No. 9). Washington, DC: Gallaudet College, Office of Demographic Studies.

Dixon, K., Pearson, P. D., & Ortony, A. (1980). *Some reflections on the use of figurative language in children's textbooks.* Paper presented at the annual meeting of the National Reading Conference, San Diego, CA.

Doehring, D., Bonnycastle, D., & Ling, A. (1978). Rapid reading skills of integrated hearing-impaired children. *Volta Review, 80,* 399–409.

Eckhoff, B. (1983). How reading affects children's writing. *Language Arts, 60,* 607–616.

Ehri, L., & Wilce, L. (1985). Movement into reading: Is the first stage of printed word learning visual or phonetic? *Reading Research Quarterly, 20,* 163–179.

Fruchter, A., Wilbur, R., & Fraser, J. (1984). Comprehension of idioms by hearing-impaired students. *Volta Review, 86,* 7–17.

Gallaudet Research Institute. (1985). *Gallaudet Research Institute Newsletter.* Washington, DC: Gallaudet College.

Gardner, J., & Zorfass, J. (1983). From sign to speech: The language development of a hearing-impaired child. *American Annals of the Deaf, 128,* 20–24.

Geers, A., Moog, J., & Schick, B. (1984). Acquisition of spoken and signed English by profoundly deaf children. *Journal of Speech and Hearing Disorders, 49,* 378–388.

Gilman, L., Davis, J., & Raffin, M. (1980). Use of common morphemes by hearing-impaired children exposed to a system of manual English. *Journal of Auditory Research, 20,* 57–69.

Giorcelli, L. (1982). *The comprehension of some aspects of figurative language by deaf and hearing subjects.* Unpublished doctoral dissertation, University of Illinois, Urbana-Champaign, IL.

Goetzinger, C., & Rousey, C. (1959). Educational achievement of deaf children. *American Annals of the Deaf, 104,* 221–231.

Griswold, E., & Cummings, J. (1974). The expressive vocabulary of preschool deaf children. *American Annals of the Deaf, 119,* 16–28.

Gustason, G. (1983). *Teaching and learning Signing Exact English.* Los Alamitos, CA: Modern Signs Press.

Gustason, G., Pfetzing, D., & Zawolkow, E. (1980). *Signing Exact English: The 1980 edition.* Los Alamitos, CA: Modern Signs Press.

Hack, Z., & Erber, N. (1982). Auditory, visual, and auditory-visual perception of vowels by hearing-impaired children. *Journal of Speech and Hearing Research, 25,* 100–107.

Hirsh-Pasek, K., & Treiman, R. (1982). Recoding in silent reading: Can the deaf child translate print into a more manageable form? In R. E. Kretschmer (Ed.), *Reading and the hearing-impaired individual* [Special issue]. *Volta Review, 84,* 71–82.

Iran-Nejad, A., Ortony, A., & Rittenhouse, R. (1981). The comprehension of metaphorical uses of English by deaf children. *Journal of Speech and Hearing Research, 24,* 551–556.

Jensema, C. (1977). Letter to the editor. *Volta Review, 79,* 180.

Jones, P. (1979). Negative interference of signed language in written English. *Sign Language Studies, 24,* 273–279.

Jordan, I., Gustason, G., & Rosen, R. (1979). An update on communication trends at programs for the deaf. *American Annals of the Deaf, 124,* 350–357.

Karchmer, M., Milone, M., & Wolk, S. (1979). Educational significance of hearing loss at three levels of severity. *American Annals of the Deaf, 124,* 97–109.

King, C., & Quigley, S. (1985). *Reading and deafness.* San Diego: College-Hill.

Kluwin, T. (1981). The grammaticality of manual representations of English in classroom settings. *American Annals of the Deaf, 126,* 417–421.

Lake, D. (1980). Syntax and sequential memory in hearing-impaired children. In H. Reynolds & C. Williams (Eds.), *Proceeding of the Gallaudet Conference on Reading in Relation to Deafness* (pp. 193–212). Washington, DC: Gallaudet College, Division of Research.

Lane, H., & Baker, D. Reading achievement of the deaf: Another look. *Volta Review, 76,* 489–499.

Lane, H., & Grosjean, F. (Eds.), *Recent perspectives on American Sign Language.* Hillsdale, NJ: Erlbaum.

Layton, T., Holmes, D., & Bradley, P. (1979). A description of pedagogically imposed signed semantic-syntactic relationships in deaf children. *Sign Language Studies, 23,* 137–160.

Lichtenstein, E. (1984). Deaf working memory processes and English language skills. In D. Martin (Ed.), *International Symposium on Cognition, Education, and Deafness: Working papers* (pp. 331–360). Washington, DC: Gallaudet College.

Ling, D. (1976). *Speech and the hearing-impaired child: Theory and practice.* Washington, DC: Alexander Graham Bell Association for the Deaf.

Ling, D. (1984). Early oral intervention: An introduction. In D. Ling (Ed.), *Early intervention for hearing-impaired children: Oral options* (pp. 1–14). San Diego: College-Hill.

Ling, D., & Clarke, B. (1975). Cued speech: An evaluative study. *American Annals of the Deaf, 120,* 480–488.

Ling, D., & Ling, A. (1978). *Aural habilitation: The foundations of verbal learning in hearing-impaired children.* Washington, DC: Alexander Graham Bell Association for the Deaf.

Locke, J. (1978). Phonemic effects in the silent reading of hearing and deaf children. *Cognition, 6,* 175–187.

Luetke-Stahlman, B. (1983). Using bilingual instructional models in teaching hearing-impaired students. *American Annals of the Deaf, 128,* 873–877.

Marmor, G., & Pettito, L. (1979). Simultaneous communication in the classroom: How well is English grammar represented? *Sign Language Studies, 23,* 99–136.

Maxwell, M. (1983). Simultaneous communication in the classroom: What do deaf children learn? *Sign Language Studies, 39,* 95–112.

McClure, A. (1977). Academic achievement of mainstreamed hearing-impaired children with congenital rubella syndrome. *Volta Review, 79,* 379–384.

Meadow, K. (1968). Early manual communication in relation to the deaf child's intellectual, social, and communicative functioning. *American Annals of the Deaf, 113,* 29–41.

Menyuk, P. (1977). *Language and maturation.* Cambridge, MA: MIT Press.

Messerly, C., & Aram, D. (1980). Academic achievement of hearing-impaired students of hearing parents and of hearing-impaired parents: Another look. *Volta Review, 82,* 25–32.

Mitchell, G. (1982). Can deaf children acquire English? An evaluation of Manually Coded English systems in terms of the principles of language acquisition. *American Annals of the Deaf, 127,* 331–336.

Mohay, H. (1983). The effects of Cued Speech on the language development of three deaf children. *Sign Language Studies, 38,* 25–47.

Moog, J., Geers, A., & Calvert, D. (1981). Conclusions. *American Annals of the Deaf, 126,* 965–969.

Moores, D. (1982). *Educating the deaf: Psychology, principles, and practices* (2nd ed.). Boston: Houghton Mifflin.

Myklebust, H. (1964). *The psychology of deafness* (2nd ed.). New York: Grune and Stratton.

Nicholls, G., & Ling, D. (1982). Cued Speech and the reception of spoken language. *Journal of Speech and Hearing Research, 25,* 262–269.

Odom, P., Blanton, R., & McIntyre, C. (1970). Coding medium and word recall by deaf and hearing subjects. *Journal of Speech and Hearing Research, 13,* 54–58.

Ogden, P. (1979). *Experiences and attitudes of oral deaf adults regarding oralism.* Unpublished doctoral dissertation, University of Illinois, Urbana-Champaign, IL.

Paul, P. (1984). *The comprehension of multimeaning words from selected frequency levels by deaf and hearing subjects.* Unpublished doctoral dissertation, University of Illinois, Urbana-Champaign, IL.

Paul, P. (1985). Reading and other language-variant populations. In C. King & S. Quigley, *Reading and deafness* (pp. 251–289). San Diego: College-Hill.

Payne, J.-A. (1982). *A study of the comprehension of verb-particle combinations among deaf and hearing subjects.* Unpublished doctoral dissertation, University of Illinois, Urbana-Champaign, IL.

Pearson, P. D. (1985). *The comprehension revolution: A twenty-year history of process and practice related to reading comprehension* (Reading Education Report No. 57). Champaign: University of Illinois, Center for the Study of Reading.

Pearson, P. D., & Johnson, D. (1978). *Teaching reading comprehension.* New York: Holt, Rinehart, and Winston.

Pintner, R., Eisenson, J., & Stanton, M. (1946). *The psychology of the physically handicapped.* New York: Crofts.

Pintner, R., & Lev, J. (1939). The intelligence of the hard-of-hearing school child. *Journal of Genetic Psychology, 55,* 31–48.

Pintner, R., & Paterson, D. (1916). A measurement of the language ability of deaf children. *Psychological Review, 23,* 413–436.

Pintner, R., & Paterson, D. (1917). The ability of deaf and hearing children to follow printed directions. *American Annals of the Deaf, 62,* 448–472.

Powers, A., & Wilgus, S. (1983). Linguistic complexity in the written language of deaf children. *Volta Review, 85,* 201–210.

Pressnell, L. (1973). Hearing-impaired children's comprehension and production of syntax in oral language. *Journal of Speech and Hearing Research, 16,* 12–21.

Quigley, S., & Frisina, R. (1961). *Institutionalization and psychoeducational development of deaf children* (CEC Research Monograph). Washington, DC: Council on Exceptional Children.

Quigley, S., & King, C. (Eds.). (1981–1984). *Reading milestones.* Beaverton, OR: Dormac.

Quigley, S., & Kretschmer, R. E. (1982). *The education of deaf children: Issues, theory, and practice.* Austin, TX: PRO-ED.

Quigley, S., & Paul, P. (1984a). *Language and deafness.* San Diego: College-Hill.

Quigley, S., & Paul, P. (1984b). ASL and ESL? *Topics in Early Childhood Special Education, 3*(4), 17–26.

Quigley, S., & Thomure, R. (1968). *Some effects of hearing impairment upon school performance.* Urbana: University of Illinois, Institute for Research on Exceptional Children.

Quigley, S., Wilbur, R., Power, D., Montanelli, D., & Steinkamp, M. (1976). *Syntactic structures in the language of deaf children* (Final Report). Urbana: University of Illinois, Institute for Child Behavior and Development. (ERIC Document Reproduction Service No. ED 119 447)

Raffin, M. (1976). *The acquisition of inflectional morphemes by deaf children using Seeing Essential English.* Unpublished doctoral dissertation, University of Iowa, Iowa City, IA.

Raffin, M., Davis, J., & Gilman, L. (1978). Comprehension of inflectional morphemes by deaf children exposed to a visual English sign system. *Journal of Speech and Hearing Research, 21,* 387–400.

Reich, C., Hambleton, D., & Houldin, B. (1977). The integration of hearing-impaired children in regular classrooms. *American Annals of the Deaf, 122,* 534–543.

Rosenstein, J., & MacGinitie, W. (Eds.). (1969). *Verbal behavior of the deaf child: Studies of word meanings and associations.* New York: Teachers College.

Ross, M., Brackett, D., & Maxon, A. (1982). *Hard-of-hearing children in regular schools.* Englewood Cliffs, NJ: Prentice-Hall.

Ross, M., & Calvert, D. (1984). Semantics of deafness revisited: Total Communication and the use and misuse of residual hearing. *Audiology, 9,* 127–143.

Sanders, D. (1982). *Aural rehabilitation: A management model* (2nd ed.). Englewood Cliffs, NJ: Prentice-Hall.

Schlesinger, H., & Meadow, K. (1972). *Sound and sign: Childhood deafness and mental health.* Berkeley: University of California Press.

Schlesinger, I. (1982). *Steps to language: Toward a theory of native language acquisition.* Hillsdale, NJ: Erlbaum.

Schulze, G. (1965). An evaluation of vocabulary development by thirty-two deaf children over a three-year period. *American Annals of the Deaf, 110,* 424–435.

Slobin, D. (1979). *Psycholinguistics* (2nd ed.). Glenview, IL: Scott, Foresman.

Stark, R. (Ed.). (1974). *Sensory capabilities of hearing-impaired children.* Baltimore, MD: University Park Press.

Stokoe, W., Jr. (1975). The use of sign language in teaching English. *American Annals of the Deaf, 120,* 417–421.

Stuckless, E. R., & Birch, J. (1966). The influence of early manual communication on the linguistic development of deaf children. *American Annals of the Deaf, 111,* 452–460, 499–504.

Taylor, L. (1969). *A language analysis of the writing of deaf children.* Unpublished doctoral dissertation, Florida State University, Tallahassee, FL.

Tierney, R., & Leys, M. (1984). *What is the value of connecting reading and writing?* (Reading Education Report No. 55). Champaign: University of Illinois, Center for the Study of Reading.

Trybus, R., & Karchmer, M. (1977). School achievement scores of hearing-impaired children: National data on achievement status and growth patterns. *American Annals of the Deaf, 122,* 62–69.

Walter, G. (1978). Lexical abilities of hearing and hearing-impaired children. *American Annals of the Deaf, 123,* 976–982.

Wilbur, R. (1979). *American Sign Language and sign systems.* Austin, TX: PRO-ED.

Wilcox, J., & Tobin, H. (1974). Linguistic performance of hard-of-hearing and normal hearing children. *Journal of Speech and Hearing Research, 17,* 286–293.

Wolk, S., Karchmer, M., & Schildroth, A. (1982). *Patterns of academic and nonacademic integration among hearing-impaired students in special education* (Series R, No. 9). Washington, DC: Gallaudet College, Center for Assessment and Demographic Studies.

Woodward, J. (1973). Some characteristics of Pidgin Sign English. *Sign Language Studies, 3,* 39–46.

# 3

# The Psychological World of the Hearing-Impaired Child and the Family

*DEBORAH S. ROSE*

$T$he emotional well-being of the hearing-impaired child has been of long-standing concern. Whether it be observations of high rates of emotional problems and poor academic and intellectual achievement (Schlesinger & Meadow, 1972) or of a common constellation of personality traits (Altschuler, 1971; Lesser & Easser, 1972), many have sought to detect and explain the effects of a preverbal hearing loss on the emotional development of the child (Altschuler, 1971; Galenson, Kaplan, & Sherkow, 1983; Galenson, Miller, Kaplan, & Rothstein, 1979; Lesser & Easser, 1972; Schlesinger & Meadow, 1972). Interventions have been recommended, the major thrusts being the auditory approach, the use of total communication with the child in school and at home, and the provision of counseling for the parents.

The experience of the parents in the "diagnostic crisis" (Schlesinger & Meadow, 1972) has been recognized, as have the issues of parental grief and loss of the perfect child (Solnit & Stark, 1961). Parental anger at and guilt over the hearing-impaired child have been demonstrated to contribute to overprotectiveness.

Crucial areas that have received less study are the interface of professionals and the child and family, the parent-child unit, and the role of hearing in preverbal emotional development.

When professionals, child, and family meet, the focus is primarily on difficulties in having the diagnosis and recommendations for amplification accepted and in implementing satisfactory educational arrangements. Failure of professionals in the prediagnostic and diagnostic phases to respond to parents' concerns that something is wrong with their child has been reported by Meadow (1968) and Sweetow & Barrager (1980). But the consequences of this failure have been viewed too narrowly— simply as a delay in providing amplification and educational interventions instead of as a potential cause of major distress and damage for the hearing-impaired child and the family.

Most studies on the impact of hearing loss on the emotional development of the child and the family have dealt with either the child or the parents. Although each of these entities does have its own developmental line, this approach omits the parent-child unit, another key factor in emotional growth. Winnicott (1975) has stated it quite succinctly, "There is no such thing as a baby" (p. 99). By this he means that, for a long time, the focus in child development was only on the infant, ignoring the fact that the infant can survive only through its relationship with a mothering person. The impact of the hearing loss on the family unit, the parents' relationship, and the siblings is also neglected.

The new field of infant psychiatry (Call, Galenson, & Tyson, 1983) is exploring the very early development of auditory functioning, the course of verbal development, the presence of other communication systems, the development of thought before and apart from the presence of language, and the subtle and very powerful interrelationship between mother and infant. From the resulting information, psychological intervention is being developed for high-risk infants. The infants themselves may have a developmental problem, such as prematurity or blindness; or they may be placed at risk because of a severe emotional disturbance in the mother. Unfortunately, disputes over which form of communication system best serves the hearing-impaired child frequently preempt fundamental research. And many of the answers to this dispute may be found only by taking a broader and deeper approach to the emotional development of hearing-impaired children. Only by drawing on these areas of knowledge can the clinician provide adequate care for the child and parents. The researcher who omits these variables compromises the validity and significance of the results.

# A Familiar Story: What Is Wrong?

Rarely does the audiologist, otolarygologist, speech pathologist, teacher, or psychiatrist have the opportunity to hear the whole story from the child and parents. Each specialist has a particular area of expertise, and providing adequate care in these sectors fills the available time. Yet much information present in the relatively neglected areas may directly impact the ones under scrutiny, thus limiting successful treatment.

What follows is a composite case report of a child and her emotionally healthy family, a whole story that is familiar in several ways. Whether it be the events and concerns that led to the diagnosis of a hearing loss, the diagnostic sequence itself, or the world into which the child and family were plummeted thereafter, what this family experiences and reports is the norm, not the exception. Perhaps the major deviation is the very positive outcome for all involved.

Interwoven with the report will be a psychiatrist's observations, questions, and concerns, based on current understandings in the areas of infant psychiatry, child development, loss and grief, and crisis and coping. The interplay of biological, psychological, interpersonal, and social factors is clearly seen.

Susan, a gregarious 12-year-old, with a moderately severe to severe hearing loss, is the third child in the G. family. Her older brother, John, is 17, and David, her other brother, is 14. Susan was supposed to be the "easy" child the pediatrician had promised Mrs. G. after the difficulties and worries of the first two.

Mrs. G's pregnancy and delivery with John were uneventful with the exception of the possibility of problems with future pregnancies because of Rh incompatability. But John has been a handful, though delightful, ever since. He was motorically precocious, crawling at 6 months and pulling the Christmas tree over onto himself. He has always craved his mother's attention, which she gave in abundance, as he was the first child and so clearly sought her involvement.

The pregnancy with David brought the problems associated with Rh incompatability. Delivery came 5 weeks early; David had respiratory distress syndrome, was on a respirator initially, and was severely jaundiced. The nursing staff and social services did not provide very much support during this difficult time. Mr. G. has a demanding job, but he was actively involved in caring for John and gave his wife emotional support during the ordeal. David came home from the hospital and continued to develop uneventfully. However, when he was 2 years old, Mrs. G. expressed her concern to her pediatrician that David's speech seemed to be somewhat delayed. To reassure her, the pediatrician reminded her that John was precocious in this area, as in many, and stated that she might be prone to be overly anxious because of David's perinatal problems. But Mrs. G. had begun to read about complications of prematurity, respiratory distress syndrome, and hyperbilirubinemia and was aware that David was at risk. To her relief, language began to proceed normally shortly thereafter.

By then Mrs. G. was pregnant with Susan; now she was well informed about the complications of Rh incompatibility. To Mrs. G.'s relief, Susan, though premature, did not have respiratory distress and was less jaundiced than David had been. Mrs. G. was delighted to be bringing home a happy, healthy "good" baby. Susan's development proceeded unremarkably; she was a very contented baby, one to whom busy Mrs. G. could offer a toy and anticipate that she would play happily for half an hour. This was markedly different from her first two children, and, although Mrs. G. savored her mellow, easy baby, at times she felt that she was not as involved with her as she had been with her first two. She thought that she might be feeling a little rejected by Susan because Susan did not seem to need her very much; but Mrs. G. brushed it off by reminding herself of the pleasures of having a "good" baby and noted that Susan seemed very responsive and full of smiles when Mrs. G. made efforts to engage her directly. When Susan was about 2 years old, Mrs. G. began to be concerned that herspeech was delayed, although she had some speech. Again Mrs. G. sought out her pediatrician, who reassured her in the same manner he had done previously. Mrs. G. agreed and thought herself to be a worrywart. When Susan did not turn around when Mrs. G. called to her in the yard, Mrs. G. told herself that children do not like to be called in by their mothers. But she could not help feeling somewhat rejected by Susan. Her worries about Susan's speech development gnawed at her; although she did her best to believe that her pediatrician was right and that her doubts were unfounded, she decided to take Susan to a speech pathologist.

# Commentary

Several areas of potential problems for Susan and her family are already present: first, the effect of the hearing loss on emotional, intellectual, and social development in Susan's life up to this point; second, Mrs. G's strain as a mother already and the impact of this on the mother-child relationship; and last, the results of denial in professionals and parents.

## Hearing and the Child's Emotional Growth

Central to an infant's development are sensory experiences that promote an optimal interest in and stimulation by the environment. These experiences lead to successful learning, emotional and cognitive integration, and comfortable and pleasurable interest in the world. Equally important are experiences that promote soothing and effective regulation of feeling-states. Hearing may have an impact in both these areas. For example, even *in utero*, different auditory frequencies lead to what we might think of as soothing or stimulation. And by one week of age, infants are moving in synchrony with the rhythm of speech. By one month of age, the infant recognizes and prefers its own mother's voice (Northern & Downs, 1978) and finds the mother's voice more soothing than her visual presence (Brazelton, 1974). Other evidence (Stern, 1983) suggests that infants come "prewired" to make certain kinds of sensory discriminations and are predesigned for abstract knowledge, such as knowing that visual events are related to sounds.

These finding suggest several things of great importance for healthy emotional development. In a world in which important sensory input is diminished or absent, there may be a diminution of the inherent pleasurable drive to become involved and learn. In addition, it may be that, as Stern (1983) suggests, an infant with a hearing loss "would be at an enormous disadvantage in constructing a cohesive unified picture of the world of human behavior" and "in comprehending the basic fabric of human behaviors that constitute emotional expressions and verbal meanings, and the material that makes school learning" (p. 12). Perhaps these problems are related to the frequent observation that people with a preverbal hearing loss are less empathic and more self-centered than the norm and show a tendency toward lower academic achievement.

An adolescent with a moderately severe to severe hearing loss and good speech described these issues, as he told of his recent experiences with a new, more powerful hearing aid. He decided to reject the aid because he heard sounds never available to him before, such as the ones he made as he sat down in a chair. Rather than finding these of interest, he felt distressed by the presence of sounds he could not identify and link with his bodily experiences. And what must a world be like with fewer soothing experiences and less ability to be in control? Although Susan was reported to be a very contented baby, often noted in children with a hearing loss (H. Schlesinger, personal communication, September 23, 1981), this is not always so. In a study by Galenson, Miller, Kaplan, and Rothstein (1979) six sets of parents, with 10 hearing-impaired infants and toddlers, reported difficulties in soothing and in establishing regular sleep-wake cycles in all of the children. Also noted in all of the children of deaf parents and five out of six of the children of hearing parents were significant delays in emotional development in several areas. These included problems with delayed attachment to mothers, deviant and sometimes abusive relationships to transitional objects (blankets and other objects normally used in a comforting and loving way), problems in separation from the mother in the second year, and lackluster, brief play. The one relatively unscathed child, who had hearing parents, had a superior mother but still had more than the usual problems with separation.

Even more remarkable is the report by Beratis, Rubin, Miller, Galenson, and Rothstein (1979), in which a 4-month-old with a mild to moderate hearing loss (probably secondary to middle ear problems) was observed to have problems with soothing and separation. By 2 months of age, his experienced mother suspected that he had a hearing loss because of lack of responsiveness to sound; by 3 months she had noted visual hyper-alertness and problems with separation; he would cry when left without visual contact with a family member. The mother reported that he was more watchful than her other children and that family friends had nicknamed him "Mr. Nosey." He needed the visual presence of someone or the television set left on in order to take a nap. At night, the lights had to be left on for him to be able to go to sleep. At 4 months of age, he was provided with amplification, which shifted his elevated hearing levels to normal. As a result, the symptomatic behaviors entirely disappeared, only to return when his hearing aids were not available for a few days at the age of 6 months. After an episode of otitis media at 7 months, the hearing loss disappeared rapidly, and his subsequent emotional development over the next 2 years of follow-up was normal and unremarkable. Lang (personal communication, March 5, 1982) reports several toddlers and young children who, after having been fitted with amplification and having begun to enjoy auditory input, developed problems with separation at bedtime if their hearing aids were removed.

These observations not only indicate difficulties in being soothed or in feeling comfortable with physical separateness but also suggest that these infants are already experiencing strains in emotional development that can lead to major widespread psychopathology. Effective soothing is one of the cornerstones for the child's image of the world as a safe and gratifying place and of himself or herself as an effective person who can get needs and wishes fulfilled. The ability to be comfortable with physical separateness, particularly when the mother is not within eyesight, means that the child has had adequate gratifying experiences with the mother. These experiences result in the child's being able to form an inner representation of the mother that supports and is present for the child when the mother is not available. The mother continues to exist for the child, even in her absence. The child feels that he or she, too, will survive and not run the risk of annihilation, even if the mother is gone temporarily. The child has "stored" internally the many ways that the mother has been a parent and can now use those identifications with her for growth and learning.

Without these capacities, represented by the capacity to be soothed and to enjoy being physically separate, the child does not have a stable, enduring sense of self and experiences chronic terror of annihilation and inability to trust others. Self-confidence is impossible, and learning and exploration of the world are markedly impaired, as seen in the play of the children in Galenson's study (Galenson et al., 1979). Memories of gratifying experiences also promote the development of frustration tolerance, the ability to wait, to anticipate, and to plan. Again development in this area seems to be taxed by the presence of a hearing loss. A college sophomore with a moderately severe to severe hearing loss and good auditory comprehension described repeated experiences of frustration in her years in school. Whenever she had a teacher who was not responsive to her auditory and written-language deficits, she opted to drop the course after a few weeks rather than feel too much frustration and get lower grades. If one were to describe an adult with the emotional problems observed in the children, that person would be seen as self-centered, mistrustful and suspicious, impulsive, unempathic, and limited in the ability to learn academically and socially. Although there is controversy about the presence and etiology of this constellation of character traits (Altschuler, 1971; Lesser & Easser, 1972), the characteristics described above for a hypothetical adult mesh alarmingly with those noted by Altschuler and Lesser and Easser. So the perceived characteristics of deaf adults, as stigmatizing as they may be, are cause for concern.

Meadow (1983; Meadow-Orlans, 1984, February), H. Schlesinger (personal communication, 1981), and Schlesinger and Meadow (1972) take issue with the validity of the observations of Galenson et al. (1979, 1983) and the lines of thought that proceed from them. They feel that the developmental difficulties seen in hearing-impaired children stem mainly from the problems and deficits in symbolic communication caused by the hearing loss; in their opinion, the use of signed communication by the family and child, beginning as soon as the hearing loss is detected, rectifies many of the psychological problems noted by others. They suggest that the other studies are faulty in design because parents were included who were unaccepting of their child's hearing loss and who did not use sign language. Although few could disagree with their recognition of the need for a way for the hearing-impaired child and the family to communicate in complex symbolic ways, their studies have some of the very same methodological problems they note in others. Many variables, such as selecting parents and children who may have been the recipients of many preventative psychological and educational interventions, are overlooked; thus, they may be presenting the results of superparents and superkids.

A longitudinal study of the emotional, cognitive, social, and language development of hearing-impaired infants is sorely needed. A model for this kind of study is that of Fraiberg (1977), who studied the development of totally blind infants, with no other known defects, over a period of several years. All observations occurred in the home, with the mother involved both as a participant with the infant and as an observer. A program of intervention was offered concurrently, in order to maximize development in the areas of human relationships, prehension, locomotion, and language. Fraiberg's interest was piqued by the observation that 25% of children with only the defect of total blindness became autistic and that many others had autistic patterns. She reasoned that this unusually high rate must come from the problems in development that they encountered very early in their lives because of their sensory defect. She noted major impediments and different developmental routes in all four areas studied: human attachments, prehension, gross motor development, and language development.

In the area of human attachments, blindness resulted in the alteration or absence of a set of signs and signals by which parents could interpret the baby's recognition of and responses to them, as well as the baby's desires and preferences. The course of smiling was different from normal; there was an absence of differentiated and modulated facial expressions. In addition, because of these differences, the parents felt that they were attempting to relate to a child who spoke an alien language. They had great difficulty experiencing that their baby recognized them, thought that they were special, and loved them. Even Fraiberg, one of the world's experts on infants with problems of attachment, noted that her responses to the blind infants were different and deficient, particularly her level of verbalization, even while knowing that the infant was blind. Separation distress was delayed, this being a consequence of the difficulty the infant experienced in achieving the concept of the mother as existing in a permanent way, not just when she was in contact with the infant. When the infant did develop separation distress, the level was much higher than usual.

In the area of prehension, it had long been noted that, without a program of intervention, blind children extended their arms at shoulder height with their fingers moving aimlessly. In the infants, Fraiberg noted that all had a marked deficit in prehension; none between the ages of 4 to 8 months reached for persons or toys not in physical contact with them, even when voice or sound cues were provided. This was interpreted to mean that vision is crucial to the normal development of the use of hands for exploration and contact. Vision must function to bring the hands together at the midline, thereby resulting in mutual fingering, transferring, and coordinate use. Vision also functions to unite the existence of a person or object with the sounds they make; this facilitates the capacities to be soothed, to feel separate, and to develop language. Even if a baby were not blind, these deficits would have major consequences for development. In the blind baby, hands must substitute for eyes as much as possible, but blindness can damage this substitute. Hands must provide the experiences that allow the baby to develop a sense of the existence and content of the world of people and objects. Even with programs of intervention, blindness delays the development of the awareness of the existence of the outer world and the capacity to unite sound and person or object.

In gross motor development, although all postural attainments were within normal limits, the kinds of mobility that normally follow the achievement of each posture (i.e., crawling follows the hands-and-knees position) were severely delayed. And until the blind baby reached for a person or object on sound cue only, there was no forward motion. This suggests that the baby first has to solve the difficult problem of conceptualizing the existence of an outer world toward which he or she wants to move, based solely on sound.

Language development, too, was delayed. Two sources were an experiential poverty and a delay in development of a self-concept, secondary to the effects of blindness on the development of human attachments. As a result, the development of language overall was retarded; even more striking was the delay, by several years, of the use of the word *I* to represent the self in language and in play. Blindness thereby continuously impeded the development of the capacity for symbolic thought.

This elegant study suggests, to those interested in the development of the hearing-impaired child, that many areas of growth may be affected adversely simply by the presence of a hearing loss and that some of the problems seen, such as those of language development, may in part be due to delays and arrests in human attachment and cognition. Only in painstaking longitudinal studies, such as Fraiberg's pioneering one, can these hypotheses and others be tested.

## Hearing and the Parent-Child Relationship

The strain on the parents and on the parent-child relationship of having a hearing-impaired child, as yet undiagnosed, can now be explored. Clearly, parents have a different kind of child with whom they must develop a relationship, although the kinds of differences are only suggested by the scant research on emotional development of hearing-impaired children. Parents have a child who speaks "an alien language" (Fraiberg, 1977) but with the additional complication that the parents and child are usually entirely unaware of the alien status. What is the impact on the parents in terms of how the parents experience themselves and consequently the infant? In what ways is one of the keystones of emotional, cognitive, and language development—the parent-infant relationship—stressed and damaged? Perhaps these questions are what Mrs. G. was alluding to when she reported that, despite her best efforts to cope and deny, she felt somewhat rejected by Susan and thought that she was less involved with her than with her other two children.

Having a child with whom one cannot establish a comfortable, satisfying relationship can evoke feelings of profound loss and inadequacy for the parent. Many of the early and ongoing satisfactions for a parent involve the experience of feeling in contact with the child, what Stern (1983) calls "communing" and "communication." "Communing" is the state of being together, of deep sharing, the forerunner of empathy. All people hunger for and need this experience repeatedly; in parents, it is a key experience for two reasons. First, empathy is the almost exclusive means of understanding and relating to the infant; parents temporarily allow themselves to empathize or identify with the infant in order to detect what the infant needs. Second, by simply being parents in the presence of one's infant, the parents have evoked in themselves very early memories of being cared for and so partially regress to a state in which the need for feeling in contact is accentuated. Who has not witnessed a parent reduced to a state of what would appear to be flamboyant, bizarre babbling if one did not know that this was simply a parent "talking" with the baby? The capacity to empathize comes, in part, from being able to read accurately the signals and signs from the child; the ability to decode and respond appropriately appears to be both prewired and learned from one's own early experiences of being the recipient of empathy.

When a misreading occurs because the signs and signals from the infant are deviant, both infant and parent feel that something is wrong and may become overtly distressed. For example, in experimental situations, if an infant is making a sound with a certain loudness and the mother responds by jiggling the baby's leg, but purposefully with less vigor (Stern, 1983), the baby will stop, look bewildered or dismayed, and may even burst into tears. Thus the parent feels fundamental distress, a sense of inadequacy and loss, from the failure to make satisfactory contact. Anger and guilt may then ensue. The sequence of inadequacy, loss, anger, and guilt may prompt in the parent a defensive withdrawal from the child so as to lessen these painful feelings. The parallel experience is present for the child. None of this distress can be beneficial for the parent-child relationship. A deaf college student talked of her pain and embarassment at feeling not in synchrony with her classmates as they asked questions of the professors. She had an interpreter and wished to ask questions, too, but worried that she would be woefully behind in the dialogue among her classmates if she did. In high school she was an excellent student, without the use of an interpreter. Because of her feelings in college, she decided to transfer to a college for the deaf, where she hoped that she would feel more able to participate in the rhythm of communications. In a psychodynamic and psychotherapeutic study of three severely hearing-impaired toddlers and their mothers, Galenson, Kaplan, and Sherkow (1983) documented the profound damage to emotional, intellectual, and social development that resulted from the presence of the hearing loss. Unfortunately, it is not possible to tease apart the various contributions. These consist of the consequences of the hearing loss on the toddler, the effect of the differently responsive child on the mother, and the impact of the mother's depression on the toddler.

## Denial in Parents and Professionals

Having developed some hypotheses about the impact of the hearing impairment on the emotional development of the child and on the parent-child relationship, we can now consider how the use of denial by the parents and professionals can be understood. What are the effects of using denial? Denial is a mechanism of defense against emotions and therefore serves to protect the user from intolerable and unmanageable levels of various feelings that are set off by a perception. The parent perceives that something is wrong either with the child's response or with the way the parent feels; the professional perceives either distress in the parent or something different about the child's responses. As any of these perceptions have potentially painful consequences, the parties involved are therefore vulnerable to experiencing a variety of intensely painful feelings. Parents may feel terror, helplessness, anger, guilt, shame, severe loss, failure, and depression; the professional may feel some of the same feelings.

The use of denial serves to obscure entirely these feelings and the perceptions from which they arise or to allow the perceptions and the attendant feelings to be admitted to consciousness in manageable doses. Total denial in the parent is certainly not the optimal path, but neither is it all bad. As Mrs. G. suggested, it allowed her to continue to treat Susan as a normal child in many ways, thereby protecting the two of them and their relationship to some degree. The feelings precipitated by discovering that one's child has a hearing loss are difficult to integrate; even if the integration is ultimately successful, the long period prior to this is stormy and disruptive for all involved. Therefore Susan and her mother may have benefited some from the protection that resulted. Total denial may protect the severely disturbed parent from becoming psychotic and unable to function; although the psychosis may ultimately lead to much-needed help, it is damaging to all those involved prior to a successful resolution. Of course, partial denial—leading to a gradual integration of feelings, realistic perceptions, and interventions—is vastly preferable. Only this course can result in the child and parents truly having their needs met.

Doctor-shopping, a term commonly embued with judgment and rejection, can now be viewed in a different light; it can stem in part from a normal need of parents to deal with their feelings in doses manageable for them. Rather than condemning and crushing denial and doctor-shopping, it is far more useful for all parties involved to interpret these as resulting from severe distress. Only then can the professional perceive what interventions need to be provided to lessen the distress to manageable levels so that the other interventions can proceed.

Denial in professionals can have no benefit other than the miniscule one of reinforcing denial in parents, with the resulting protection from disruption then experienced, to some degree, by the parents. On the other hand, the damage from the use of denial by professionals can be severe and long-lasting. The denial has at least two sources: minimal education about hearing loss and discomfort aroused by having to inform parents of an incurable and difficult problem. The training of most professionals has habitually overlooked the area of hearing loss. Not only does this lack of training lead to ignorance, which decreases sensitivity to signs of hearing loss, but it also makes the professional vulnerable to frightening misconceptions and to a feeling of inadequacy that may be defended against by denying the possibility of hearing loss.

Sweetow and Barrager (1980) demonstrated the great frequency with which the diagnosis was missed and the persistence needed by parents in order to obtain adequate diagnosis and treatment. Mendelsohn (1981), a parent-professional, presents a powerful account of her and her family's responses to having a deaf child, both before and after diagnosis. Until the diagnosis of deafness was made when the child was 3 years old, Mendelsohn was plagued with feelings of inadequacy and self-blame as a mother, and her marriage was sorely taxed. Although the family repeatedly brought up the possibility of hearing loss with several professionals, the diagnosis was rejected. Reassurances by the professionals only served to heighten the parents' negative feelings and led to individual isolation because each felt foolish and ashamed for having any worries about their child or themselves. The correct diagnosis brought relief. In a report by Meadow (1968), three parents describe critical and attacking comments by physicians when the parents suspected a hearing loss. At a time when the child and parents most need help and are already suffering from a sense of inadequacy and isolation, critical and harsh responses from the professionals to whom they have turned further damage their self-confidence. This leads to mistrust and disillusionment with health care providers. It is most often with this background that parents arrive in the audiologist's and otolaryngologist's office, about to receive the diagnosis of an incurable hearing loss in their young child.

# The Story Continues: Diagnosis, Devastation, and Relief

Mrs. G. took Susan to the speech pathologist for several months but felt discomforted by the professional's failure to do an audiogram during this time. As time passed, Mrs. G.'s distress became intolerable and could no longer be denied. Despite the obstacles she encountered, she insisted that the pediatrician refer Susan for a hearing test when the child was 3 years old. Mrs. G. regarded this as a great achievement for her because she was in awe of physicians and had a devalued image of herself; she was usually quiet and unassertive and kept her distress and dissatisfactions to herself.

As she approached the first appointment with Dr. T., the audiologist, Mrs. G. felt mistrustful; after all, Mrs. G. had been referred to Dr. T. by the pediatrician, and she no longer had the total confidence in him that she formerly had. She found Dr. T.'s approach to be direct, clear, and supportive throughout the process of history-taking and audiologic testing. The medical examination was done by an otologist.

It had not occurred to Mrs. G. to have her husband come with her and Susan to the consultation; most of the three children's medical needs had been attended to by Mrs. G. alone. Only much later, after significant changes in her own personality and characteristic ways of doing things, brought about by her successful emotional growth following the diagnosis of Susan's hearing loss, would Mrs. G. recognize the need for both parents to be present and involved during the whole diagnostic and habilitation process. Mrs. G. alone heard Dr. T.'s diagnosis of Susan's moderately severe to severe mid- to high-frequency hearing loss. Dr. T.'s explanation was clear and to the point; she did not burden Mrs. G. with too much information for her to incorporate, particularly taking into consideration Mrs. G.'s emotional state. Mrs. G. was stunned by the diagnosis, although it was one that she had long expected. She did not look upset and did not cry, a response that could have lulled Dr. T. into a false sense of ease had she not been sensitive to and aware of the characteristic initial responses of parents upon receiving such news. Dr. T. was also well aware of her own wish not to have to be the bearer of such a distressing diagnosis. Later Mrs. G. remembered that Dr. T. had been emotionally supportive not only by not burdening Mrs. G. with too much information to digest but also by recognizing and verbalizing Mrs. G.'s feelings and reassuring her that these would be understandably present at this time. Dr. T. also wanted Mrs. G., Mr. G., and Susan to return within 3 days in order to discuss the diagnosis further, begin habilitation, address emotional concerns, and answer rapidly emerging questions. Dr. T. knew that the diagnosis had precipitated a crisis for the family and did not want them to feel abandoned by the professionals, which families often feel when not seen frequently and intensively immediately after the diagnosis is presented to them. But, although Mrs. G. liked Dr. T. and her handling of the diagnostic crisis, she still felt mistrustful and disillusioned with professionals and wanted to provide herself with reassurance and restoration of trust by getting a second opinion.

When Mr. G. came home from work that night, Mrs. G. burst into tears; it was then that she realized how devastated she felt. Although she was an experienced mother and had been through some very difficult experiences with her children, beginning with their births, she felt entirely unequipped for Susan's problem. She realized that she had never known anyone with a hearing loss among her entire family and friends and had always thought that hearing loss was synonymous with "deaf and dumb," an idea that terrified her. She felt that she was suddenly living with a stranger, someone with whom she had very limited means of communicating; she felt that she had little experience in common with her daughter and that this problem would grow worse as the years passed. How would she know how to be a mother to Susan? Mr. and Mrs. G. sought out a large audiology center several miles from their home. Although distressed about Susan's diagnosis, they also felt a sense of relief. The discomfort and worry that had been nameless for so long was now identified. Despite her questions about how she would be able to mother Susan, Mrs. G. felt that she now knew what the problem was; her basic confidence in her judgment was restored. She no longer felt the self-doubt and feeling of rejection she had lived with so long with Susan. Nor did she feel helpless and in the dark; she had questions and things she could learn. With the second opinion confirming that of Dr. T., Mrs. G. also began to experience the return of trust in professionals; but the idealization of professionals at the expense of her own self-esteem and judgment was gone forever. She felt a swelling of self-esteem and relished the realization that she had been assertive and demanding, with a resulting positive outcome. Her old posture of withdrawal no longer seemed appealing or functional.

The family returned to Dr. T. to begin habilitation and to have Susan provided with amplification. There was so much to learn, and Dr. T. seemed to be the only source of information in the beginning. Susan's response to amplification caused ripples of surprise in the family. Within a few minutes of having put the aids on, Susan looked puzzled; she scanned the room, searching for something. Finally she reached out to touch the air-conditioning vent and pointed to her hearing aid. The family realized that she was hearing the high-pitched whistle in the air-conditioning system that they had learned to ignore. When Susan began to speak, she looked startled and clapped her hands over her ears. Her own voice sounded shockingly loud to her. Half an hour later, with the family seated for dinner at their favorite restaurant, Susan seemed wide-eyed with surprise as the waiter spoke. The family suddenly understood that Susan had never been able to hear the soft-spoken waiters in the noisy restaurant before. The dinner was remarkable in other ways. Toward the end, Mrs. G. noticed that she felt relaxed and not exhausted. As she wondered why, she realized that all of the family had not been straining to talk loudly enough to make themselves heard to Susan and get her attention. Susan's voice was no longer loud and penetrating. Mrs. G. was becoming aware of the impact of the hearing loss on Susan and on the family's relationship with Susan. Susan adjusted to the aids fairly easily. She liked the increased auditory input and contact. But she also was uncomfortable with unfamiliar sounds, complained about how noisy it was, and initially removed the aids several times each day when she wanted to return to her old familiar world.

For Mrs. G. waves of feelings of devastation continued, as did the sense of profound doubt about being able to mother Susan adequately. During the first several months, Mrs. G. wished that Dr. T. lived next door, so that Mrs. G. could run over several times daily with the questions and worries that seemed endless. She went to the public library and, despite a thorough search, was able to turn up very little. Dr. T. made herself very available; she encouraged Mrs. G. to ask questions and seek information. She wanted Mrs. G. to be an active participant in Susan's habilitation and knew that not only would this increase Mrs. G.'s knowledge but that this would also help to repair the damage to the mother-daughter relationship that was the usual outcome of having a child with a hearing loss. Mrs. G. would lose the feeling of helplessness and inadequacy that she had experienced and would also feel able to communicate with her child again. In this setting Dr. T. could also point out to her the different responses of a hearing-impaired child and show the progress that Susan and Mrs. G. were making, which would have been missed by Mrs. G. or any unskilled observer. Dr. T. was aware that the child experiences the change in the relationship with the mother in a mixture of ways, from feelings of pleasure resulting from the increased attention from the mother to feelings of frustration and resentment at the demands and intrusions.

Mrs. G. began to feel involved and effective in contrast to her early experiences with Susan, in which she had felt more distant and out of tune than she had with her other children. As Dr. T. pointed out Susan's responses, Mrs. G. began to review her experiences with Susan over the years, and small things that had felt troubling—but had been denied or ignored—suddenly made sense. Mrs. G. felt an enormous sense of relief at being able to empathize with her daughter. She felt that a large part of her relationship with Susan had returned to her, which helped to lessen the grief that she had felt since the diagnosis was made. She wondered whether she had perhaps felt the sense of loss and grief from early in Susan's infancy, when she had first had a sense of something not being right, a subtle lack of attunement and gratification. Dr. T. facilitated Mrs. G.'s ability to empathize with Susan by talking with her about what Susan's experience was like; she also provided an audiotape that replicated how persons with different degrees of hearing loss would experience normal speech; Mrs. G. was stunned by the degree of difficulty that even a person with a mild hearing loss has. But then she remembered how she herself labored to hear when congested from allergies or a cold. Now she could feel Susan's hearing loss herself, to some degree.

Support for Mr. and Mrs. G.'s feelings came not only from Dr. T. but also from the parents of a child with a similar hearing loss, whom Mr. and Mrs. G. had met through Dr. T. As a result, Mrs. G. felt less alone. This was part of Dr. T.'s goal; she had seen many parents who, because of their sense of helplessness, inadequacy, and disillusionment at this time, became totally dependent on a professional who, in turn, fostered this attachment and derived gratification from being treated as omnipotent and omniscient. This kind of relationship inhibits self-esteem and independence in the parents and child; the development of a rich, involved, strong, and realistic family interaction is prevented in these cases by the presence in everyone's mind of the "all-knowing" professional. With the background that Susan's parents now had, they decided to begin Susan in a preschool with a mixture of hearing-impaired and normal hearing children. Susan was thrilled by the sight of other children wearing hearing aids and was endlessly curious about their aids; she took her own aids out less often and seemed happier with herself.

# Commentary

This is an important point at which to pause and reflect on the the G. family who, out of devastation, has grown and even begun to triumph.

## Devastation, Grief, and Disillusionment

The seed of triumph is in Mrs. G.'s ability to let herself experience the feeling of devastation. Despite all the forces supporting her impulse to deny her feelings, the fundamental need of all parents to experience a gratifying reciprocal relationship with their child won out. Accompanying her ability to let herself experience the feeling of overwhelming loss that is devastation, Mrs. G. was also able to admit her disillusionment with her pediatrician, yet another severe loss. Although no one would wish for anyone to have to suffer a loss, being able to run the risk of and tolerate loss is essential for emotional growth; positive change also brings loss by definition. One cannot take the chance of growing if loss is too frightening; instead, one is left limited and rigid, often trying to impose these restrictions on others in one's life also.

What loss is experienced by the parents of a hearing-impaired child? Solnit and Stark (1961) conceived of the loss in two ways—namely, "loss of the ideal child," of which every parent carries an image, and loss as a single, one-time experience that may nevertheless take a long time to resolve. Olshansky (1962) has conceptualized it instead as a "chronic grief," one that parents experience again and again as they encounter the child in the millions of events in daily living over the years, particularly at points of transition in the child's life. This latter formulation fits the descriptions of parents and audiologists more adequately than the single-loss perspective. The child does not die, resulting in a single-event loss; instead, the child continues to live, and the parents and child have an ongoing relationship. In addition, the parents experience a lessening of the usual rewards of parenting, such as having a child who meets their own standards of success as an adult.

Unless one thinks of the loss and grief as a frequent and repetitive experience, the grief of the parents, as it reappears, will be viewed as pathological. Viewing the grief as pathological leads to lack of support for the parents' normal grief, although unrelenting or pervasive grief does signal a pathological process and requires appropriate professional intervention.

The loss experienced by the parent is then seen not only as the "loss of the ideal child" but also as the loss of the gratifications of the parent-child relationship and as the loss of some of the memories of the parents' own early gratifications as the child in the parent-child unit. With loss of both sets of early parent-child memories, the foundation for emotional survival and relationship is gone. Optimally, the parent experiences this sense of loss only for short bursts of time and can call on other experiences and memories. Obviously, the support and caring of others at this time are essential; others replace in an ongoing way what was lost and provide a more realistic assessment of what actually remains than the devastated parent alone can perceive. The parents also get real rewards from the child, as the child benefits from interventions and is not limited in achievements by the attitudes of the parents.

The disillusionment with professionals is yet another great loss. This comes from two sources: the real failures of professionals and the need of parents to project their own feelings of failure and mistrust onto professionals. Many people will normally attempt to relieve themselves of an uncomfortable feeling by projecting it onto the outside world; parents of children with a hearing loss are no different from others and may try to restore their sense of confidence in their own feelings by projecting their mistrust onto the professionals with whom they must deal. When professionals actually fail their patients and become untrustworthy at this difficult time, the situation becomes much more complicated. Viewed from this perspective, doctor-shopping is not something devious or disturbed but an attempt to deal with damaged trust. Verbalization by the professional of the various concerns leading to the parents' problems with trust can lead to enormous relief for the parents and to the foundation for a solid relationship between parents and professionals. This, too, is gratifying to the parents and repairs experiences of loss.

## Intervention and Triumph

Now that we have explored the issues facing parents and professionals as they meet at the point of diagnosis, what can be said about psychological interventions that are invaluable at this time? One intervention encompasses all others—namely, helping parents realize that their feelings can be understood and mastered. There are several ways in which this needs to be done. By having knowledge of any parent's usual experience and the normal ways in which a parent handles it, the professional can listen to whatever the parents say and *verbalize* their feelings for them. In the midst of a crisis, verbalization of feelings enables a person to deal successfully with them. Feelings cannot be truly mastered if they are not within conscious awareness. When the feelings are made conscious by verbalization, they lose some of the discomfort and power they have when they are unconscious and therefore inaccessible to a person's more mature thought processes. Even if the feelings are those of anger or resentment toward a child, they lose some of their impact on the bearer when they are seen as only verbalized feelings, not as dangerous, forbidden impulses. The verbalization of these feelings by the professional also lets the parents know that these are feelings of which one can speak. The professional must let the parents know that these are usual and expected feelings and that one would be surprised if these emotions were not there. Accompanying the verbalization, the professional must have an interest and curiosity about the parents' experiences; the latter must be viewed without judgment and criticism. The parents will sense these positive attitudes and become more observant and introspective themselves.

Professionals have a tendency to burden parents with information, particularly during the diagnostic crisis. This tendency may reflect ignorance of the presence and effects of a crisis; it may also be an attempt by the professional to deny or fill the void caused by the devastation. Unfortunately, this approach is doomed to failure at best; most likely the parents will see it as a failure of the professional to provide the understanding and support they need so badly. Information given at the time of crisis will be missed or misinterpreted, a problem that can come back to haunt all those involved. While there is reason to have hope for the child and the family, professionals may try to force this attitude on the parents by providing too much information and expecting too many decisions. No one likes to be the bearer of bad news, but this is not the way for professionals to handle their own distress of being in that position.

The use of euphemisms is also to be avoided, for they indicate an inability by the parents or the professional to face the truth, either because they are too weak and fragile or because the truth is unbearable for all. For example, Mendelsohn (1981) was told that her profoundly deaf son had a "hearing problem" and that she needed to "put an auditory trainer on him"; or parents are also taught to call hearing aids "beepers" when talking with their children.

Having developed the basis for a trusting, working relationship with the parents, the professional then needs to teach them about the impact of the hearing loss on their child's responses. When these altered responses have been identified, the professional must help the parents to become aware of their misinterpretations of these, such as feeling rejected when the child seems to ignore them. In actual interactions with their child, parents need to be shown the ways to make effective contact with the child and to learn how the child communicates a positive response.

In addition, parents need to learn that many of the child's emotional tasks are made more difficult or different by the hearing loss. The child must recurrently deal with the question of bodily intactness and adequacy. The goal is, as some young adults with severe hearing losses have stated it, for the children to have a sense of themselves as people who happen to have a hearing loss and resultant language problems rather than as inadequate, defective people. The young infant presented with hearing aids early on may come to feel that the aid is part of his or her body image; this is helpful in long-term adjustment. But it is at least interesting, if not important, to wonder about what the infant and small child's psychological experience must be of a body part and sensory input that can be detached and removed. Lang (personal communication, March 5, 1982) observed an infant, fitted with amplification at 5 months, who put his finger in his ear whenever the aid was removed, perhaps restoring the lost tactile sensation of the aid. Fraiberg (personal communication, June 6, 1981) recommended providing amplification as early as possible so as to help make the aid part of the normal body image. On the other hand, a toddler is likely to experience the aid as an intrusion on his or her newly developed autonomy and need for control over the body. This can lead to rejection of the aid and a struggle between parents and child. By being aware of the importance of body control to the toddler, parents can approach the toddler more gently. In addition, creative approaches to important emotional issues for the toddler can be developed. An excellent example of this was the solution of a mother of an 18-month-old girl with a newly diagnosed profound hearing loss. The child refused to wear the aids. The mother recognized the eagerness with which her child wanted to identify with her in all ways. So the mother sat her daughter on the dresser while the mother put on her own earrings. Having made this a slow and fascinating process, the mother then proceeded to put "earrings"—the hearing aids—on her daughter. The bulk of the struggle was circumvented in this manner.

Later the child will wonder about the cause of the loss and often will verbalize the feeling that it is unfair. As a child is wont to blame others for problems and to use "magical" thinking to explain the sources of problems, the child may think that if the hearing aids are removed, then the hearing loss will go away. The child feels different and abnormal and is relieved and delighted to see others wearing aids. Fargo-Lathrop (personal communication, October 27, 1984) describes the excitement of toddlers when they first see others wearing aids at the audiologist's office. The toddlers often readily approach these strangers to show them they also wear aids. These contacts support the child's normal process of identification. Identification helps people to acquire new and enriching skills and images of themselves. These experiences increase the child's sense of adequacy and wholeness.

A child also needs help in solving the problem of developing an inner sense of the mother's enduring presence and availability, even when she has left the room. At this point, the child no longer has visual contact and, because of the hearing loss, is deprived of the reassuring auditory information that lets the child know of the mother's presence in the vicinity. With such a child, a mother might play repeated games of separation and return, helping the child to gain a sense of the mother's continuing existence. She would also need to let the child know, by using other sensory modalities, that she was leaving and would return, so that the child would feel prepared and not surprised. Other sensory modalities also need to be supplemented in order to provide the stimulation essential for normal development. These senses should be used to substitute for the soothing and maternal attunement that hearing normally provides. The professional must encourage the parents to play the leading role in observing and understanding these daily emotional problems and in finding their own uniquely suited solutions. Fraiberg's (1977) work with blind children demonstrates the many developmental problems caused by blindness and the interventions devised to facilitate normal development. Meadow-Orlans (1984, February) presents a review of other early interventions as well as approaches devised for use with older children. With a positive experience behind them, the child and the parents now have the basic psychological equipment with which to deal with the successive stages.

# Up to the Present: Learning What We Need to Help

Mrs. G. found herself left with many questions about how to relate to Susan; she was surprised because she thought that she had already resolved these with her two older children. Instead she struggled with issues of how to deal with her child and the outside world and how to handle the sibling relationships. Thankful that she was already an experienced mother, with two older children with whom she felt successful and confident, she reflected on how much more insecure she might feel if Susan had been her first child and if she did not have the knowledge gained from experience that she and a child could weather most experiences successfully. Still, she was startled by her temptation to treat Susan differently from the ways in which she had treated her prior to the diagnosis and the ways in which she had dealt with her other children. Although Susan had happily been riding her tricycle in the driveway for a few months, now Mrs. G. was concerned that Susan might not be careful about cars or so frightened about not being able to hear her mother that she would not want to be out of eyesight. The neighbors compounded Mrs. G.'s response; when they found out about Susan's hearing loss, they wanted to put a sign at the end of the street warning drivers that there was a deaf child on the street. When she saw her older children roughhousing with Susan or teasing her, as they would each other or their friends, she wanted to rush in to stop them. But Dr. T. kept reminding Mrs. G. that Susan was first a child and, only after that, a child with a hearing loss, and that she must be treated with that in mind. The teachers supported this viewpoint also. "It's a rough world out there," Mrs. G. thought to herself, and she realized that Susan would be prepared to cope and fit in only if she lived in the real world with real relationships like everyone else. If Susan did not have the opportunity to experience normal everyday relationships and the love and difficulty that come with them, how could she possibly deal with the even more challenging problems accompanying her hearing loss! Based on this realization, Mrs. G. dealt more successfully and calmly with Susan; she no longer intervened in most of the teasing and squabbling among the children, and Susan was expected to participate in the household functions in the same way the two older children had. This seemed to lessen the resentment Mrs. G. had noticed in the older children, beginning with the diagnostic process and Mrs. G.'s increased time commitment to Susan. Mr. and Mrs. G. became used to the quieter, less taxing Susan and had almost forgotten the effort required to communicate with her before she was fitted with hearing aids. But when Susan forgot her hearing aids at a friend's home where she had gone swimming, Mrs. G. was frantic to get them back. She was clearly having difficulty in communicating with Susan, and Susan's piercing noisiness was almost more than Mrs. G. could stand.

Continuing with the basic approach to Susan that they had evolved, Mr. and Mrs. G. wanted to try to mainstream Susan in kindergarten. Dr. T. was very supportive of this idea and helped Mrs. G. to learn about the school system and relevant legislative issues. Dr. T. knew that lack of necessary supports in the school districts were frequently the undoing of otherwise successful mainstreaming. So Mrs. G. acquired yet another area of expertise, the special education laws, which helped once again to lessen the sense of helplessness and inadequacy she had felt with Susan. She discovered that Susan was entitled to have a teacher's aide in the classroom, but it was only after she showed a copy of the legislation to the district head of special education that she was believed. She felt that it was best to provide the aide for Susan quietly, as someone for the whole class, since Susan was already struggling with feelings of being different. Instead of the neighborhood school Mrs. G. chose the one in the district that housed the program for hearing-impaired children in addition to regular classrooms. This program would serve many functions. Susan would be provided with daily sessions with hearing and speech therapists, and she would be on a campus in which students with hearing aids were a familiar sight to both teachers and students. Mrs. G. knew that Susan would also feel a sense of relief and support at seeing other children with hearing aids. Seeing adults wearing aids had helped Susan and the family to deal with her periodic question, "Will I have to wear hearing aids when I grow up, or will I outgrow them like David did his braces?" Mrs. G. interviewed the possible teachers to determine who would be most suitable for Susan, encouraging them to discuss openly any discomfort with having a hearing-impaired child in their classroom; if they did, she decided it was best not to have Susan in that class. She also volunteered in the class so as to keep close tabs on how all parties were faring and to provide information and assistance to the teacher as readily as possible. To her delight, things went reasonably smoothly, much better than she had anticipated. Susan did have to struggle to follow the directions and participate in class discussions, and helping her took a lot of time and energy. Friendships developed gradually, with some of the children being able to tolerate Susan's tendency to miss parts of conversations or rules of games and generally to react to the ongoing action more slowly than the other children. Susan also had a tendency to blame her hearing aids for the reticence of some children to play with her, but her parents patiently discussed this with her.

Each year, Mrs. G. gave a talk and demonstration on hearing loss and hearing aids to the class. Much to her shock, as she was standing outside the second-grade classroom, the mother of a hearing-impaired child who was new in the class unknowingly began to complain to Mrs. G. about this person who was to talk to her son's class about hearing loss and hearing aids. The mother felt that this would only humiliate her son and wanted to hide his hearing loss as much as possible. She talked about how difficult it had been when he was an infant and toddler; they would go shopping, only to have people stop and stare at her son and his aids. One older woman said angrily, "Why do you take a child like that out in public?" This reminded Mrs. G. of the time when a man criticized her at the supermarket for having Susan's hair in a ponytail, revealing her hearing aids, as well as when her father asked whether Susan's hearing loss and aids would lessen the possibility of her marrying. She remembered the response of some friends at a time when she still felt the devastation and grief acutely and had hungered for support. They commented on how much more pleasant Susan was to be around now that she had been fitted with hearing aids, which made her less noisy and less active, never considering that her unpleasant behaviors were signs of Susan's hearing loss and not those of an undisciplined child. She could still feel the sting from these insensitive comments and wished that she did not have to endure these painful feelings. But then she thought to herself, "Everyone must have their own feelings, regardless of what they are." She had heard this at a workshop for parents of hearing-impaired children. This had been a revelation to Mrs. G. and a source of enormous comfort and strength ever since.

Mr. G. attended all the workshops and conferences; although he kidded his wife about her activism, he was pleased with the changes she had undergone and was very supportive. He and Susan had a close relationship and shared many activities, such as soccer and YMCA activities. He had met another father of a hearing-impaired child, a boy who was then in high school, who had discovered the importance of the everyday parent-child activities that a parent would enjoy with any child. As the father put it, "We didn't play enough baseball." Mr. G. was aware that this was an all too common experience; many families seemed to be more concerned that their child's speech sounded "normal" so as to hide the hearing loss if at all possible. Play, the child's version of learning and working, was limited, and repetitious drills filled the nonschool time. In addition, the range of academic material was narrowed, and much time was spent on overly simple work.

As fourth grade approached, Mr. and Mrs. G. thought about enrolling Susan in the neighborhood school. Susan herself was eager to do so; she had a few friends in the neighborhood and felt comfortable academically. The whole family realized that this would be an important transition and one that would require even more effort on the parents' and Susan's part. The special education teachers would not be as available in the new school whenever Susan needed help; and the neighborhood teachers were not used to having hearing-impaired students in their classrooms. Still, Mr. and Mrs. G. recognized the importance to Susan's development of more socialization with her peers. Adolescence was approaching, and Susan's parents knew the importance of peer relationships in adolescence, as their home was often filled with teenagers talking endlessly to one another behind closed bedroom doors or occupying the telephone for hours. They could feel their older children shifting their dependency and need for relationships onto peers and away from them, as is needed to enable the adolescent to separate from the family and develop new, intimate, adult relationships. They had heard from other parents, in groups for parents of hearing-impaired children, of the social isolation that often began in early adolescence, when issues of body image and peer pressure are so strong. This even occurred among the students at a school for the hearing-impaired, in which the students who appeared more "deaf and dumb" than the rest were rejected by the others. They had also learned that commonly the adolescent experimented with going without hearing aids and that they ought to be prepared emotionally for this occurrence. Very few students had been mainstreamed in Susan's district, so little information was available from other parents, by now the major source of assistance for Mr. and Mrs. G. They did not how know they would handle adolescent rejection and Susan's feelings about her hearing loss in this new stage, but they felt that what they had provided Susan with—an ability to function successfully in everyday settings and interactions and thus a realistic sense of self-esteem—would stand her in good stead. They had supported her acceptance and expression of her feelings and thoughts. Consequently, when difficulties did arise, she would not have the added pain of feeling ashamed and guilty for whatever emotions she had and for wanting to share the burden of pain and anger with others. Otherwise shame and guilt could lead her to withdraw unnecessarily. The parents felt prepared in fundamental ways because they no longer dreaded the unknown as they had before; they had found that they could survive and conquer devastation; they had the resources and skills, as well as the support of many other people, as they entered this stressful period.

Susan had fairly solid self-esteem, was able to weather some of the teasing and rejection that occurred because of her hearing loss, and felt pleased with her ability to participate and succeed in the usual activities of children.

# Commentary

We have followed the G. family from the time of mainstreaming in kindergarten up to the beginning of adolescence. A major theme throughout this span of years is the development of Susan's physical, emotional, and intellectual autonomy. By this is meant the growth of a healthy self-concept and set of skills that allow the child to move gradually from the world of the family into the ever-expanding one of friends, school, work, and intimate relationships with others. An adult described as having the constellation of personality traits noted in the deaf (Altschuler, 1971; Lesser & Easser, 1972), whether or not one thinks this description is entirely accurate, is someone who has not successfully developed emotionally or intellectually. Families of hearing-impaired children often fret over which world their children will choose—that of the hearing-impaired subpopulation or that of the hearing population. Regardless of what these children decide to do, it is essential that they make these choices on the basis of what they genuinely wish and are in reality able to accomplish rather than from the need to protect a shaky self-concept and inadequate experience in the world. A high school student with a moderately severe to severe loss talked about this problem when she described insisting that a friend of hers, who was deaf, try to order her own food at a restaurant rather than not trying in order to avoid her feelings of inadequacy and shame. She thought that her friend's speech was adequate to make herself understood, and she knew that this was the way for her friend to acquire self-confidence and the capacity to take care of herself and participate as fully as possible in the world. Mr. and Mrs. G. grappled successfully with many difficult issues that directly affect autonomy and self-esteem. These include overprotection; father-child, sibling, and marital relationships; the response of the outside world; schooling; and peer relationships.

## Overprotection

Overprotection has usually been attributed to unconscious anger and guilt in the parents, leading them to have a wish for and therefore a fear of harm coming to the child. Although this certainly can be a major factor as parents struggle for many years with feelings of loss, pain, and therefore resentment, other elements play an important role also. Mrs. G. had lost her confidence as a mother, which made the world seem a less predictable place and one she would not be able to deal with adequately. She tried to protect herself from these feelings by limiting Susan's contact with the world. Professionals who provide parents with effective emotional interventions, education, and skills, as Mr. and Mrs. G. were, can do much to reverse this loss. Instead, all too often children may be wrenched away from their parents by educators who are angry and contemptuous toward the parents for their overprotectiveness and who are going to teach the parents how to treat their children the correct way. This only increases the feelings of loss and inadequacy, thereby worsening the situation. In addition, the unconscious, guilt-laden resentment stemming from the loss increases, also fueling the overprotectiveness.

Other factors leading to protectiveness are the resentment and jealousy from siblings and insensitive responses from others outside the immediate family. Not only is resentment created among siblings by the additional parental involvement that a hearing-impaired child requires, but also insensitive and hostile attitudes arise from the uncomfortable feelings that the siblings and others may have about the disability. People find it frightening and shameful to have contact with someone who appears different or defective; it serves as a painful reminder of one's own concerns about these issues, and as a result of the discomfort people often feel angry. So an older brother may want his hearing-impaired sister not to play with him and his friends or may ask his mother not to put her hair into braids, thereby revealing the hearing aids. Strangers may make hurtful comments and recoil. An effervescent deaf college student recalled trying out for cheerleader in junior high. When she succeeded, some said she was chosen because she was deaf. One girl repeatedly tormented her; although she knew it was because of the girl's own emotional problems, she decided not to continue the next year.

Schools may also overprotect. A young woman who was mainstreamed in fourth grade described the lack of appropriate expectations for her behavior at the district school for the hearing-impaired. Physical expression of anger among the students was allowed, so verbal expression was not required. She felt that it took her 2 years after mainstreaming to learn appropriate ways of communicating and behaving, 2 years that were filled with bewilderment, rejection by students and teachers, humiliation, and feelings of inadequacy.

Many children feel that the most effective way to deal with rejection is to be open to others about the hearing loss and its manifestations as soon as possible after meeting someone. This opens the topic to discussion and questions rather than leaving the new acquaintance puzzled about what is wrong and feeling that all discomfort must be denied. The directness lessens the possibility of avoidance and rejection by others.

## Shame and Hurt

The family's wish to be spared painful feelings may cause parents to want the hearing-impaired child to speak with no indication of the disability. Parents can develop a strong desire to hide the manifestations of the hearing loss, undermining the possibility of a successful adaptation for all involved. The child feels the parents' rejection and shame of the impairment. The child is then burdened with more difficult feelings to handle and with the loss of necessary resources to deal with life—namely, self-esteem, helpful parents, and recognition, instead of the denial of reality. The parents lose in the same manner. The marital relationship is taxed simply by having a child with a problem; the addition of troubled and inadequate ways of coping with the feelings increases the strain. Fathers are vulnerable to being excluded from a successful relationship with the child. Professionals often overlook the need for the father's involvement, thereby reinforcing this development. The mother and child become an inappropriately intense unit, excluding the rest of the world. Some of this comes simply from the time and educational demands of the child, with the problem of who will meet them. Most often in our society it is the mother who does so.

## Schools

Schools can be an invaluable resource, furthering the successful adaptation of the hearing-impaired child in the world. Often they succeed at this task, increasing the child's self-esteem, intellectual and emotional skills, and peer relationships. Mr. and Mrs. G. demonstrated excellent ways of handling these issues. Some of their encounters with the school district and with other parents reveal the common problems parents and children experience and the guidance needed from professionals to solve them. The school setting, whether it be a school for the deaf or the local junior high school, needs to be given careful scrutiny. Some of what has formerly been attributed to intellectual and emotional problems stemming from a hearing loss may be more accurately related to problems in the school setting. Schlesinger and Meadow (1972) have decried the boring, repetitious, limited academic fare many hearing-impaired students are offered. A college student connected some of her academic limitations to an overemphasis in her earlier schooling on acquiring lipreading proficiency, with a relative neglect of reading and vocabulary skills; in her experience, this problem is widespread. Feinstein (1983) describes a therapy group for deaf adolescent boys in which much of their behavior appeared to be very self-centered, competitive, and disruptive; but his interpretation changed after examining the group setting and the school as a whole. He found that the school had been inadvertently structured to minimize social interaction among the students and, as a result, part of the self-centeredness and competition represented the boys' hunger for relating with peers. Using sign language also made it difficult for more than dyadic (between two people) communication to occur in a group setting, again increasing the boys' seeming inability to function in a healthy manner. Feinstein demonstrates the complexity of understanding certain deviant behaviors and the necessity of approaching these without bias. A deaf college student who decided to transfer to a college for the deaf from a university setting in which she had had to rely on an interpreter realized that, by having to use an interpreter, she could never participate in the class to her own satisfaction. She was often out of step in the class interchanges and felt inhibited and withdrawn.

## Other Hearing Losses, Other Children, and Their Families

A child with a moderate to moderately severe loss and a family that dealt successfully with the impairment have been presented. Many of the experiences and issues are the same, regardless of the degree of a child's hearing loss. But some are different, depending on the degree of the loss.

In children with a mild hearing loss, the diagnosis is often missed and mislabeled. The child is seen as having a behavior problem. Parents and professionals are commonly reluctant to provide amplification, fearing that the child will be identified as having a hearing loss and will look different because of wearing aids. They want the child to be spared the emotional and social problems that attend having a hearing loss and wearing hearing aids. This decision may come from lack of knowledge and understanding by parents and professionals or may arise from the adults' wish to protect themselves from their own uncomfortable feelings. Even if hearing aids are used, not infrequently the use is erratic and inconsistent. Unfortunately, the focus is commonly shifted to the child's learning and interpersonal problems, and the child is seen as inattentive, restless, hyperactive, immature, or a slow learner. Lang (personal communication, June 10, 1985) described the case of a high school freshman who sought amplification because he had a known mild hearing loss and felt that it was limiting his academic achievement. Even when the hearing loss is identified, many parents try to provide help for the secondary difficulties in learning and avoid dealing with the underlying hearing loss. On the other hand, the children can seem very bright and outgoing because they monopolize conversation, especially with adults, in an effort to avoid having to listen or because they are unaware someone else is talking. Because the manifestations of the hearing loss seem subtle compared to those of a child with a much greater loss, parents may have an opportunity to recognize the impact only when the child who uses amplification regularly goes without it.

At the other end of the spectrum is the child with a severe to profound loss. As an infant, the child often seems unresponsive, and parents can carry a deep-seated fear that something is profoundly wrong with their child. These parents are also usually faced with a major choice very early in the habilitation process—that is, which system to use for communication. This can be a very difficult choice. In addition, partly from the distress resulting from this difficulty, parents may lose the flexibility needed to reevaluate as they and the child proceed. They may be unable to change course, even when it is clearly indicated. This difficulty has been known to result in a child being left without a functional communication system. A college freshman described having had to learn sign language beginning in college so that he could use an interpreter in his classes; he had not clearly needed sign language earlier in school because lectures had not contained any information not present in textbooks, and his academic performance had been outstanding. Parents, needing to deny this as the problem, may then, as with children with a mild loss, focus instead on the behavior problems resulting from the lack of a communication system.

Parents may not like the sound of the speech of their severely hearing-impaired child and so may go to signing to avoid having a child who talks, thereby depriving the child of the world of auditory input and speech. As a result, they also never really face and resolve their own feelings. Correspondingly, a child with a severe loss who has a strong desire to communicate verbally but who must struggle and work very hard to do so may be viewed by the educational system as denying the hearing loss and be pressured to use signing.

Clearly, a family's responses to the hearing impairment can range from successful adaptation to failure caused by denial of any of the many aspects of having a child with a hearing loss. Even terribly difficult situations involving a child with a profound loss can have very positive outcomes because of the contributions of the child, the parents, and others. Conversely, the outcome of a child with a mild loss can be disastrous.

# Summary

When a hearing-impaired child and the family come to any professional, much has already occurred that can profoundly affect the success of the intervention and the relationship with the family; and far more is yet to be experienced by all the participants. Yet professionals rarely have the time to tap into, or perhaps have not understood, the wealth of information and experience that the child and family bring. It is only by listening that accurate interventions and revision of incomplete and inaccurate concepts occur. From the ongoing experiences with the child and family, the professional learns both new solutions and new questions that need to be answered.

# References

Altschuler, K. (1971). Studies of the deaf: Relevance to psychiatric theory. *American Journal of Psychiatry, 127,* 97–102.

Beratis, S., Rubin, M., Miller, R., Galenson, E., & Rothstein, A. (1979). Developmental aspects of an infant with transient moderate to severe hearing impairment. *Pediatrics, 1,* 153–155.

Brazelton, T. B. (1974). Origin of reciprocity in the mother-infant interaction. In M. Lewis & L. Rosenblum (Eds.), *Origins of behavior* (Vol. 1, pp. 49–76). New York: Wiley.

Call, J., Galenson, E., & Tyson, R. (Eds.). (1983). *Frontiers of infant psychiatry* (Vol. 1). New York: Basic Books.

Feinstein, C. (1983). Early adolescent deaf boys: A biopsychosocial approach. In M. Sugar (Ed.), *Adolescent psychiatry* (Vol. 2, pp. 147–162.). Chicago: University of Chicago Press.

Fraiberg, S. (1977). *Insights from the blind.* New York: Meridian Books, New American Library.

Fraiberg, S. (Ed.). (1980). *Clinical studies in infant mental health: The first year of life.* New York: Basic Books.

Galenson, E., Kaplan, E., & Sherkow, S. (1983). The mother-child relationship and preverbal communication in the deaf child. In J. Call, E. Galenson, & R. Tyson (Eds.), *Frontiers of infant psychiatry* (Vol. 1, pp. 136–149). New York: Basic Books.

Galenson, E., Miller, R., Kaplan, E., & Rothstein, A. (1979). Assessment of development in the deaf child. *Journal of the American Academy of Child Psychiatry, 18,* 128–142.

Lesser, S., & Easser, R. (1972). Personality differences in the perceptually handicapped. *Journal of the American Academy of Child Psychiatry, 11,* 458–466.

Meadow, K. (1968). Parental response to the medical ambiguities of congenital deafness. *Journal of Health and Social Behavior, 9,* 299–309.

Meadow, K. (1983). Attachment behavior of deaf children with deaf parents. *Journal of the American Academy of Child Psychiatry, 22,* 23–28.

Meadow-Orlans, K. (1984, February). Psychosocial intervention with deaf children. Manuscript submitted for publication.

Mendelsohn, J. (1981). The parent-professional: A personal view. In L. Stein, E. Mindel, & T. Jabaley (Eds.), *Deafness and mental health* (pp. 37–47). New York: Grune and Stratton.

Northern, J., & Downs, M. (1978). *Hearing in children* (2nd ed.). Baltimore: Williams and Wilkins.

Olshansky, S. (1962). Chronic sorrow: A response to having a mentally defective child. *Social Casework, 38,* 190–193.

Schlesinger, H., & Meadow, K. (1972). *Sound and sign: Childhood deafness and mental health.* Berkeley: University of California Press.

Solnit, A., & Stark, M. (1961). Mourning the birth of a defective child. In R. Eissler, A. Freud, H. Hartmann, & M. Kris (Eds.), *The psychoanalytic study of the child* (Vol. 16, pp. 523–537). New York: International Universities Press.

Stern, D. (1983). Implications of infancy research for clinical theory and practice. *Dialogue, 6,* 9–17.

Sweetow, R., & Barrager, D. (1980). Quality of comprehensive audiologic care: A survey of parents of hearing-impaired children. *Asha, 22,* 841–847.

Winnicott, D. W. (1975). *From paediatrics to psycho-analysis.* New York: Basic Books.

# Recognizing Children with Language Disorders

## PATRICIA R. COLE

$Q$uestions about hearing are likely to arise when a child has difficulty learning to talk, responds inconsistently to speech and other sounds, or experiences academic problems. An audiologist may be one of the first professionals whose assistance is sought when a child's speech, language, or learning behavior is a source of concern. As key members of a team of professionals who assess and treat communication disorders, an audiologist's responsibilities do not end with a description or diagnosis of hearing functioning. Audiologists should recognize symptoms of other disorders and assist families in finding the appropriate source of help for their children.

Other chapters in this book focus in detail on the etiologies and evaluation and treatment strategies for hearing-impaired children. The purpose of this chapter is to provide information to assist in recognizing children with other language and learning disorders and in making referrals so that appropriate assessment and management can be obtained.

To recognize children who need in-depth evaluation and possible special management to facilitate language learning and use, one must be familiar with normal language acquisition and with symptoms of communication disorders. This chapter will provide basic information about (1) the importance of identifying deficits in communication, (2) dimensions of language and communication to be considered, (3) normal and disordered patterns of language acquisition in preschool children, (4) symptoms of communication disorders in school-age children, (5) procedures for screening for disorders, and (6) interpreting information to families and making referrals for further evaluation or treatment.

# Identification: Why Is It Important?

A child's most important achievement is learning to communicate effectively with other people. Language is a vital part of a larger communication system, which also includes the integrated use of facial expressions, body movements, gestures, nonlinguistic vocal patterns, and other behaviors that signal meanings to other people. While most children learn language through normal daily experiences, some fail to progress at an expected rate or in the predicted patterns. Compared to their age peers, their ability to communicate is restricted, and all aspects of their functioning may be affected adversely.

It is the challenge and the responsibility of specialists in communication disorders to recognize children who are not progressing normally and to provide evaluation and intervention at an early age or assist them in receiving these services. To recognize the importance of early intervention, one should consider the important roles of language in the life of a young child.

## Language and Cognitive Development

*Language acquisition and cognitive growth are interrelated.* Concepts are formed through mental representations and categorization of stimuli and experiences. Learning to use a linguistic code effectively requires conceptual knowledge of objects and object relationships, an understanding of people and their experiences and relationships, and an organized knowledge about sequences of events that are related on the basis of temporal contiguities (Rice, 1984). Recent studies suggest that atypical language acquisition may be related to the onset of specific cognitive abilities (Bates, Benigni, Bretherton, Caminoni, & Voltena, 1979; Snyder, 1981, 1984a, 1984b), or it may be a part of a broader representational deficiency (Johnston, 1982b). If the language-deficient child has significant disruptions in cognitive development, remediation programs may be necessary not only to enhance language acquisition but also to facilitate learning in other areas.

Certain components of conceptual organization are influenced by language. Regarding the categorization of objects, Schlesinger (1974) states, ". . . by learning the meaning of words the child learns how to categorize the entities these words stand for" (p. 145). Ervin-Tripp (1975) and Bowerman (1981) observed that certain social distinctions and socially important concepts are introduced through language and have no nonlinguistic correlates; therefore, development of these concepts is dependent on language acquisition. Evidence that language is an organizing mechanism for categorizing experiences and is necessary for awareness of certain social concepts leads to the conclusion that failure to acquire language normally interferes with some aspects of cognitive growth.

## Language and the Fulfillment of Material Needs

*Language helps children fulfill material needs and desires.* From an early age children request objects, ask for assistance in performing actions or obtaining objects, seek permission to do things, and demand certain services that fulfill a need or desire (Halliday, 1973, 1977). Language allows children to communicate their wishes more efficiently and effectively than they can with nonlinguistic actions, and those with ineffective language use are less able to make their needs and desires known.

## Language and Interpersonal Growth

*Language helps children control other people.* From the onset of speech, children use language to direct people to do certain things and not to do others. They issue commands, warnings, threats, or promises in order to control someone else's actions, and they learn to present arguments that influence other people's attitudes, beliefs, and decisions. Without language, children have much less influence and control over other people.

*Language influences children's social interactions.* Children use language to establish and maintain relationships with other people. Halliday (1973) states: "Even the closest of the child's personal relationships, that with his mother, is partly and, in time, largely mediated through language; his interaction with other people, adults and children, is very obviously maintained linguistically" (p. 5). To function successfully, children must learn to adapt their behavior to meet the demands of a variety of social situations and interpersonal encounters. An important part of language acquisition is learning to alter both what is said and how and when it should be said in order to accomplish one's intended purpose and to be acceptable socially (Rees, 1978).

Children with language disorders often have problems in social adjustment (Donahue, Pearl, & Bryan, 1982; Simon, 1985). They may have difficulty establishing and maintaining interpersonal relationships because they cannot initiate and maintain conversation or because their manner of speaking is offensive. Their behavior may be judged as inappropriate because they do not use language in a way that is acceptable in a given situation.

## Language and Self-Identity

*Language assists children in establishing self-identity.* Children use language to express their awareness of themselves, separate from other people (Rees, 1978). Through verbal expression, they reveal their attitudes and feelings and define their attributes and their perceptions of their status in the world. Without effective use of language for self-expression, a child's self-identity and feelings of self-importance may suffer.

## Language and Learning

*Language permits children to exchange information with other people.* Children can check on the accuracy of their own perceptions by verbalizing their ideas and gaining a response from another person, and they can use language to ask someone for information they do not have (Brown, 1973; Halliday, 1977). Through verbal exchanges, children learn from the experiences of another person, and they can provide new information to others, although the use of language for the latter purpose is infrequent in the early stages of language development.

Children with spoken language disorders have fewer opportunities to learn from other people, particularly when new information is presented verbally and pertains to items or events outside the immediate situation or to abstract ideas or feelings. Without the use of language as a tool for learning, children must learn from their own experiences or from events that they personally observe.

*Spoken language influences the learning of written language.* Academic success is largely dependent on a child's prior mastery of spoken language. Pick (1978) emphasizes the important relationship between reading and spoken language: ''. . . all the models of reading that have been proposed to date acknowledge explicitly that the language that children have acquired prior to formally learning to read is an important basis for what it is that they learn when they learn to read'' (p. 107).

Having language deficits places preschool children at risk for difficulties in learning written language when they reach school age. Richardson (1979) states, ''We know that one of the earliest indications of possible school difficulty is delay in the acquisition and use of language'' (p. 76). From a study of adolescents who as preschoolers had been diagnosed as having language disorders, Aram, Ekelman, and Nation (1984) report that the language deficits persisted. Aram et al. state, ''. . . for most of this group, the language disorders recognized in the preschool years are only the beginning of long-standing language, academic, and often behavioral problems'' (1984, p. 240).

Language deficits in school-age children cause poor academic and social performance, since achievement and adjustment in an academic situation place great demands on cognitive and linguistic functioning. In a review of the literature on dyslexia, Vellutino (1979) notes that language deficits are common in children with reading disorders. Donahue et al. (1982), Goodman (1982), Simon (1985), Snyder (1986), and Wiig and Semel (1980) point out underlying communication problems that accompany learning disabilities in school-age children. Children who have disorders in language content, form, or use are almost certain to suffer in academic achievement and in peer relationships. Academic remediation or personal counseling programs for language-disordered children are not likely to be successful without special attention to associated communication disorders.

# Dimensions of Speech and Language

The term *language* refers to a set of verbal symbols that human beings use to codify ideas and experiences, usually for the purpose of communicating with someone else. Bloom and Lahey (1978) identify the major components of language and their interrelatedness in the following statement: "Language consists of some aspect of *content* or meaning that is coded or represented by linguistic *form* for some purpose or *use* in a particular context" (p. 11). Language content is the *semantic* component of language and includes the meanings coded by single words and by word combinations. Language form is the *syntactic* component of language. It includes rules for combining words into grammatical utterances as well as grammatical morphemes, such as linguistic markers to indicate number, time, location, etc. Language use is the *pragmatic* component of language. Examples of the pragmatic aspects of languages are signaling intentions, such as demanding, requesting, or inquiring; engaging in conversation or dialogue; and adapting language content and form to fit the context.

Children learn to talk because of the advantages they gain through speaking. Language use—the pragmatic component—is at the core of language development. Children are motivated to learn language form and content because these components enhance their ability to use language effectively.

Certain *prelinguistic* communicative behaviors provide a foundation for language acquisition. Interaction routines between infants and adults become systematic and are a framework for subsequent linguistic development. Learning to share focus on a common referent, to engage in goal-oriented acts, and to use conventional signals to indicate intentions are precursors to the learning of language. By tracking prelinguistic development, one can predict whether an infant is progressing normally toward a readiness to learn a linguistic code of communication. To determine whether communication skills are age-appropriate, one should look at prelinguistic communicative behaviors in infants and at language use, form, and content in children who have begun to talk.

# Patterns of Language Development in Preschool Children

To recognize language disorders, one should have an understanding of the prelinguistic underpinnings of language and of the normal rate and patterns of language development. The following discussion provides an overview of some of the major achievements that precede language and of observable steps in language learning and use that occur after children begin to talk. Professionals responsible for recognizing disorders in the development of language and communication skills can identify infants and children in need of more in-depth evaluation or remedial programs by comparing the behavior of the child to the behaviors of his or her normally developing age peers.

## Prelinguistic Development

From birth, infants engage in activities in a social context that includes siblings, parents, and other caregivers. Through these interactions, they learn to take part in systematic social interactions that are devoid of content but serve several important functions relative to later development of meaningful communication behaviors. Infants who do not achieve these prelinguistic goals are not progressing normally toward a readiness to learn language. The following information about normal prelinguistic development is drawn from information presented by Bradley (1978), Brown (1973), Bruner (1978), deVilliers (1984), Halliday (1973, 1977), McCormick (1984), Sachs (1978, 1984), Snow (1977, 1984), Snyder (1984a, 1984b), Sugarman (1984), Uzgiris (1981), Uzgiris and Hunt (1975), and Wilcox (1986).

Within the first 2 months, infants attend to certain types of stimuli. These include vocal behaviors, such as high-pitched vocalizations, exaggerated intonation patterns, and changes in rhythm and speed of vocalization. Nonvocal stimuli that often capture the infant's attention include exaggerated facial expressions and head movements and positioning the child face-to-face with another person so that they have direct eye contact. In interacting with the child, adults usually combine vocal and nonvocal behaviors, giving the child opportunities to integrate these two forms of input in a social context. The primary function of these early interactions is to engage the child in interpersonal events. An infant's failure to respond to vocal and/or nonvocal stimulation at an early age may indicate sensory or perceptual deficits. A nonresponsive infant should have further evaluation and may need to be in a specially planned infant stimulation program.

At about 3 months of age, infant-parent coactions become important. Joint activities, such as covocalization, mutual gaze, and posture-sharing, encourage infants to share experiences with other people and serve an emotional bonding function. At first, infants take part in covocalizing or other coactions only if the parent initiates an activity and the infant then joins in. Later, children show a pleasurable awareness of coactions by continuing an activity when another person joins them. These joint activities are primitive forms of interactional communication and prepare the child to learn more advanced interactional schemes.

Infants who do not participate in joint activities may not recognize the relationship between their own and another person's actions and probably will not learn to engage in more complex forms of interaction. While coactions decrease as infants mature and engage in alternate action routines, these early joint activities are an important phase in the infant's progress toward learning language.

Between 4 and 8 months of age, infants begin to perceive their actions in relationship to the effects on the external environment. They begin to repeat actions in order to recreate results, and they differentiate between their own and someone else's actions and between an object and its movement or location. As these skills develop, the infant starts to participate with another person in alternate exchanges. At first the parent must imitate the infant's act in order to get the infant to repeat it. Later, the infant will imitate an action initiated by another person, provided it is an action already in the infant's repertoire. These alternate action exchanges become social games in which both child and partner have a part to play in maintaining the interchange.

During this stage of development, infants show increased attention to objects they can act on, such as mobiles. When their actions cause the mobile (or other object) to move, they learn to repeat that action to recreate the results. This behavior shows that the child is learning that his or her actions can cause changes in the environment, a realization that is an important prerequisite to language learning and use.

Infants who do not learn to engage in alternate action routines or to repeat actions to recreate results may not have progressed cognitively to a point where they differentiate between themselves and other people or between objects and their movement or location. They may not be learning that their actions bring about reactions. Failure to acquire these concepts is a barrier to effective language learning.

Soon after 4 months of age, infants begin to notice another person's line of attention. Parents can direct the child's attention by moving objects, placing a tempting object near the child, creating sound near the item of focus, or directional gesturing. Infants soon begin visual cross-checking to determine whether they and the other person are attending to the same item. Joint attention and responding to signals of line of regard are necessary in order for the child to learn referential language, communicative behaviors indicating location, and conversational skills. Infants who do not acquire these skills are not progressing normally toward a readiness to use language effectively.

At 6 to 8 months of age, infants begin to produce a greater variety of vocalizations and to increase the frequency of vocalization. Infants frequently babble when alone, which may be the beginning of self-reinforcement in the language-learning process. Infants whose vocalizations do not increase in variety and frequency may have motor deficits that prevent their producing various vocal patterns, or they may not monitor their own vocalizations so that there is no pleasurable feedback.

Around 8 to 10 months of age, infants show a rapid increase in behaviors intended to achieve certain goals. As they learn that other people have actions that are separate from their own, they begin to engage in an exchange mode of interaction. They demand an object from someone, give it back to that person, then demand it again. Through such interchanges the infant is learning role reversal, which serves as a basis for subsequent learning of reciprocal interactions in which the child and another person engage in an activity with complementary roles.

At about 10 to 12 months of age, infants begin to employ another person to assist in accomplishing a goal. They learn new ways to achieve their purposes and new forms of communicating in order to reduce the uncertainty in the outcome of their actions. Rather than crying or whining as they have in the past, they use more specific acts, such as pointing, to convey their intentions. These actions represent initial steps in learning conventional communication acts and are an early phase in the pragmatic aspects of language acquisition. A child's use of these elementary yet conventional signals increases his or her success in achieving a goal and serves to motivate the child to learn language, since language use will further reduce the likelihood of misinterpretation of intent.

Infants who do not learn progressively more conventional nonverbal ways to communicate their intentions will not learn to use verbal communicative symbols normally, since the use of linguistic devices to communicate is an extension of the use of nonlinguistic communication acts. Infants who persist in more primitive behaviors—such as crying or yelling, rather than using more definitive signals like pointing—may require special assistance in learning language.

Because the sequence and rate of normal development in the prelinguistic period are known, we can provide special programs to assist the child in moving toward a readiness to learn language. Infants who are not progressing normally or older nonverbal or low-verbal children should be referred for evaluation of their developmental status. If prelinguistic development is inadequate, special programs can be provided to enhance the child's progress.

## Linguistic Development

Linguistic and related communication behaviors develop in predictable rates and patterns. The following overview of language development is taken from information provided by Bloom and Lahey (1978), Bowerman (1981), Brown (1973), deVilliers (1984), Gordan and Ervin-Tripp (1984), Halliday (1973, 1977), Leonard (1986), McCormick (1984), McNew and Bates (1984), Rees (1978), Sachs (1984), Snow (1984), Snyder (1984a), and Wilcox (1986). Audiologists and other professionals who serve young children should be familiar with normal developmental patterns so that they can recognize children with atypical communication skills.

*12 to 18 Months.*   Around their first birthday, most children begin using conventional linguistic forms to express intentions they previously expressed nonlinguistically. Initially they vocalize or verbalize and gesture simultaneously to request objects or assistance, control actions of other people, express their own feelings, call attention to themselves, initiate or maintain social interactions, and refer to objects or persons. Language becomes a functional tool for communicating with other people. Children's early verbalizations most often relate to changing or new items, actions, or conditions in the immediate situation.

In the 12- to 18-month period, young children become more assertive participants in familiar social situations. Their effectiveness and persistence as communicators increase as they become more aware that they can bring about change in their surroundings. They use more words and learn other more refined and conventional signals to make their intentions clear. They begin to alter the loudness and intonation patterns of their vocal and verbal acts to reflect their feelings or attitudes.

During the 12- to 18-month period, children's imitations of other people's linguistic and nonlinguistic behaviors become more frequent and more closely approximate the model. They begin to follow one-step directions and to respond to requests for actions. They also become more involved in the social environment, laughing when others laugh, raising the loudness of their vocalizations when others are speaking loudly, and pouting, crying, or whining in concert with other people.

*18 to 24 Months.*   Vocabulary increases and speech intelligibility improves between 18 and 24 months of age. Children's use of jargon decreases during this age period. While gestures or other nonlinguistic acts still may be used to assist in communication, children become increasingly able to exercise control and to express feelings linguistically. Their utterances usually refer to items, people, or actions with which they are directly involved and which are in the immediate context.

During the single-word phase of development, children observe several basic conversational rules. They usually take turns in speaking, and they may use verbal acts (''hey'' or ''look'') or nonverbal behaviors (touching or lining up in front of the listener) to gain the listener's attention.

As children near their second birthday, they begin using two-word phrases to express intentions that were earlier communicated through single words and gestures. They begin asking for certain information, using utterances such as "What's that?" or "Where cookie?"

***24 to 30 Months.*** Children's use of connected utterances increases in frequency and variety soon after their second birthday. Two-word phrases are common, with word order being the primary syntactic device for signaling meaning. Most of their utterances are associated with their own activities, observable conditions or events, or familiar people and routine activities. They continue to use language to satisfy their needs, express their attitudes, engage in interpersonal exchanges, control other people, and comment on changing or new aspects of the immediate environment. While they rarely use language to inform others, they may make statements about items, people, or events in order to check on their own perceptions or to direct another person's attention.

At about the age of 2, children begin calling the name of the listener to gain his or her attention, indicating that they are beginning to monitor conversational interactions. However, they rarely engage in dialogue, and they do little to maintain conversations initiated by someone else.

Children make more discriminating use of verbal input after their second birthday. They respond more consistently to verbal requests or commands, and they begin to answer yes/no questions that include words they know and pertain to familiar people, objects, and events. They increasingly refute what someone else says, either by refusing to comply with a request or by disagreeing with an assertion.

***30 to 36 Months.*** Speech intelligibility improves to about 75% during this age period. Children expand utterances into three-word phrases, and they begin using progressive verb inflections: -*s* to mark plurality, *in* to mark location, and *no* or *not* to indicate negation. Their vocabulary continues to expand both in number and types of words used, and they gain in the ability to control their environment and to assert themselves through talking. While their comments are usually tied to the immediate context, verbalizations related to imaginative play increase, and they more frequently talk about prior or future events.

Between 2 and 3 years of age, children begin to take more responsibility for maintaining dialogue. More often they expect a response to verbalizations addressed to someone else and acknowledge when they are addressed by another person. Increasingly they maintain a topic across conversational turns by preserving the topic of the prior speaker.

Children's responsiveness to what is said improves during this age period. They answer questions about actions ("What is Daddy doing?"), item labels ("What's that?"), and location ("Where are you going?" or "Where's the book?"). They also respond to indirect forms of request and to more complex verbal instructions or explanations.

*36 to 48 Months.*   After the age of 3, children begin to use four- and five-word sentences and rarely have to resort to nonverbal acts to communicate effectively. While speech articulation may continue to vary from adult patterns, their speech is almost always intelligible, even to unfamiliar listeners. Syntax continues to improve. Soon after their third birthday, children use copular forms of *to be*, possessive markers, *can't* or *don't* to indicate negation, and prepositions to signal location or directionality. They begin to ask *wh-* questions, although they may fail to transpose word order, producing question forms such as "What that is?" By their fourth birthday, grammatical skills have improved significantly. They use correct regular and irregular past tense forms (although overgeneralizations such as "runned" for *ran* may continue to appear). They use verb inflections to indicate person and number, contractible and uncontractible auxiliary and copular verbs, articles, and a variety of forms of negation. By age 4, children use compound and complex sentence forms rather than a series of simple sentences.

Among the most significant changes in children's language between 3 and 4 years of age are the improvements in conversational skills. They both preserve the topic and use grammatical forms, such as the same verb forms and appropriate referential pronouns, to tie their responses to the prior speaker's utterance. They also begin using grammatical ellipsis as a conversational tool. With these increased skills, children are able to maintain the flow of conversation so that they engage in dialogue more frequently and with greater success.

Another major change in conversational skills between 3 and 4 years of age is children's increasing ability to alter what they say and when and how they say it, taking into consideration the prior knowledge and the relative social status of the listener. They begin to provide more detailed information when they perceive that information essential to appropriate interpretation is not available to the listener, and they less often state the obvious. By the age of 4, children also begin to alter linguistic form to suit their social role relative to the listener. They learn to use indirect rather than direct forms of request, and they more often use polite terms, such as *please* and *thank you*, in order to achieve their goals.

Between 3 and 4 years of age, children begin using conversational narratives. Three-year-olds use narratives to report on events or to give new information to a listener, which is the beginning of their use of language to inform. However, 3-year-olds generally complete their narratives in a single conversational turn and may not demand a response from the listener. They rarely attempt to engage in extended verbal exchanges about their own or another person's narratives.

*48 to 60 Months.* After their fourth birthday, children's speech is rarely unintelligible. They show an increased interest in and ability to talk about prior or future experiences, and they use language to give new information to others. In conversational narratives, they usually begin with a comment to gain the listener's attention (''Know what?'' or ''Guess what I did!''). They also use linguistic forms to orient the events in their narratives with respect to time. Between 4 and 5, children increasingly use language to persuade others and to justify their requests or actions. They structure their statements in an effort to influence the listener's interpretation, and they show a greater reliance on their conversational partner's responses to direct their continued explanations.

Between 4 and 5 years of age, children show greater sensitivity to the status and needs of the listener, modifying content and form to accommodate the listener's needs and capabilities. As a respondent in dialogue, their responses are almost always appropriate in both topic and form. They become more effective conversationalists, although they may not participate beyond one or two conversational turns unless the topic is of special interest to them.

## Symptoms of Communication Disorders

Certain behaviors or developmental patterns suggest that a child probably has a communication disorder and may need special help. Through direct observation or from reports of parents or others familiar with the child, the alert professional should recognize behavioral patterns that are significant indicators of disorders. Based on recognized patterns of normal communication development, the following behavioral patterns usually indicate problems to which additional attention should be given. The behaviors listed relate primarily to disorders in the acquisition and use of interactional communication abilities and are often reported as sources of concern. Certainly this is not an all-inclusive list of aberrant communicative behaviors, and the occasional occurrence of these behaviors may not be clinically significant. The following list may be useful to professionals in recognizing behaviors symptomatic of communication disorders in children.

**Birth to 3 Months**

1. Inconsistent or no response to sound or novel events in the immediate environment

2. Frequent fussiness or irritability, with little or no positive response to comforting from other people

3. Consistent lethargy and unresponsiveness rather than increasing interest and responsiveness to environment

4. Little or no vocalization in interactions with others

5. Failure to track another person's movement within the infant's visual field

**3 to 6 Months**

1. Little or no increase in attention to other people's attempts to interact through vocal and nonvocal interactions (focus on another person, quieting or showing excitement when caretaker approaches, etc.)

2. Failure to join into familiar vocal and nonvocal actions with another person (coactions)

3. Little or no differential vocalization in states of pleasure, dissatisfaction, or anger

4. Little or no anticipatory response to familiar objects or people (bottle, approach of caregiver, etc.)

5. Failure to begin simple turn-taking activities

**6 to 9 Months**

1. Little or no participation in alternate-action routines (cooing, hand movements, etc.)

2. Little or no response to another person's efforts to comfort or satisfy infant's needs (cuddling, comforting vocalizations, etc.)

3. Little or no response to another person's efforts to direct attention (pointing, following visual line of regard, movement of object of attention, etc.)

4. Failure to repeat actions to recreate results (moving mobile, vocalizing to other person, etc.)

5. Little or no increase in frequency and variety of vocalization

**9 to 12 Months**

1. Failure to engage in goal-oriented activities (removing an obstacle to reach a specific object, hitting an object to make it move, yelling to gain another person's attention, etc.)

2. Failure to engage in systematic turn-taking routines (handing objects back and forth, dropping a block for someone else to pick up, etc.)

3. Undifferentiated whining or crying rather than more specific communicative acts (pointing, pulling a person toward a desired item, shaking head or turning away to indicate rejection, etc.)

4. Failure to begin using conventional signals to control other people (waving bye-bye, vocalizing to gain another person's attention, etc.)

5. Failure to express anger or displeasure when a desirable object is taken away

6. Failure to express affection to familiar people (hugging, cuddling cheek-to-cheek, etc.)

7. Failure to anticipate events from familiar signs (eating when placed in high chair, excitement when caregiver gets out stroller, etc.)

**12 to 15 Months**

1. Little or no increase in effective communication behaviors incorporating conventional signals (directional pointing, handing cup to caregiver when thirsty, pulling caregiver to item to direct attention or gain assistance, etc.)

2. Little or no alterations in vocal patterns to indicate pleasure, anger, or other feelings

3. Limited combining of vocalization and gesture to request objects or control other people

4. No intelligible words

5. Little or no increase in variety of speechlike vocal patterns

6. Failure to recognize own name or names of a few familiar people or objects

7. Failure to engage in simple play routines

## 15 to 18 Months

1. Failure to follow familiar one-step commands

2. Failure to use some intelligible words meaningfully

3. Failure to assert self into social activities with familiar people

4. Limited repertoire of vocal patterns

5. Failure to act to control other people and to assert own feelings

6. Failure to improve vocal and nonvocal imitative skills

## 18 to 24 Months

1. Failure to increase reliance on intelligible words to communicate

2. Persistence of jargon as the primary vocal pattern

3. Failure to make nonlinguistic communicative acts more specific and conventional (definitive pointing and gesturing, waving, pouting expressions, etc.)

4. Failure to initiate interpersonal interactions

5. Failure to respond to simple comments or requests

6. Failure to assert self to gain attention or express feelings (increasing loudness of vocalization to gain attention, rejecting with "no," etc.)

7. Failure to acknowledge utterances of another person (looking to speaker, vocalizing or other response when spoken to)

## 24 to 30 Months

1. Continued reliance on gestures or actions without significant increase in intelligible speech

2. Limited use of linguistic forms to control others, ask for objects or assistance, enter into interpersonal interactions, attract attention, express own feelings

3. Failure to ask and to answer simple questions ("What's that?" "Where's Mommy?")

4. Failure to comment on items or events, both in the immediate environment and not immediately present

5. Failure to express negation

6. Disregard for or failure to comprehend familiar comments or requests

7. Frequent echolalic speech or inappropriate use of memorized phrases

### 30 to 36 Months

1. Frequent unintelligible speech

2. Reliance on gestures to communicate

3. Reliance on single words rather than two- and three-word phrases to communicate

4. Few or no comments about items or events not immediately present

5. Failure to *initiate* verbal interactions

6. Disregard for or inappropriate response to familiar requests, commands, and comments

7. Failure to answer "What" and "Where" questions appropriately

8. Echolalic speech

### 36 to 48 Months

1. Poor speech intelligibility

2. Telegraphic speech or frequent omissions of words in connected speech

3. Utterances limited to two or three words in length

4. Failure to carry on meaningful, short conversational exchanges

5. Little or no adjustment of speaking patterns to fit listener and to provide clarification if the message is not understood

6. Inappropriate response to requests, commands, questions

7. Failure to learn frequently heard songs, rhymes, TV commercials, etc.

8. Failure to play "pretend" games, either when playing alone or with others

### 48 to 60 Months

1. Failure to talk meaningfully about prior experiences or anticipated events

2. Failure to use language to justify behavior, to state reasons for actions or events, or to persuade others

3. Inappropriate or unrelated comments in conversational exchanges

4. Failure to follow two-part commands and to answer questions appropriately

5. Failure to use language to ask for new information

6. Communication in which intended meaning is difficult to ascertain because child rambles from topic to topic, uses unusual word order or word combinations, or uses overly general rather than specific referential words

7. Inappropriate pronoun usage

8. Frequent inattention or inappropriate response to what others say

9. Reliance on physical contact to initiate or respond in social interactions

10. Tendency to be unusually withdrawn in social situations with peers and/or with adults

While some of the behaviors in the above list may occur occasionally in children who are developing normally, the persistence of these behaviors usually indicates disordered development. Children for whom these behaviors are characteristic should be referred for in-depth evaluation of language so that appropriate remediation can be initiated if deemed appropriate.

# Symptoms of Communication Disorders in School-Age Children

Normally developing children are effective communicators by the time they reach school age. They usually understand what other people say, and if they do not understand, they ask for clarification. Their speech is easily understood, and they are successful conversationalists. They use language with ease and effectiveness in interpersonal exchanges and to express their feelings, attitudes, and beliefs. School-age children rely on language as a tool for learning. They benefit from hearing about the experiences of other people, and they gain new information from verbal explanations. They use language to provide information to other people, and they adapt what they say and how they say it so that it fits the age, background, and relative social status of the listener. By school age, children have acquired the basic language system used in their environment.

Children continue to expand their knowledge and use of language through the teen-age years. Comprehension and expression of complex and abstract ideas expand, and they learn to use figurative language. They increasingly learn to adjust the form, content, and manner of speaking so that they more effectively accomplish their intentions. Well into adulthood, vocabulary expands, and adaptations in language behavior are made to accommodate the goals and roles of speakers.

Experts in language and its disorders are able to identify changes in school-age children's language behavior and to recognize atypical patterns of language learning and use. These changes in development are neither as dramatic nor as readily observable as are developmental changes in preschool children. A discussion of the progression in language acquisition in older children is beyond the scope of this chapter, since that information is not essential to the audiologist responsible only for recognizing children who need in-depth evaluation by an expert in language disorders.

Although audiologists need not be expert diagnosticians of language disorders, they should be aware of behavioral symptoms that suggest atypical language learning and use. The following listing of behaviors often noticed in school-age children with language disorders includes information from Donahue et al. (1982), Garnett (1986), Goodman (1982), Johnston (1982b), Menyuk (1983), Pick (1978), Simon (1984), Snyder (1986), and Wiig and Semel (1980).

### Spoken-Language Comprehension

1. Often requires more than one explanation or visual demonstration to understand verbal explanations or instruction

2. Responds inappropriately to questions or comments

3. Has difficulty learning from verbal explanations

4. Often ignores what others say or has a short attention span for verbal stimuli

5. Misses the point of what is said

6. Rarely catches on to jokes or other forms of verbal humor

7. Is overly literal in interpreting what is said

8. Does not learn new words as readily as peers do

9. Is forgetful, or has poor memory for what is said

10. Avoids verbal games or activities

## Spoken-Language Expression

1. Poor speech intelligibility

2. Gestures or visual clues necessary to convey a point to another person

3. Rambling or nonspecific in verbal explanations so that meaning is difficult to ascertain

4. Difficulty recalling names of people or items, either to respond to questions or to give explanations

5. Errors in word order and/or grammar

6. Limited vocabulary

7. Frequent misuse of words

8. Difficulty in clarifying intended meaning when listener misunderstands or asks for clarification

9. Verbalizations inappropriate or irrelevant in the verbal or nonverbal context

10. Overusage of rote or ritualistic verbal patterns

## Academic Performance

1. Difficulty learning phonics or other early reading and spelling skills

2. Inconsistent reading and spelling performance

3. Poor memory, either for rotely learned or for meaningful material

4. Limited reading comprehension, with or without adequate word-calling skills

5. Difficulty recognizing the major theme of what is read

6. Difficulty inferring meaning beyond what is contained in the written text

7. Heavy reliance on memorizing material, with difficulty applying or generalizing from what is memorized

8. Significant discrepancy between reading, spelling, or language arts and math performance

9. Difficulty in written expression, including both poor spelling, grammar, punctuation or capitalization, and inadequate content

10. Short attention span

**Social Behavior**

1. Immature social behavior

2. Difficulty adapting to new or changing social situations

3. Overly aggressive, either physically or verbally

4. Unusually shy or withdrawn (''a loner'')

5. Difficulty taking part in verbal exchanges with peers

6. Misses the point of jokes, teases, or peer-group jargon

7. Often fails to interpret or adapt behavior based on another person's signals of irritation, distress, etc.

8. Difficulty adapting behavior so that it is appropriate for the social context

9. Abnormal affective behavior

10. General difficulty in relating to peers and/or adults

While most children display some of the above-mentioned behaviors at times, when they occur on an ongoing basis or are of consistent concern to parents or teachers, they likely indicate a disorder of some nature. Because language influences all aspects of a child's learning and adjustment, abnormalities in spoken language, academic performance, and social and interpersonal adjustment may be the result of a communication disorder. Children who have difficulties in these areas should have an evaluation of language skills to determine whether remedial assistance is indicated.

# Screening for Language Disorders

Audiologists or other professionals who screen children for language disorders must determine whether each child's communication behavior is adequate or whether reported or observed behavior suggests the likelihood of a communication disorder. The purpose of screening is to determine whether additional assessment is needed, not to make a diagnosis or to give a detailed description of the nature and the extent of the disorder. If the child's development or behavior suggests atypical functioning, referral for a comprehensive evaluation is indicated.

The audiologist or other professional may rely on observed or reported information about a child's behavior in order to make a judgment about the adequacy of communication skills. The primary sources of information about the child's learning and use of language are reports from parents or others who are familiar with the child and direct observation of the child in communication situations that are as nearly normal as possible. Either of these sources may provide information sufficient for recognizing significant symptoms of disordered communication. However, a more accurate determination is likely if information from more than one source is considered.

## Interviewing Parents

Rarely is a child brought to a professional for an evaluation unless the parents or other familiar adults have specific cause for concern. When parents seek assistance from an audiologist or speech-language pathologist, they usually have questions about their child's communication behaviors.

Because parents usually know their child better than anyone else and can provide information that may not be available through direct observation in a clinical setting, they should be made aware that their contributions are an important part of the assessment process. Clinicians can gain valuable information about a child's communication patterns by listening to parents and by asking questions that prompt parents to describe the child's daily behavior. Early in the assessment period the clinician should take the time to interview the parents, listening carefully and following up with questions that assist the parents in providing a full description of the child's communication behavior.

Asking open-ended questions that encourage the parents to talk about their concerns often brings out pertinent descriptive information useful to the clinician. Questions such as ''What concerns about Tommy caused you to bring him to see me?'' usually are appropriate for opening an initial interview. Should the parent respond that he or she is not worried but that the evaluation was recommended by someone else (teacher, babysitter, physician, etc.), ask for a description of the behaviors that caused the other person to be concerned. It may be appropriate to follow with more focused questions, such as ''How does Tommy respond when someone talks to him?'' ''How does Susan let you know what she wants you to do?'' It is important to remember that the clinician's goal is to get from the parent a picture of the child's regular communication behavior. It is also important to remember, and often to remind parents, that the clinician is not asking the parent to diagnose a problem but rather to provide information that will permit the clinician to make a judgment about whether a problem exists.

Once a description of the child's current behavior is given, it is usually instructive for the clinician to gain information about the child's history. This information may be obtained from parents as well as from other adults who have known or provided services to the child.

## Obtaining a Case History

Information about conditions or events that may have had an adverse effect on development or functioning can assist in identifying children who are either at risk for or are experiencing communication disorders. Family history, prenatal conditions, the child's condition at birth, prior or current medical conditions, developmental patterns, social/emotional status, and academic progress should be explored to identify conditions that place the child at risk or suggest abnormalities in communication skills.

Ramey, Trohanis, and Hostler (1982) identify the following three at-risk categories, which are not mutually exclusive:

1. *Established Risk.* Ramey et al. (1982) use this category to refer to infants ''. . . whose early appearing and aberrant development is related to diagnosed medical disorders of known etiology and which have relatively well known expectancies for developmental outcomes within specified ranges of developmental delay'' (p. 8). A child with Down's syndrome would fall within this category.

2. *Environmental Risk.* Ramey et al. observe that ''When the life experiences of a biologically sound infant are limited to the extent that, without corrective intervention, they impart a high probability for delayed development, the infant is at environmental risk'' (p. 8). Severely neglected, malnourished, or abused children may be in this category.

3. *Biological Risk.* According to Ramey et al., this category refers to infants who have ''. . . a history of prenatal, perinatal, neonatal and early development events suggestive of biological insult to the developing nervous system and which, either singly or collectively, increase the probability of later appearing aberrant development'' (p. 8). Anoxia, low birth weight, metabolic disorders, and central nervous system dysfunction are among the conditions in this category.

Certainly all children with one or more of these at-risk factors will not have communication disorders, and the absence of such factors does not guarantee normal development and functioning. However, when a parent is concerned about a child's development and behavior, a history that includes conditions often associated with communication problems may contribute to a decision to refer the child for more in-depth assessment.

The at-risk factors suggested by Ramey et al. (1982) provide categories based on identification of the cause of aberrant behavior or patterns of development. Often no causal factors can be identified, and determination of potential communication disorders must be made on the basis of reported or observed deviations in development or behavior. Children who appear to be atypical should be referred for more thorough assessment, whether or not the probable cause for a disorder can be identified. The common characteristics of disorders described earlier in this chapter may assist the clinician in recognizing children whose development or behavior indicates a need for more in-depth assessment.

In obtaining pertinent background information, several areas should be explored to determine whether the child is in an at-risk category or whether current conditions may be contributing to disruptions in development. Areas to be considered include family history, prenatal conditions, birth history, medical history, developmental history, social adaptation, and academic achievement.

*Family History.*   A family history of developmental, emotional, intellectual, medical, or educational difficulties increases the likelihood that a child will experience abnormalities in development or functioning.

*Prenatal Conditions.*   Any abnormal conditions or events affecting a woman during pregnancy increase the chances that the child will have a handicapping condition. Viral illnesses, chemical abuse, inadequate nutrition, accidents, or severe emotional stress may have an adverse effect on the unborn child.

*Birth History.*   Handicapping conditions are more likely to be present in premature children or in those with low birth weight than in full-term infants of normal birth weight. Prolonged or precipitous labor and any condition causing anoxia or respiratory distress increase the chances that the child will experience developmental disabilities. Descriptions of the child's condition immediately following birth may suggest some abnormalities. Disruptions in establishing a normal breathing pattern, jaundice, or unusual difficulties in sucking or swallowing may indicate abnormalities that later result in disordered development.

***Medical History.*** Abnormalities in development and behavior are more likely in children who have physical anomalies, chromosome disorders, sensory deficits, metabolic disturbances, or neurological dysfunction. A history of seizures, prolonged high fever, severe and prolonged diarrhea, viral diseases, head injuries, and poor nutrition increases the child's risk of having disorders in development and learning.

Of particular interest to audiologists is the possible adverse effect of prolonged or recurrent otitis media on the development of language and communication abilities. Friel-Patti, Finitzo-Heber, Conti, and Brown (1982) note: ''The presence of fluctuating changes in hearing means that the young child must deal with conflicting and inconsistent information on which to base his language learning. Indeed one would suspect that the presence of a chronic conductive hearing loss during the first two years of life would pervade all aspects of rule acquisition in oral language learning . . .'' (p. 104). Friel-Patti et al. found that young children who had recurrent middle ear infections in the first 18 to 24 months of life were more likely to show a delay in language development than were a matched group of children who had experienced no more than one ear infection up to that time. Others have expressed concern that intermittent disruptions in auditory input during crucial prelinguistic and early verbal stages may have a detrimental effect on auditory perception and the development of language and cognitive abilities (Bricker & Schiefelbusch, 1984; Gottlieb, Zinkus, & Thompson, 1979; Katz, 1978) and on later learning of written language (Sloan, 1980). Audiologists and physicians who serve young children with middle ear pathologies should be aware that recurrent otitis media may place a child at risk for disorders in oral and written language.

***Developmental History.*** The age and pattern of development of nonverbal and verbal interactional behaviors, motor skills, cognitive abilities, and social behavior contribute important information about the normalcy of the child's development. Overall delay or irregular rates or patterns across various areas of development generally indicate that the child is not progressing normally and may need special assistance.

McCormick (1984) outlines normal developmental steps in cognitive, interactional, and language behaviors in children from birth to 4 years of age. Halliday (1973, 1977) gives information on prelinguistic and interactional communicative development. Uzgiris and Hunt (1975) provide scales to assist in evaluating children's early development. Shane (1981) and Bricker and Schiefelbusch (1984) describe oral-motor development associated with normal and abnormal acquisition of speech. Sources such as these can be tapped by clinicians who need additional information about normal developmental patterns.

Atypical development should trigger referral for an in-depth assessment of functioning. Early intervention may eliminate or reduce the deleterious impact of disorders on the child's behavior and learning. A "wait and see" approach often leads to increased negative impact on the child's learning and adjustment.

*Social Adaptation.* Prior or current difficulties in social adjustment may be caused by inadequate language learning and use. Behaviors that may be diagnostically significant were discussed earlier in this chapter. When attempting to determine whether a child needs further assessment or treatment, clinicians should gather information about the child's social behavior.

*Academic Achievement.* As was discussed earlier in this chapter, problems in academic peformance may result from weaknesses in language. Since some aspects of language growth in school-age children may not be apparent to lay persons, basic language deficits may not be recognized without the assistance of a professional with expertise in language learning and use. Additionally, many persons do not recognize the close relationship between spoken and written language and therefore may not look at spoken-language skills when a child experiences difficulty in written language. When academic difficulties are a source of concern, it is usually wise to recommend that a child have an in-depth language assessment.

Case history information may be obtained in written form by asking parents to complete a case history form or by getting written reports from others familiar with the child. This information is useful, but it is wise to discuss the child's history with parents or other familiar adults rather than relying solely on written data.

## Observing Children's Behavior

Observing a child in communication interactions provides clinicians data to assist in determining whether the child's communication skills are adequate or whether those skills are either questionable or clearly inadequate. Information gained through parent interviews and case histories assists in making that determination, but a skilled clinician gains valuable insights through direct observation of the child's communication behavior.

Clinicians usually have only a few minutes to observe the child, so their judgments about the adequacy of the child's language skills are based on a limited sample of behavior. It is important that this sample reflect as accurately as possible the child's typical communication patterns.

In observing infants, it is very important to have a parent or other familiar caregiver involved. They know the interaction routines familiar to the infant and therefore are more likely to elicit typical interactional behaviors. Infants in a drowsy state are not likely to enter into social routines, even with familiar adults. Under these conditions, clinicians must rely on reports from parents or caregivers to find out about the infant's interactional behaviors.

With young children, the context and procedures of the sampling situation influence the child's language behavior. Language elicited in highly structured events is often not typical of the language the child uses in normal communication situations. Miller (1978) states, ''. . . the more structured the elicitation session, the less varied the resultant langauge in terms of the variety of structures and meanings expressed'' (p. 293). Therefore, question-and-answer formats, picture or item naming, or similarly structured activities are not likely to elicit language behaviors that are typical for the child.

This author prefers to carry out screenings with preschool children in a free-speech context in which the children are engaged in play activities they enjoy. It is usually preferable to have a child interact during play with parents, siblings, or peers, with the unfamiliar clinician at least initially acting as a noninvolved observer. This type of setting is more likely to place the child at ease, and it gives the clinician an opportunity to observe the interactional behaviors of the child and of those who communicate with him or her on a daily basis. Since adults and older siblings often unconsciously adapt their behavior to meet the child's needs, clinicians can gain insights into the child's communication skills by observing the way familiar adults and siblings adjust when dealing with the child.

If clinicians are directly involved, they should join in the child's activities and attempt to elicit language as a part of the playing rather than putting the child "on the spot" through direct questions and answers. By becoming a part of the child's activities, clinicians increase the likelihood that the child's behavior in the screening situation will be typical of behavior in the day-to-day situation.

With older children conversations or narratives may be useful resources for obtaining language samples. Older children more commonly take part in conversational exchanges and use narratives in communication interactions, so their behavior in these activities may reflect their typical communication patterns. As with younger children, a less structured format is more likely to elicit greater variety and complexity in language use.

If parents or familiar others have identified certain aspects of communication behavior that concern them, clinicians can manipulate the situation so that these behaviors are called for in the screening situation. If parents participate in or observe the screening session, clinicians should ask them during or after the session whether the child's behavior is an accurate reflection of the behavior they see at home. If the parents have not been present, clinicians should describe the behavior they observed, asking whether this behavior is a reasonable representation of the child's usual language and communication behavior.

While observing the child's communication behavior, the clinician may note both adequate and inadequate or questionable communication skills. Notes should reflect the judgments and examples of behaviors on which these judgments are based. Some clinicians prefer to use a checklist of normal and abnormal behaviors, marking the items observed and noting specific behaviors in the area marked. Others take notes about significant behaviors they observe. For example, notes may include "points to indicate wants; pats mother's arm to get her attention; frowns when scolded; screams when brother takes a toy away; names body parts touched by mother; picks up toys when mother says item label but not when function is stated." Through a series of statements such as these, clinicians familiar with normal and abnormal behaviors for a child in a certain age range can determine which aspects of behavior appear to be adequate and which are questionable or inadequate. It is important to remember that the purpose of screening is to determine whether more in-depth evaluation should be recommended. The clinician is not expected and should not attempt to diagnose the disorder or to recommend treatment on the basis of a screening evaluation.

# Giving Interpretations and Recommendations to Parents

Clinicians are more likely to be successful in communicating with parents if they keep in mind the parents' concerns and perspectives about their child. Generally it is important for clinicians to begin by reminding the parent that they have not done a thorough evaluation of language and therefore cannot give a diagnosis or in-depth description of the child's language. However, they have listened to what the parent described, have observed the child, and want to share their judgments about the child's communication skills.

Once these parameters have been established, it is often useful to establish a common point of reference by restating a concern the parent has expressed and to move from there into the clinicians' observations and recommendations. For example, the clinician may say: ''You told me earlier that you notice that Peggy often does not answer when people talk to her. In watching her playing with her brother, I noticed that she responded when he talked to her about something she was playing with at the time and pointed to or held up the object he was talking about. However, she usually did not respond if he talked about something outside the room and if he didn't show her the object. Many times children don't answer when they don't understand what the other person means. I suspect this is what Peggy is doing. Unless he showed her what he was talking about, she didn't seem to know what he meant. I think testing should be done to look closely at how well Peggy understands what people say. I share your concern about her not responding to what people say to her, and I think we need to look at this more carefully. If understanding what people say is a problem, she can have therapy to improve her ability to understand speech. I will give you the names of several speech-language pathologists who work with children Peggy's age and can help in finding out more about Peggy's understanding of language. They also know how to help her improve in this area if they find that she needs special help.''

It is likely that further discussion and possibly more examples of observed behaviors will be needed to ensure that the parents understand and are comfortable with the clinician's judgments and recommendations. Certainly the clinician should observe the parents' reactions, clarify information if the parents look puzzled, and ask whether the explanation makes sense to them.

In the example given above, several important aspects of the explanation should be pointed out. First, the clinician began by stating a concern that the parents had expressed. This is important because it focuses the discussion on a behavior that is familiar to the parents. Second, the clinician describes the specific behavior observed and pertinent aspects of the context so that the parents can picture the event. Third, the clinician suggests the possible cause of the behavior and points out to the parents the significance of the difference in the child's response under one condition versus the response under a different condition. Fourth, the clinician relates these response differences back to the behavior that had concerned the parent. Fifth, the clinician makes a specific recommendation for action on the part of the parent to address the problem and states the reason for the recommendation. Sixth, the clinician gives specific suggestions for where help may be sought and encourages the parent to follow the recommendation by pointing out that once the problem has been defined in greater detail, help is available.

Contrast the previous example of an explanation to parents with the following: "Based on my observations, I suspect that Peggy has an auditory comprehension disorder. Her responses seem to be based on visual clues rather than verbal stimuli. She needs testing of comprehension skills by a speech-language pathologist."

In this second example, the clinician has not related the reported observation to the parents' previously identified concern. Since parents probably are not familiar with terms such as "auditory comprehension problem," "visual clues," "verbal stimuli," and "testing of comprehension skills," this explanation is likely to be confusing or meaningless to them. The clinician did not give examples of behaviors and events on which the conclusions were based, so the parents will not have a familiar frame of reference for understanding what the clinician means. Explanations that are confusing or meaningless may frighten or frustrate parents and certainly increase the likelihood that they will not follow through on the recommendations for additional testing. Effective and knowledgeable clinicians are able to present interpretations and recommendations so that parents understand what is meant and know what course of action they should take.

# Summary

Audiologists frequently are among the first professionals to see children whose communication skills are in question. In addition to describing these children's auditory functioning, audiologists should recognize symptoms of language disorders and make referrals for in-depth evaluations of language when communication abilities are questionable or clearly inadequate. Audiologists need not be experts in evaluation, diagnosis, or treatment of language disorders. However, as key members of a team of specialists with expertise in communication disorders, they should be able to carry out screening evaluations, to recognize symptoms of communication disorders, and to refer families to appropriate sources of assistance.

Prelinguistic development provides the foundation for language learning, and recognition of disordered development in infants is both possible and important. Knowledge of normal patterns of development in infants and of symptoms of disordered development is important for professionals who serve infants. Often later problems in language learning can be reduced or avoided if disordered development is identified and appropriate remediation is begun early.

Preschool children follow predictable and observable patterns of language learning. By comparing children's behavior with expected developmental patterns and by recognizing symptoms of disordered behavior, audiologists can identify those who are not progressing normally. If a child's disorder is identified and appropriate services are provided early, the adverse impact on later functioning may be reduced or eliminated. Professionals who serve preschool children should therefore be familiar with both normal and abnormal developmental patterns.

School-age children with communication disorders may display problems in verbal comprehension or expression, in social adjustment, and in academic achievement. Professionals who screen school-age children should recognize common symptoms of language disorders. Since language deficits may adversely affect all areas of functioning, identification and treatment of language dysfunction is often vital to the child's future progress.

Professionals may rely on parents' reports of current behaviors, case history information, and observations of the child in screening for language disorders. While any of these sources may be sufficient to recognize the need for further evaluation, the clinician's judgment is likely to be more accurate if it is based on information from more than one source. Clinicians should gain expertise in interviewing parents, interpreting background information, and observing children's behavior so that they can screen effectively.

Identifying problems and recommending further evaluation is useless if parents do not understand the meaning and importance of the clinician's statements and recommendations. Skill in interpreting judgments to parents should be a high priority for audiologists and other professionals who work with infants and children. Clinicians should not consider their job complete or their services effective unless they communicate effectively with the families of the children they serve.

# References

Aram, D., Ekelman, B., & Nation, J. (1984). Preschoolers with language disorders: 10 years later. *Journal of Speech and Hearing Research, 27,* 232–244.

Bates, E., Benigni, L., Bretherton, I., Caminoni, L., & Volterra, V. (1979). Cognition and communication from 9–13 months: Correlational findings. In E. Bates (Ed.), *The emergence of symbols: Cognition and communication in infancy* (pp. 36–47). New York: Academic Press.

Bloom, L., & Lahey, M. (1978). *Language development and language disorders.* New York: John Wiley.

Bowerman, M. (1981). Cross-cultural perspectives on language development. In H. Triandis (Ed.), *Handbook of cross-cultural psychology* (pp. 149–177). Boston: Allyn and Bacon.

Bradley, D. (1978). Parameters of communication with infants and young children. *Allied Health and Behavioral Sciences, 1,* 550–566.

Bricker, D., & Schiefelbusch, R. (1984). Infants at risk. In L. McCormick & R. Schiefelbusch (Eds.), *Early language intervention* (pp. 243–265). Columbus, OH: Charles E. Merrill.

Brown, R. (1973). *A first language: The early stages.* Cambridge, MA: Harvard University Press.

Bruner, J. (1978). From communication to language: A psychological perspective. In I. Markova (Ed.), *The social context of language* (pp. 17–48). New York: John Wiley.

deVilliers, J. (1984). Form and force interactions: The development of negatives and questions. In R. Schiefelbusch & J. Pickar (Eds.), *The acquisition of communicative competence* (pp. 193–236). Austin, TX: PRO-ED.

Donahue, M., Pearl, R., & Bryan, T. (1982). Learning-disabled children's syntactic proficiency on a communicative task. *Journal of Speech and Hearing Disorders, 47,* 397–403.

Ervin-Tripp, S. (1975). Speech acts and social learning. In K. Basso & H. Shelby (Eds.), *Meaning in anthropology* (pp. 107–130). Albuquerque: University of New Mexico Press.

Friel-Patti, S., Finitzo-Heber, T., Conti, G., & Brown, K. (1982). Language delay in infants associated with middle ear disease and mild, fluctuating hearing impairment. *Pediatric Infectious Disease, 1,* 104–109.

Garnett, K. (1986). Telling tales: Narratives and learning-disabled children. *Topics in Language Disorders, 6,* 45–56.

Gottlieb, M., Zinkus, P., & Thompson, A. (1979). Chronic middle ear disease and auditory perceptual deficits. *Clinical Pediatrics, 18,* 725.

Goodman, K. (1982). Revaluing readers and reading. *Topics in Language and Learning Disabilities, 1,* 87–93.

Gordan, D., & Ervin-Tripp, S. (1984). The structure of children's responses. In R. Schiefelbusch & J. Pickar (Eds.), *The acquisition of communicative competence* (pp. 215–321). Austin, TX: PRO-ED.

Halliday, M. A. K. (1973). *Explorations in the functions of language.* New York: Elsevier North Holland.

Halliday, M. A. K. (1977). *Learning how to mean: Explorations in the development of language.* New York: Elsevier North Holland.

Johnston, J. (1982a). The language-disordered child. In N. Lass, J. Northern, D. Yoder, & L. McReynolds (Eds.), *Speech, language and hearing* (pp. 211–230). Philadelphia: W. B. Saunders.

Johnston, J. (1982b). Narratives: A new look at communication problems in older language-disordered children. *Language, Speech, and Hearing Services in Schools, 13,* 144–155.

Katz, J. (1978). The effects of conductive hearing loss on auditory function. *Asha, 20,* 879–886.

Leonard, L. (1986). Normal language acquisition: Some recent findings and clinical implications. In J. Costello & A. Holland (Eds.), *Handbook of speech and language disorders* (pp. 543–578). San Diego: College-Hill Press.

McCormick, L. (1984). Review of normal language acquisition. In L. McCormick & R. Schiefelbusch (Eds.), *Early language intervention* (pp. 35–88). Columbus, OH: Charles E. Merrill.

McNew, S., & Bates, E. (1984). Pragmatic bases for language acquisition. In R. Naremore (Ed.), *Language science* (pp. 67–105). San Diego: College-Hill Press.

Menyuk, P. (1983). Language development and reading. In T. Gallagher & C. Prutting (Eds.), *Pragmatic assessment and intervention issues in language* (pp. 82–114). San Diego: College-Hill Press.

Miller, J. (1978). Assessing children's language behavior: A developmental process approach. In R. Schiefelbusch (Ed.), *Bases of language intervention* (pp. 269–318). Austin, TX: PRO-ED.

Pick, A. (1978). Perception in the acquisition of reading. In F. Murray & J. Pikulski (Eds.), *The acquisition of reading: Cognitive, linguistic, and perceptual prerequisites* (pp. 99–122). Baltimore: University Park Press.

Ramey, C., Trohanis, P., & Hostler, S. (1982). An introduction. In C. Ramey & P. Trohanis (Eds.), *Finding and educating high-risk and handicapped infants* (pp. 1–36). Austin, TX: PRO-ED.

Rees, N. (1978). Pragmatics of language: Applications to normal and disordered language development. In R. Schiefelbusch (Ed.), *Bases of language intervention* (pp. 191–268). Austin, TX: PRO-ED.

Rice, M. (1984). Cognitive aspects of communicative development. In R. Schiefelbusch & J. Pickar (Eds.), *The acquisition of communicative competence* (pp. 141–189). Austin, TX: PRO-ED.

Richardson, S. (1979). Myth-communication. In A. Simmons-Martin & D. Calvert (Eds.), *Parent-infant intervention: Communication disorders* (pp. 73–87). New York: Grune and Stratton.

Sachs, J. (1978). The adaptive significance of linguistic input to prelinguistic infants. In C. Snow & C. Ferguson (Eds.), *Talking to children: Language input and acquisition* (pp. 51–61). New York: Cambridge University Press.

Sachs, J. (1984). Children's play and communicative development. In R. Schiefelbusch & J. Pickar (Eds.), *The acquisition of communicative competence* (pp. 109–140). Austin, TX: PRO-ED.

Schlesinger, I. (1974). Relational concepts underlying language acquisition. In R. Schiefelbusch & L. Lloyd (Eds.), *Language perspectives—Acquisition, retardation, and intervention* (pp. 129–151). Austin, TX: PRO-ED.

Shane, H. (1981). Decision making in early augmentative system use. In R. Schiefelbusch & D. Bricker (Eds.), *Early language: Acquisition and intervention* (pp. 210–233). Austin, TX: PRO-ED.

Simon, C. (1984). Functional pragmatic evaluation of communication skills in school-age children. *Language, Speech, and Hearing Services in Schools, 15,* 83–97.

Simon, C. (1985). The language-learning disabled student: Description and therapy implications. In C. Simon (Ed.), *Communication skills and classroom success* (pp. 1–56). San Diego: College-Hill Press.

Sloan, C. (1980). Auditory processing disorders and language development. In P. Levinson & C. Sloan (Eds.), *Auditory processing and language: Clinical and research perspectives* (pp. 91–119). New York: Grune and Stratton.

Snow, C. (1977). The development of conversation between mothers and babies. *Journal of Child Language, 4,* 1–22.

Snow, C. (1984). Parent-child interaction and the development of communicative ability. In R. Schiefelbusch & J. Pickar (Eds.), *The acquisition of communicative competence* (pp. 69–107). Austin, TX: PRO-ED.

Snyder, L. (1981). Assessing communicative abilities and disabilities in the sensorimotor period: Content and context. *Topics in Language Disorders, 1,* 31–46.

Snyder, L. (1984a). Cognition and language development. In R. Naremore (Ed.), *Language science* (pp. 107–145). San Diego: College-Hill Press.

Snyder, L. (1984b). Communicative competence in children with delayed language development. In R. Schiefelbusch & J. Pickar (Eds.), *The acquisition of communicative competence* (pp. 423–478). Austin, TX: PRO-ED.

Snyder, L. (1986). Developmental language disorders: Elementary school age. In J. Costello & A. Holland (Eds.), *Handbook of speech and language disorders* (pp. 671–700). San Diego: College-Hill Press.

Sugarman, S. (1984). The development of preverbal communication: Its contribution and limits in promoting the development of language. In R. Schiefelbusch & J. Pickar (Eds.), *The acquisition of communicative competence* (pp. 23–67). Austin, TX: PRO-ED.

Uzigiris, I. (1981). Experience in the social context: Imitation and play. In R. Schiefelbusch & D. Bricker (Eds.), *Early language: Acquisition and intervention* (pp. 187–212). Austin, TX: PRO-ED.

Uzgiris, I., & Hunt, J. (1975). *Assessment in infancy.* Urbana: University of Illinois Press.

Vellutino, F. R. (1979). *Dyslexia: Theory and research.* Cambridge, MA: MIT Press.

Wiig, E., & Semel, E. (1980). *Language assessment and intervention for the learning disabled*. Columbus, OH: Charles E. Merrill.

Wilcox, J. (1986). Developmental language disorders: Preschoolers. In J. Costello & A. Holland (Eds.), *Handbook of speech and language disorders* (pp. 643–670). San Diego: College-Hill Press.

# PART II
## *Diagnosis*

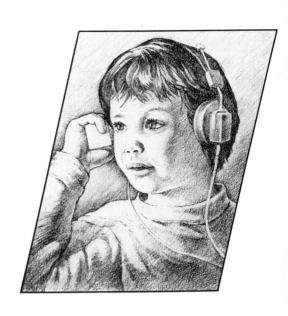

*I*t is safe to say that most hearing-impaired adults come to the audiologist through their own motivations to learn of the nature of their auditory deficits so that steps can be taken to lessen the effects of these deficits. As a rule, the pediatric patient is an unwilling or unwitting participant in measures related to diagnosis of a hearing loss. It is generally agreed that the assessment of hearing disorders in children is often different from, and more difficult than, evaluations of disorders in adults. With adults, evaluation begins from the audiologist's point of view. With children, audiologists must be sensitive enough to select methods that tap their patients' interests whenever possible.

Because of their ages and the nature of the handicap, many children do not cooperate during behavioral measurements of hearing. In Chapter 5 Charles Berlin and Linda Hood describe the use of objective tests that have been developed to determine or infer hearing sensitivity and the status of the middle ear system. The term *objective* in this context means that the patient offers no subjective response to a stimulus; it is generally agreed that a great deal of experience and expertise may be required in interpreting some of these tests.

A large number of even very young children can be persuaded to cooperate during voluntary hearing tests. William Hodgson, in Chapter 6, focuses on some of the procedures for the very young child. In Chapter 7, Ross Roeser and Wende Yellin review the procedures used in testing children with pure tones. This review of the tests available and the authors' own suggestions for their use are contemporary and useful. In Chapter 8 I discuss the values and methods used in speech audiometry with children.

# 5

# *Auditory Brainstem Response and Middle Ear Assessment in Children*

*CHARLES I. BERLIN*
*LINDA J. HOOD*

$A$s yet there is no absolutely objective physiologic test of the "moment of hearing." In a philosophic sense we still do not understand the concomitants of the "moment" of sound awareness and/or classification. We do, however, have at our disposal many physiologic tools that allow us to infer with some precision the status of the middle ear, cochlea, and auditory pathways of the lower brainstem. In this

Work on this chapter was supported by NIH NS-07058, the Lions of Louisiana, and KAM's Fund. The authors wish to thank Vibha Brown for her assistance with the manuscript.

chapter we will discuss two of the most commonly available techniques for objective assessment of audition, the auditory brainstem response (ABR) and middle ear measurement.

There are excellent summaries on the background and application of these two techniques that include considerable attention to their history and technology (Jacobson, 1985; Jerger, 1984; Northern & Downs, 1984). This chapter instead will focus on a "how we do it" approach to show how the techniques complement one another and to assist the audiologist in making pediatric patient-management decisions.

# The Auditory Brainstem Response: History

We were first able to record the compound action potential of the synchronous discharge of the human eighth nerve around 1960 (Ruben, Knickerbocker, Sekula, Nager, & Bordley, 1959). This recording was done without the use of computers, in the operating room, with an electrode placed on or near the round window and very intense pulses generated in the sound field. Powerful preamplifiers picked up the electrical activity from the vicinity of the round window of the cochlea and displayed it on an oscilloscope screen. The response was small and difficult to see when the stimulus intensity fell much below 90 to 100 dB peak equivalent sound pressure level. With the advent of portable averaging computers, it became possible to extract that electrocochleographic response from the background noise and view it as it diminished in response to progressively weaker stimulation. Some clinics and laboratories were ultimately able to record the response via needle electrodes at the promontory or electrodes in the ear canal at levels approximating normal detection thresholds.

Then two separate laboratories discovered the auditory brainstem response almost at the same time. Sohmer and Feinmesser, in Israel, were recording electrocochleograms and attempting to study them from the surface of the scalp. They picked up a multiwave response and classified it as a special form of "surface electrocochleography" (Sohmer & Feinmesser, 1967). Therefore, they approached ABR as a special case of electrocochleography. In contrast, Jewett, while studying glial potentials during a postdoctoral stay with Galambos, uncovered a set of potentials that were essentially ignored for a number of years thereafter. The findings were published at about the same time as the Israeli observations

(Jewett, Romano, & Williston, 1970; Jewett & Williston, 1971), but personal communication suggests that Jewett's data had been collected and stored well before anyone had any notion of their significance.

# What Is the ABR?

The auditory brainstem response represents the synchronous discharge of first- through sixth-order neurons in the eighth nerve and brainstem. It is a very small response, approximately 0.1 of 1 millionth of a volt in amplitude, and in order to be seen it must be extracted from the background interference. In this case background interference represents any other electrical signals going on at the same time, such as the cortical EEG, the electrocardiogram, the electrical potentials of muscles and neural groups being used, as well as radio frequencies and the 60 Hz rise and fall of electrical fields around outlets in the wall. (*A note on so-called 60 Hz interference:* Because any electrical field that crosses a wire will induce a current in it, it is important that the undesired electrical fields from power conductors in the wall or from other sources be cancelled out as much as possible and the desired response be extracted as efficiently as possible from the background.) In order to reduce interference we rely on several important techniques:

1. *Filtering.* We rely on the principle that the ABR is made up of electrical frequencies that can be characterized. In our experience the dominant frequencies of the ABR are between 100 and 3000 Hz. Therefore, the first step for separating the ABR from the background interference is to filter it properly. We therefore recommend filters on the input side of the ABR equipment to be set at a bandpass of 100 to 3000 Hz.

2. *Computer averaging.* The second principle we depend upon is that the ABR will be time-locked to the stimulation and will always occur at essentially the same time, all the time, following the presentation of a brief stimulus. This time-locked registration permits the use of an averaging computer that extracts the desired signal from the background noise by a process of summation. Each time a stimulus is given, the computer starts its analysis and continues that analysis for a period of approximately 10 to 12 milliseconds after stimulation. If the synchronous discharges occur in the proper time frames, they are added proportionately to the number of passes that the computer makes at the data. Since the desired response is buried in the noise,

we also depend on the principle that the noise will not be as time-locked to the stimulus as the response. Mathematically we add the response to the signal-plus-noise in such a way that the noise adds as the square root of the number of passes. Figure 5.1 shows how a tiny response buried deep within the noise can be extracted from that signal-plus-noise background as the number of sweeps increases.

3. *Common-mode rejection.* The third technique we use to extract the signal from the noise is called common-mode rejection. With this technology the response, which is embedded in the interference, is passed through two electrodes simultaneously and presented to an amplifier that subtracts the contents of one electrode from the other. Since the undesired noise usually reaches both electrodes with common amplitude and phase, but one electrode has the desired signal at somewhat larger amplitudes, the resultant subtraction leaves *mostly* signal and little residual noise.

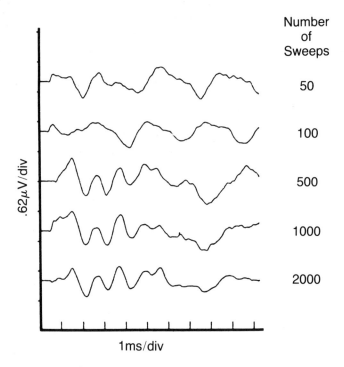

**Figure 5.1.**   The effect of computer averaging on extraction of the ABR from background noise. The normal five-wave complex emerges around 500 sweeps in this example.

# The ABR Response

Figure 5.2 shows the appearance of a normal auditory brainstem response from a normal 2-year-old child. When the intensity is around 75 dB above normal threshold we see a five-wave complex that has a very orderly relationship between each of the waves. While the waves do not exist in the brain (that is, what looks like a wave on the computer screen is in fact a sum of the electrical activity of many fibers discharging around the same time after stimulation), the intervals between each wave are predictably about 1 millisecond. As will be seen later, in very young children below 8 months of age those intervals are somewhat longer, reflecting the immature nature of the nervous system and perhaps even the cochlea. The response seen here is acquired at high intensities and then at progressively lower intensities until no response is seen. As the intensity of the stimulus drops, the shape of the five-wave complex changes and only a single bump is left down near threshold (Figure 5.3). Eliciting such a synchronous discharge to a very faint pulse is used as ''proof'' that the peripheral auditory system is working normally. We will show why this is a valid assumption only in part and that some other procedures need to be used to cross-check that assumption.

# When to Use ABR Testing

ABR testing should be used when one desires a noninvasive, safe, benign approach in very young infants, children, adults, or mentally or multiply handicapped individuals who cannot participate in voluntary audiometry. The ABR procedure is especially ideal if one wishes to know the sensitivity of each cochlea separately (it is far superior to sound-field audiometry in that respect), to know bone conduction results with or without masking, to obtain some form of low-frequency sensitivity estimate, and to gain insight into the neural integrity of the auditory brain in any given patient. It should *not* be used in lieu of an audiogram in patients who can give voluntary responses but is quite useful as an additional test that gives some idea of the neurologic maturity of the auditory brainstem; the voluntary pure-tone audiogram in such a case should be normal. Note that in the presence of hydrocephalus the ABR can be obliterated despite normal hearing; absence of an ABR should be interpreted with great caution under those conditions (Kraus, Ozdamar, Heydemann, Stein, & Reed, 1984).

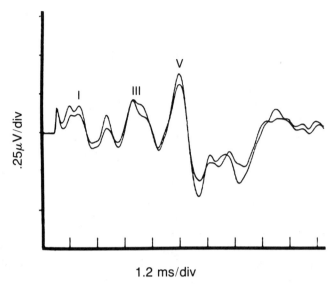

1.2 ms/div

**Figure 5.2.**   ABR obtained from a normal 2½-year-old child. Latencies of Waves I, III, and V for positive polarity pulses presented at 75 dB HLN and 27.7 pulses per second are 1.58, 3.84, and 5.95 milliseconds, respectively.

## What Constitutes a Complete ABR and Why

An ABR is obtained only when the stimulus is brief enough or has a rapid enough onset that many units in the eighth nerve and brainstem discharge simultaneously and synchronously. The need for a brief onset stimulus to elicit the ABR causes a special problem: that is, any acoustic stimulus will contain a broad spectrum of energy if the onset of that stimulus is brief. Thus, if we restrict onsets to less than 1 millisecond, for example, the spectral content of a pulse is mandatorily broad; the slower the onset, the narrower the spectral content becomes. This phenomenon is summarized in Figure 5.4, which shows three important principles about the acoustics of brief signals: (1) they generate broad frequency responses, (2) there is an electrical null at a frequency of 1/duration of the pulse (e.g., Figure 5.4 shows a brief 100 microsecond pulse with a null at 10 kHz, whereas a 200 microsecond pulse would have a null at 5 kHz and a 500 microsecond pulse at 2 kHz), and (3) the transducer used adds its own

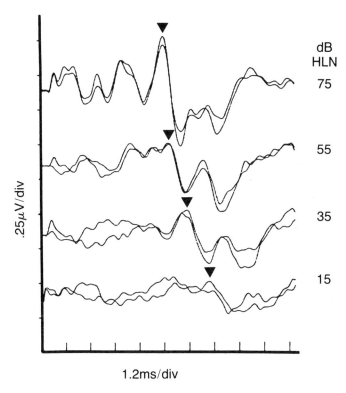

**Figure 5.3.** Changes in the ABR as a function of intensity. Wave V latencies increase from 5.95 to 6.33 to 7.05 to 8.20 milliseconds as the intensity decreases from 75 to 55 to 35 to 15 dB HLN, respectively.

characteristic "signature" to the pulse. Once the electrical pulse hits the transducer, the transducer "rings and resonates" at its own natural frequency, superimposing a spectral "signature" onto the electrical impulse. Figure 5.4 shows that sequence in a standard audiometric earphone. As one can see from that sequence, the pulse has most of its energy in the range from 2000 to 4000 Hz. Therefore, if one uses only the most common 100 microsecond pulse as a stimulus, then patients with audiograms A, B, and C shown in Figure 5.5 will all give poor and probably absent ABRs. Needless to say, the management of those three patients, all other things being equal, is quite different. Similarly, audiograms D, E, and F in Figure 5.5 are all different, yet the ABR to a brief 100 microsecond pulse alone will most likely look normal even at low intensities (Glattke, 1983). Therefore, one step in a complete audiologic ABR must include some low-frequency stimulation either at 500 Hz or a similar frequency. We will discuss how to acquire and use such data later in this chapter.

Similarly, it is quite possible that a conductive hearing loss and/or mixed hearing loss can so delay or desynchronize the ABR so as to confuse the tester into believing there is a peripheral sensorineural loss. For reasons that will become clear later in the chapter, we strongly recommend bone conduction if there is any abnormality in the ABR. Thus, our protocol for a complete ABR in a young child includes responses to air-conducted pulses, to 500 Hz tonebursts or the equivalent, and to bone-conducted pulses. Naturally if the ABR to a pulse alone is normal, it is quite likely that there is peripherally normal sensitivity, but there is much more of a guarantee when bone-conduction and 500 Hz responses are also normal. Normal tympanometry and normal acoustic reflex thresholds also help to establish and confirm the normal peripheral sensitivity. Even more important, an absent ABR that might likely occur to a pulse alone in the presence of audiograms A, B, and C (Figure 5.5) could be misinterpreted as severe to profound deafness. Either the wrong hearing aid or, in some cases, no hearing aid might be recommended without full under-

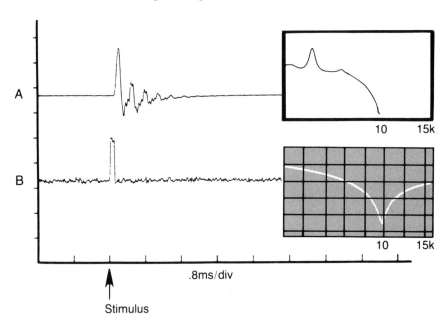

**Figure 5.4.** Time (*x* axis) by intensity (*y* axis) plots of the acoustic (A) and electrical (B) responses of a 100 microsecond pulse. Insets represent the frequency (*x* axis) by intensity (*y* axis), or spectral, plots.

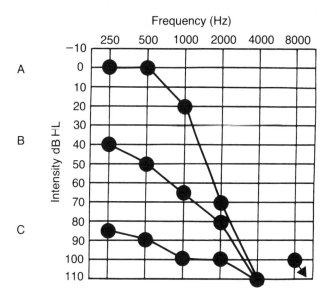

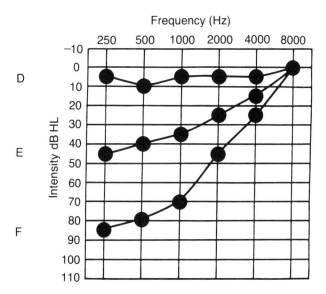

**Figure 5.5.** Audiograms that will yield a poor or absent ABR to a 100 microsecond pulse (A, B, C) and audiograms that will usually show a normal ABR to the same type of stimulus (D, E, F).

standing of the nature of the peripheral hearing impairment. Here again combined use of the ABR with tympanometry and reflexes might reveal a sloping hearing loss by virtue of a slope in the reflex threshold. As we shall see, the complete ABR is enhanced by the use of and interpretation with immittance audiometry.

# How to Conduct ABR Testing

## Necessary Equipment

A commercially available system that can generate pulses and tonebursts and has air- and bone-conduction transducers is highly recommended. As a result of our experience with collapsing canals, shifting phones, and complications requiring masking and as a result of viewing many records over the years that have been contaminated by electrical artifacts interfering with both the cochlear potential and the eighth-nerve action potential, we strongly recommend the use of *insert* earphones. Properly selected, these earphones have a broad spectral characteristic but, because of their nature as insert devices, prevent collapsible canals, minimize the need for masking during air-conduction testing, and introduce a very helpful sound travel delay between the onset of the stimulus and its arrival at the ear. This travel delay, which varies from 0.4 to 0.9 of a millisecond based on the distance from the earphone to the tympanic membrane, helps to separate the electroacoustic artifacts from the physiologic responses acquired from the ear itself. If insert phones are to be used in operating room recordings, we encourage their use in the clinic as well, so that the same spectrum presented to the ear during clinical assessment can be used in the operating room to monitor the ABR during procedures around the eighth nerve and cerebellar-pontine angle. Intraoperative monitoring, of course, is not a common procedure in children but is just one of the many circumstances under which we encourage users to employ insert earphones.

## Settings

Our recommendations for filter settings, rates, pulse durations, and windows are summarized in Table 5.1. The rationale for our selections are based on the literature and our clinical experience. In our use of conden-

## TABLE 5.1
### Test Parameters We Use to Obtain Auditory Brainstem Responses to Air-Conduction Pulses, Air-Conduction 500 Hz Tonebursts, and Bone-Conduction Pulses

| Test Type | Stimulus Parameters | | | | | Recording Parameters | | |
|---|---|---|---|---|---|---|---|---|
| | Type | Duration | Polarity | Rate | | Window | Filter | Sweeps |
| Air-Conduction Pulse | pulse | 100 $\mu$s | positive | 27.7/s | | 12 ms | 100–3K | 1,000–2,000 |
| Air-Conduction 500 Hz Toneburst | toneburst 2-1-2 cycle or 1-0-1 cycle envelope | 10 ms 4 ms | alternating | 27.7/s | | 20 ms | 30–1500 | 1,000–2,000 |
| Bone-Conduction Pulse | pulse | 100 $\mu$s | alternating | 27.7/s | | 12 ms | 100–3K | 1,000–2,000 |

sation pulses we differ from many of our colleagues. Some (e.g., Picton, Woods, Baribeau-Braun, & Healey, 1977) prefer alternating polarity pulses for the very defensible reason that the (onset of) stimulus artifact and its amplitude are for the most part cancelled. However, Coats and Martin (1977) have shown that in the presence of high-frequency hearing loss it is often dangerous to use alternating polarity pulses. Similarly, it is quite physiologic and defensible to use rarefaction pulses. We, in fact, started using rarefaction pulses because of our early experience with electrocochleography. The rarefaction pulse pulls upward on the cochlear partition, and, at least at the basal turn, the phase-angle of high-frequency responses is pretty much coherent with the phase-angle of the stapes and its displacement. However, again in the presence of high-frequency hearing loss, the rarefaction pulse seems to be less efficient in eliciting a large Wave V than the condensation pulse. Rarefaction pulses tend to elicit a larger and slightly earlier Wave I whereas condensation pulses elicit a larger and slightly later Wave V. For the most part, while there is some disagreement in the literature as to what an ideal pulse is, few disagree that the 100 microsecond pulse has been wisely selected for its electroacoustic characteristics (see the earlier discussion of electrical and acoustic nulls at 1/duration of the pulse).

## Data Collection

We encourage two-channel, four-electrode recordings, but one-channel, three-electrode recordings are often quite satisfactory. Electrodes are placed in position around the head with the hot or G-1 electrode at the vertex and the two reference G-2 electrodes at the mesial surface of each earlobe. (Here we use a convention to describe the electrodes suggested by Hallowell Davis. He rightly reasons that there are no "reference" or "hot" electrodes in these recordings since both electrodes are active. Instead he suggests we name the electrodes G-1 and G-2 to represent the grid voltages of the old vacuum tube nomenclature and thereby delineate which side of a common-mode rejection amplifier is getting which electrode. In this way a G-1 electrode is the electrode that goes to that portion of the common-mode rejection amplifier which eventually produces a vertex positive upward polarity. In the Canadian and European literature it is often common to see vertex positive displayed downward.) The ground electrode is placed at the nasion. In the special case of an infant, where the fontanelles are not closed, we recommend that the G-1 electrode be placed on the forehead at the hairline.

Children under 3 months of age usually fall asleep after feeding, but children 6 months and above often require chloral hydrate sedation. Chloral hydrate is given (in dosages according to *The Physician's Desk Reference*) in our practice with an otolaryngologist or otolaryngology resident in attendance. In the 19 years we have been doing outpatient evoked potentials with sedation we have had *three* complications out of 422 patients following the use of ketamine, and *no* complications in any of the remaining 960 patients in our logs following the use of chloral hydrate. We have had some "paradoxical responses" following chloral hydrate, in which some children get hyperactive and/or fail to sedate. However, there have been no life-threatening complications, and the procedure is considered benign and virtually without risk. After the child falls asleep, tympanometry and reflexes are ideally accomplished since, if the test is done after completion of the ABR, there is often a tendency to have positive air pressure in the middle ear as a result of snoring or occasionally crying. Once immittance is completed, the electrodes are put in place and impedances are sought that are below 10,000 ohms (preferably below 5,000 ohms) and are ideally as equal as possible between all electrodes. At this point the earphones are put in place, and one of a number of strategies may be introduced depending upon the intended application of the ABR.

One of the most effective applications is the initial use of binaural pulses. In the binaural mode brief pulses generate the largest possible ABRs in contrast to the monaural mode. Therefore, Jerger, Oliver, and Stach (1985) have recommended using binaural stimuli in a descending mode until normal sensitivity is reached. At that point evidence is clear that at least one ear has normal synchrony at or near the voluntary thresholds in the range from about 1500 to 4000 Hz. At that point if the intensity of the stimulus is increased by about 10 dB to one ear at a time, then evidence can be obtained with respect to the symmetry of the two ears. If neither ear has a peripheral hearing impairment at the basal turn, then normal and symmetrical latencies will be obtained in both ears. However, if one ear is impaired, then a threshold search can be made for that ear with an ascending strategy. In children with normal peripheral sensitivity in that narrow range, data can be acquired in only four "runs": (1) binaural run at high intensities, (2) binaural run at threshold levels, (3) monaural right run at 10 dB above the previous record, and (4) monaural left run at 10 dB above the previous record. That minimal battery can give the audiologist enormous insight into the integrity of a peripheral auditory system in less than 10 minutes, assuming a stimulation rate of approximately 27 pulses per second and 1,200 sweeps per run. Since we recommend a total of two repetitions for each low-intensity run, then relatively little time is needed to establish a coherent sensitive response at low intensities.

The strategies we use in our clinic have evolved from our 1968 experience with electrocochleography where we used sound-field speakers and recorded from one ear at a time. In our current mode we do single-ear stimulation in 20 dB steps until we fail to get a response or until a 15 dB hearing level is reached by air conduction. Again, each run is repeated for consistency. Whether or not there is a normal pulse-evoked ABR, we then follow the pulse stimulation with a 500 Hz toneburst stimulation using a 2 millisecond rise/fall stimulus, which we recognize has considerable spectral "splash." While responses to this signal at high intensities contain cochlear elements that are derived from basal activity, responses seen at low intensities (35 to 40 dB HLN) are almost certainly from more apical structures. The evidence for this conclusion is compelling: the latencies are long (9 to 13 milliseconds) and the audible spectral content of the tonebursts focuses in the range from 450 to 550 Hz. While it has been said with great assurance that it is difficult to get low-frequency information because of the spectral splash of these low-frequency signals, it is important to keep in mind that when one reaches low intensities, only the peak of the spectrum is audible and synchronous response to low-intensity signals clearly suggests good low-frequency sensitivity.

In performing low-frequency toneburst assessment we change the filters to accommodate lower-frequency biologic activity; the bandpass filters are set at 30 to 1500 Hz. We also use an alternating toneburst and sometimes have to decrease the sensitivity of the input amplifier to prevent artifactual saturation of the preamplifier. Put another way, when one opens up the computer to lower-frequency inputs, including 60 Hz interference and muscle movement, it is often difficult to avoid tripping the artifact reject mechanism of the computer. This requires either deactivating the mechanism or desensitizing it slightly.

If and when there is an abnormal brainstem response to either air-conducted pulses or 500 Hz tonebursts, we make it a practice of conducting an alternating-polarity bone-conduction stimulation. When one stimulates standard bone-conduction oscillators with a 100 microsecond pulse, the resultant spectrum is considerably different, both in power and frequency content, from the air-conducted spectrum acquired in a TDH-39 phone. The bone-conducted spectrum is closer to 1000 Hz (Schwartz, Larson, & DeChicchis, 1985), and the nominal hearing level readings for air-conduction pulses on the dials of most ABR units do not apply. That is, a 95 dB dial reading on many instruments rarely exceeds a 45 to 55 dB true hearing level when using a bone transducer. Some units based on programmable computers make the necessary adjustments, but the dynamic range available is quite limited. The novice should approach the use of bone conduction with caution and become familiar with the problems of ABR by bone conduction. We strongly recommend the use of alternating-polarity pulses to minimize the artifact and encourage the acquisition of a number of bone-conduction oscillators for specific use with the ABR units. The common practice of using an audiometric bone-conduction oscillator as an ABR bone-conduction tester leads to poorly calibrated audiometric oscillators, with distortion and disrupted calibrations. The high-intensity stimulation generated by pulsatile inputs tends to break down the bonding of the oscillators and introduces distortion as well as calibration error.

During bone-conduction testing, we used to routinely place the oscillator at the frontal bone, generalizing from our audiologic experience with adults. This may well have been a tactical error. In young infants, before the fontanelles are closed, much better bone-conduction responses are obtained from the mastoid than from the frontal bone; therefore, we have changed our practice to use the mastoid air spaces and the skull configuration of infants to our advantage. Masking is used whenever there are potential differences between the ears that need to be resolved.

The combined use of ABR with tympanometry and reflexes generates an extremely powerful test of middle ear and brainstem functions simultaneously.

# Case Studies

## Case 1

Case 1 is a 3-month-old baby who was referred to us in 1974 from out of state by an obstetrician and gynecologist. His granddaughter seemed to be unresponsive to environmental sounds, and both he and his daughter were concerned that the child might be hearing-impaired. Local specialists had said that no valid hearing testing could be done at such a young age and that they should wait until the child was 6 to 8 months of age for more dependable behavioral testing. This was not satisfactory to them, so they were sent to our institution. At the first ABR testing, we obtained the tracings seen at the top of Figure 5.6. A cadre of medical students was observing our earliest application of ABRs, and at this time we were using only air-conducted pulses. When we got the flat line seen in the top two traces, we ran the mother as a control and proudly showed the observing medical students how we were able to diagnose hearing impairment in the young child. One astute young medical student was impressed but curious, and asked, "Dr. Berlin, is this a conductive or sensorineural loss?" I was about to answer that it was a sensorineural loss when common sense told me that I really didn't know! At that point we did our first bone-conduction ABR and, much to our surprise, found nearly normal responses. This case first taught us 12 years ago the necessity of using bone conduction in all infant testing where normal data are not obtained by air conduction.

## Case 2

Case 2 demonstrates the ABR test strategy we use today. This 1½-year-old male was referred to us by an astute pediatrician because of a history of middle ear fluid and the family's concern over his hearing. Behavioral responses to speech stimuli were obtained in sound field at intensity levels between 30 and 40 dB HL, suggesting a mild hearing loss in the better ear (or possibly both ears). Immittance tests yielded Type B tympanograms, decreased static compliance, and elevated or absent acoustic

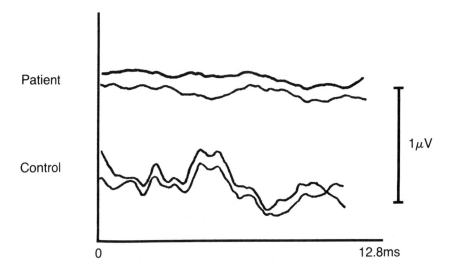

**Figure 5.6.** Case 1 (upper tracing). ABR obtained from a 95 dB HLN air-conducted pulse. Shown in the lower tracing is an ABR obtained from a normal hearing subject.

reflexes. While these results suggested a bilateral conductive hearing loss, the ABR was used to define the problem more accurately. Latency-intensity functions for air-conduction pulses showed responses at 55 dB HLN and above for the left ear and 45 dB HLN and above for the right ear (Figure 5.7). Toneburst responses were obtained at levels 20 to 30 dB poorer than normal while bone-conduction responses were obtained at normal levels. Results thus suggested a mild to moderate conductive hearing loss, greater in the higher frequencies, with slightly poorer hearing in the left ear. Normal bone-conduction thresholds were consistent with both the case history and the tympanometry and acoustic reflexes; medical treatment was pursued.

## Case 3

Case 3 provides an example of what we use as a "normal reference." This is a 2½-year-old male with normal hearing sensitivity. As shown in Figure 5.8, clear responses to air-conduction pulses were observed for each ear at 15 dB HLN and above, responses to tonebursts were present at 35 dB HLN and above, and bone-conduction responses were present at 25 dB HLN and above. Results such as these are observed in normal hearing adults and in children who subsequently have been shown to have normal hearing sensitivity with normal middle ear function. Thus, they constitute "normal function" for the evoked potential protocol presented in these case studies.

## Case 4

In contrast to the above cases showing normal hearing or conductive hearing losses, we have also found sensory hearing losses in infants and have been able to begin amplification and habilitation programs soon thereafter. Case 4 is a 4-month-old infant who was referred to us because of unresponsiveness to environmental sounds. Attempts to elicit behavioral responses to speech and noise in sound field resulted in no observable response at high intensities. Impedance testing indicated normal (Type A) tympanograms, but acoustic reflexes could not be elicited due to excessive movement. ABR testing was completed with the child sleeping without sedation. Air-conducted pulse stimuli presented at 85 dB HLN at 27.7 stimuli per second resulted in the presence of Waves I, III, and V with prolonged interwave latencies, which is normal for the age of this infant (Figure 5.9). A latency-intensity function to air-conducted pulses

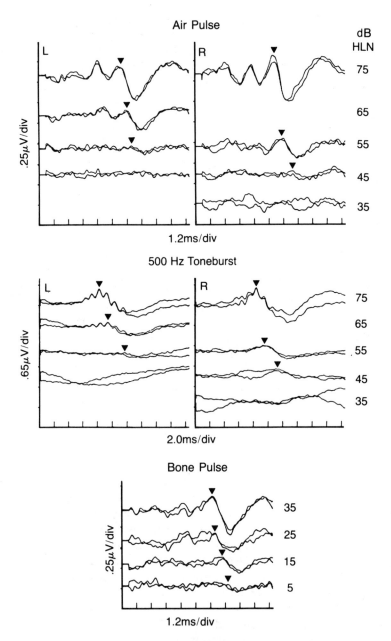

**Figure 5.7.**   Case 2. ABRs obtained using an air-conducted pulse, a 500 Hz toneburst, and a bone-conducted pulse from a 1½-year-old male with a bilateral conductive hearing loss.

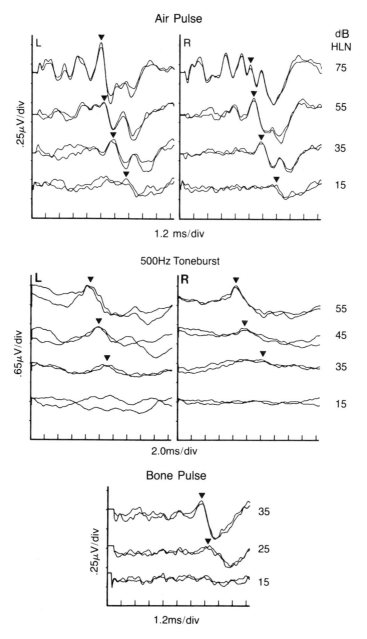

**Figure 5.8.** Case 3. ABRs obtained using an air-conducted pulse, a 500 Hz toneburst, and a bone-conducted pulse from a 2½-year-old male with normal hearing.

showed responses at 55 dB HLN and above for the right ear but only at 85 dB HLN for the left ear. Responses to air-conducted 500 Hz tonebursts were observed at 85 dB HLN for the right ear, and no clear response was evident for the left ear. Bone-conducted pulse responses were obtained at 55 dB HLN, well above normal. Based on these findings, we were able to define a moderate, fairly flat, bilateral sensory hearing loss with poorer hearing in the left ear. This child was seen again 2 months later for a repeat ABR (a procedure we use, among others, to evaluate possible central nervous system immaturity effects on the test results). Results were similar, and the child was then referred for amplification and initiation of an appropriate habilitation program.

### Case 5

Case 5 demonstrates another application of the same protocol. This patient is a 13-year-old developmentally delayed male who lacked speech and language and was unable to be trained to respond reliably on behavioral audiometric tests. ABRs to air-conduction pulses, 500 Hz tonebursts, and bone-conduction pulses were within normal limits for each ear (Figure 5.10). Immittance tests showed normal tympanograms and static compliance. Contralateral and ipsilateral acoustic reflexes were present at normal levels for each ear, and reflex decay was negative. These test results thus suggested that speech and language absence in this patient was not related to a peripheral hearing loss. However, it is important to recall that the possibility of a cortical or thalamic auditory disorder cannot be ruled out based on a normal ABR. We are currently studying middle latency responses (MLR) as well; however, MLR utility in infants and developmentally delayed individuals may require special consideration of test parameters. The discussion of these issues is beyond the scope of this chapter, but we recommend the work of Goldstein (e.g., Goldstein & Rodman, 1967) and Ozdamar and Kraus (1983) for further information on MLR.

# Middle Ear Assessment: History

The original work on middle ear impedance measurement by Metz (1946) was an exercise in applied engineering and physiology, designed to clarify the nature of middle ear mechanics. Through combinations of accidents

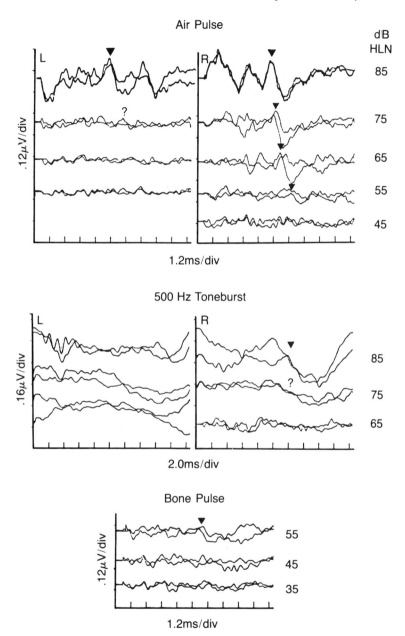

**Figure 5.9.** Case 4. ABRs obtained using an air-conducted pulse, a 500 Hz toneburst, and a bone-conducted pulse from a 4-month-old male with a bilateral sensorineural hearing loss.

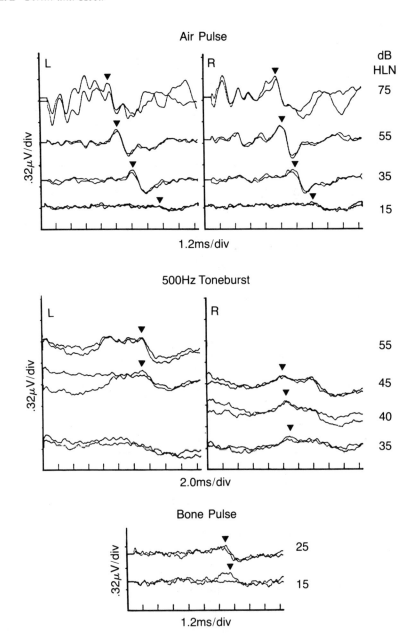

**Figure 5.10.** Case 5. ABRs obtained using an air-conducted pulse, a 500 Hz toneburst, and a bone-conducted pulse from a 13-year-old developmentally delayed male with normal hearing.

in technological limitations and convenience, it became common in the late 1960s and 1970s to measure not the impedance of the ear but, in fact, its elastic reactance or stiffness at just one frequency (220 Hz). This statement requires some explanation. The impedance (i.e., the acceptance or rejection of energy) of any mechanical system is for the most part frequency dependent. When one studies a system's mechanical response to a signal of 100 Hz, for example, the reactance measured is essentially controlled by the stiffness of the system; the stiffer the system, the harder it is for low frequencies to move it. Conversely, if one uses a frequency such as 2500 Hz, the result is controlled by the mass of the system; the more mass, the more resistance to high-frequency motion. The combined effects of mass reactance, elastic reactance (stiffness), and frictional resistance yield the total impedance of mechanical systems to motion. Knowledgeable users in this area are aware that they are measuring the mechanical properties of the ear only around the frequencies of the probe tones being used. Single-frequency bridges use probe tones that are usually 220 Hz and therefore reflect elastic reactance almost exclusively.

While these procedures are not objective measures of hearing, they do afford reasonably precise measures of mechanical and electrophysiological properties of the ear that can be used to great diagnostic advantage. When the tests were first applied, it was thought that they would give unequivocal objective assessment of middle ear effusion, tympanic membrane perforation, or even ossicular anomalies. While subsequent literature (Feldman & Wilber, 1976; Popelka, 1984) questions this simple interpretation, there is no doubt that the technique is both useful and productive, although it is much better for predicting the presence of normal ears than it is for pointing out the presence of pathology (Wright, McConnell, Thompson, Vaughn, & Sell, 1985).

# What Is Middle Ear Assessment?

Excellent reviews of the principles and techniques used in middle ear assessment are available elsewhere (e.g., Jerger, 1975; Popelka, 1981; Silman, 1984; *Ear and Hearing*, 1984). The essential factors to keep in mind are that the values being measured reflect the mechanical properties of the entire auditory path from the external ear to the stapedial footplate; flexible external ear tissues and partly formed and immature canal wall configurations can give spurious results, so great care must be taken in the application of middle ear assessment in very young babies. This does not mean, however, that the techniques should not be used. For example, in a 1-month-old baby, a normal tympanogram and reflexes at normal levels are highly likely indications that there are no middle ear pathologies and that the child is not suffering from severe sensorineural loss.

In contrast, a normal-appearing tympanogram with absent reflexes may suggest profound sensorineural loss but may also be a misleading result caused by flexible ear canal wall geometry, which simulates a normal tympanogram to a 220 Hz tone and obscures severe middle ear disease or malformations. Thus in very young babies normal-appearing tympanometry to a 220 Hz tone with absent middle ear reflexes must be interpreted with great care, whereas normal tympanometry with normal reflexes virtually always means normal middle ear function.

There are basically four parts to middle ear assessment using commonly available devices:

1. The measurement of acoustic immittance and static compliance
2. Tympanometry
3. Middle ear muscle reflex assessment, which includes a number of subtests
4. Eustachian-tube function tests

# The Measurement of Acoustic Immittance and Static Compliance

Any physical structure has mechanical characteristics of acceptance and rejection of energy that are properly referred to collectively as *impedance*. Impedance is the total opposition to oscillatory motion equal to the square root of the sums of the squares of the resistance and reactances in the total system. *Immittance* is a recently evolved neologism, ostensibly a combination of *admittance* and *impedance* and hence with no referent in traditional mathematics or physics. It has become common to refer to only a portion of that information, such as "acoustic impedance" or "static compliance" and to convert those quantities into an "equivalent volume." There is a search for a fixed relationship between a given immittance value and the condition of a single structure in the ear, which unfortunately does not exist. The values measured at the entrance to the ear represent a complex combination of mechanical characteristics of many structures;

therefore, results must be interpreted with caution and knowledge of the underlying mechanics. In the measurement of acoustic immittance a probe tone (most commonly 220 Hz or 660 Hz) is impressed against the tympanic membrane, and the amount of tone reflected is measured relative to a precalibrated standard. An air pump is used to lock down the structures of the tympanic membrane and ossicular chain, both with positive and negative pressure. The compliance of these structures is acquired by comparing their reflective properties when the system is locked down to the reflective properties when the system is at normal atmospheric pressure. When a tympanogram (as shown in Figure 5.11) is generated, the values on the flat portion of this graph represent primarily the immittance of the canal alone. The measurement at the peak of the tympanogram usually represents the immittance of the canal plus the immittance at the tympanic membrane, which represents the immittance of the tympanic membrane and all the structures medial to it. When one subtracts the ear canal immittance from the peak tympanogram immittance, one acquires what has been commonly called "static immittance" or, conversely, "static compliance." It must be remembered that this value represents the mechanical properties of the system only in response to the probe tone used. Jerger, Anthony, Jerger, and Crump (1974) showed that normal equivalent volumes for adults in response to a 220 Hz probe tone range from 0.39 to 1.30 cc.

# Tympanometry

The derivation of static equivalent volume represents the subtraction of the value at the peak of the tympanogram from the value at either extreme. Therefore, it is a simple matter to describe tympanometry as the plotting of immittance values under positive, normal, and negative air pressure. Unfortunately, this is an artificially simple and misunderstood procedure primarily based on problems of terminology. Furthermore, the tympanogram can be expressed in many different terms and formats. For purposes of demonstration, we will outline normal tympanograms using the most commonly applied single-frequency probe (220 Hz); however, the reader is referred to Shanks (1984) for a lucid, scholarly, thorough review of the utility of using multiple-frequency probes and measuring more than simply elastic reactance at one frequency.

In the most commonly employed system, Jerger's tympanometry coding system describes five types of tympanograms: Type A, Type $A_s$,

Type $A_D$, Type B, and Type C. Each of these tympanograms is said to be associated with common anomalies of middle ear structures. For example, the Type C tympanogram is associated with negative pressure in the middle ear, Type B with fluid or debris in the middle ear, Type $A_S$ with abnormal stiffness of the middle ear, and Type $A_D$ with abnormal flaccidity. The Type A tympanogram is said to be associated with normal middle ear structures but is in fact seen often in otosclerosis as well as in young babies whose ear canals flex in response to air pressure changes, giving spurious results on a 220 Hz tympanogram.

Sprague, Wiley, and Goldstein (1985) noted that tympanometry and acoustic reflex measures in neonates and infants under 1 month of age had not been outlined in a way sufficient for general use. It was only by using a 1200 Hz probe that it was observed that neonatal acoustic reflex thresholds approximated those of adults (Bennett & Weatherby, 1982). Sprague et al. (1985) examined frequency patterns, reliability, and ear-to-ear symmetry for tympanometry and measured the ipsilateral and

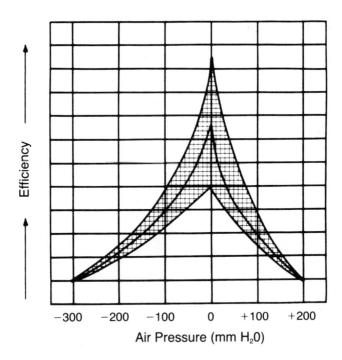

**Figure 5.11.** A normal tympanogram.

contralateral acoustic reflex characteristics in neonates. They found that the difference between acoustic immittance at the pressure extremes and maximum acoustic immittance was larger for the 220 Hz probe tone than it was for the 660 Hz probe tone (they used a Grason-Stadler 1723 bridge). Most of the ears had a notch at 0 millimeters of pressure, often exceeding the limits of the equipment in its depth. A double-peaked tympanogram was most characteristic of infant ears when a 220 Hz probe tone was used, and a single-peaked tympanogram was seen when a 660 Hz probe tone was employed. Exactly the reverse was seen in adults; that is, double-peaked tympanograms occur frequently with 660 Hz probes, and single-peaked tympanograms are most common with 220 Hz probes. Notched tympanograms are common for high-frequency probe tones in adults because the adult middle ear is stiffness-dominated up to about 1000 Hz; in contrast, a notched tympanogram suggests that the infant neonatal ear has a resonant frequency between 220 and 660 Hz. As we said earlier, the collapsibility of the infant ear canal and the existence of a resonant frequency work together.

Margolis and Shanks (1985) also conclude that a low-frequency probe tone may be more useful for tympanometry in neonates while a high-probe frequency is necessary for acoustic reflex measurement. These authors rightfully conclude that neonatal tympanograms really reflect complex interactions of external and middle ear properties and that, until more data are acquired from diseased neonatal ears, it is difficult to establish tympanogram abnormalities. In the 2- to 4-month range, however, there seems to be enough structural integrity of the external ear canal to support adultlike tympanometric patterns obtained with low-frequency probe tones.

# Middle Ear Muscle Reflex Assessment

The acoustic reflex threshold test demonstrates the lowest intensity of an acoustic stimulus at which a change in middle ear immittance can be measured. This change usually occurs when the stimuli used are from 70 to 100 dB HL for pure tones and from approximately 65 to 70 dB HL for broad-band noises. The reflex can be recorded either from the same ear that is being stimulated with sound or from the opposite ear simultaneously. Jerger, Harford, Clemis, and Alford (1974) showed that any differences between ipsilateral and contralateral reflex measures are due to neuromuscular events.

We encourage both ipsilateral and contralateral reflex recordings in infants and young children, with probably the most useful data being acquired from ipsilateral recordings. The absence of a reflex to an ipsilateral stimulus in the presence of normal tympanometric shapes strongly suggests peripheral hearing loss. We would also encourage the use of nonacoustic reflex elicitation (stroking of the tragus or eyelid) to rule out the absence of the stapedius muscle or some other occult obstructions to valid measurements (Djupesland, 1975). Probably the most useful data to be obtained in this case is the presence of an acoustic reflex in the ear with the immittance probe; conductive or severe to profound sensorineural pathology could not exist in an ear with this condition. Therefore, the use of middle ear measurements along with evoked potentials constitutes a strong pair of diagnostic tools to extract middle ear or cochlear disorders.

# Eustachian-Tube Function Tests

Often negative pressure can be seen tympanometrically in that the most compliant portion of the ear is found at around -150 to -200 millimeters of water pressure. Crying or swallowing will "pop the ear" and equalize the pressure in young children. Givens and Seidemann (1984) summarize eustachian-tube function tests succinctly and discuss their utility in clinical service.

# When to Use Middle Ear Assessment

We make it a practice of using immittance measures on virtually every patient who comes into the clinic. There are occasionally patients who cannot be tested and also some patients whose test data cannot always be interpreted unequivocally.

The tests are most effective for screening for middle ear pathology, screening for the presence or absence of normal middle ear muscle reflexes, and screening for facial nerve function.

The tests are best used in conjunction with ABR and/or a full audiologic test battery, but in children and infants they can be used extensively for cross-checking clinical observations. For example, it is highly unlikely that a patient who has no response behaviorally to sound is physiologically deaf if he or she has reflexes at levels between 70 and 80 dB HL. Conversely, a child who appears to give responses behaviorally in the range of 20 to 30 dB, and has normal tympanometry but *no reflexes*, is still highly suspect for deafness. Physiologic cross-evaluation with other procedures including ABR would be strongly encouraged; in such a case we reiterate the importance of nonacoustic reflexes if tympanometry is normal and reflexes are absent. Middle ear measurements then are powerful cross-checks for behavioral observations. The enigmatic patient who is said to have auditory problems by families and other clinicians but who shows normal behavioral audiograms may show abnormalities in the ipsilateral versus contralateral reflex evaluations and/or in reflex decay. A knowledge of the reflex arc here helps the interpretation of results. An absent reflex is *not* an acceptable variant of normal, as is so often transmitted in the oral tradition; many audiologists have been taught erroneously that absent middle ear muscle reflexes are common and should not be an area of concern. In fact, there are a few people who show no middle ear muscle reflexes because they lack stapedius muscles. No one really knows the full extent of this anomaly, but, by using a nonacoustic stimulation (a puff of air to the eyelid or a gentle rub of the fingertip or wisp of cotton in the anterior tragal region), we can reveal the function of the stapedius muscle. If there is a contraction to nonacoustic stimulation but no contraction to acoustic stimulation, this is not a normal variant and should be considered a pathologic sign. Thus we use reflexes on virtually every patient and try to integrate the reflex results with the general pattern of behavioral audiometry and ABR.

# How to Conduct Middle Ear Assessment

The ear should be examined for obstructions, tori, cerumen, or other obstacles as well as perforations of the tympanic membrane. We enjoy a productive working relationship with our otolaryngology group and usually have each infant seen by an otolaryngologist just before any audiologic test procedures.

The single most important steps for us are the acquisition of a seal and of course the acquisition of reflex data. Since each device has a somewhat different sealing mechanism and reflex testing mechanism, it is difficult to give useful instructions on exactly how to perform an immittance test. It is simply more productive to advise that, where possible, both ipsilateral and contralateral reflex data be obtained and compared to one another. Reflex decay and SPAR (Sensitivity Prediction from Acoustic Reflexes) are useful adjuncts to the basic procedures and are acquired if time and conditions permit (Jerger, Burney, Mauldin, & Crump, 1974).

# How to Interpret Middle Ear Tests

The results of the tests must be interpreted in context with all the other data. First, it should be recalled that there are three requisite conditions for the observation of a middle ear muscle reflex using one of the commonly available commercial immittance units:

1. The middle ear must be normal (operationally defined here as displaying a Type A tympanogram).

2. The stimulus must discharge many single units strongly and synchronously. That is, the stimulus must be clearly audible to the subject and in fact loud, although loudness per se is not a key requisite to elicit the reflex. (*Proof*: a "loud" 4000 to 8000 Hz tone often fails to discharge enough fibers to elicit a reflex contraction of the stapes even in a normal hearing subject.)

3. The reflex arc must be intact. The reflex arc involves the ipsilateral cochlea, the eighth-nerve, cochlear nucleus, and the contralateral medial nucleus of the trapezoid body, the medial superior olive to the facial anastomosis, and the seventh (facial) nerve to the stapedius muscle. Ipsilaterally the pathway moves from the cochlear nucleus to the ipsilateral medial superior olive, then down the seventh nerve.

For example, if a child were to show a normal Wave I latency on the ABR, and perhaps even normal Waves II and III, but only ipsilateral reflexes and not contralateral reflex contractions, we should conclude that there might be an interruption in the reflex arc around the IVth ventricle. Case 6 shows just such an anomaly: the first three waves from the ABR are intact, but only ipsilateral reflexes can be observed (Figure 5.12). The patient died of a gliomatous process in the brainstem that served to obstruct the reflex arc for the contralateral reflexes and desynchronized the auditory brainstem response of fourth- through fifth-order neurons.

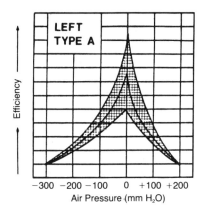
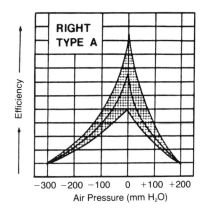

## Acoustic Reflex Thresholds

|       | 500 | 1000 | 2000 | 4000 | Hz      |
|-------|-----|------|------|------|---------|
| **LEFT** | A   | A    | A    | A    | Contra  |
|       | 70  | 80   | 85   | 90   | Ipsi    |

|        | 500 | 1000 | 2000 | 4000 | Hz      |
|--------|-----|------|------|------|---------|
| **RIGHT** | A   | A    | A    | A    | Contra  |
|        | 80  | 80   | 85   | 90   | Ipsi    |

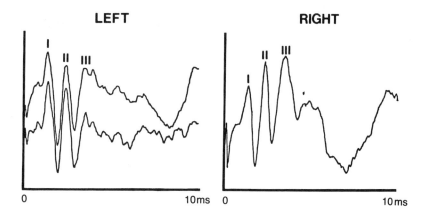

**Figure 5.12.** Case 6. Tympanograms, contralateral and ipsilateral acoustic reflex thresholds, and air-conducted pulse ABRs obtained from a patient with a brainstem disorder.

Conversely, if a child were to show normal middle ear reflexes at all levels, failed to respond to sound, and failed to develop speech and language normally, we might consider as possible diagnostic options bilateral peripheral cochlear loss with recruitment, or perhaps rostral brainstem or even cerebral disease. Naturally there are many other options, including autism and mental retardation, but the presence of the reflexes rules out profound peripheral deafness and is clearly compatible with either a normal high-intensity ABR or a normal ABR at low intensities. Note, however, that many neurologic test stations use only one level of pulse presentation (usually around 80 dB HLN, or about 115 dB peak SPL), which can often produce a normal-looking ABR despite the presence of severe peripheral cochlear hearing loss. It is for these, as well as many other reasons, that we recommend a latency-intensity function ABR, which compares consistently and uniformly with both ipsilateral and contralateral middle ear muscle reflex tests. The importance of this internal consistency and the validity of the cross-check cannot be overstressed (Hayes & Jerger, 1981).

# Summary

The anatomy and physiology of the auditory system, especially around the area of the IVth ventricle, are such that interrelationships between the ABR and immittance measures yield powerful and productive indices of auditory function (Hannley, Jerger, & Rivera, 1983). The practical application of these interrelationships is especially productive in the assessment of infants and difficult-to-test children. This chapter has shown how, when, and why we do auditory brainstem response and immittance studies on the pediatric population in our care, and how and why bone conduction as well as 500 Hz toneburst stimuli should be used during ABR in conjunction with the more commonly applied high-intensity air-conducted 100 microsecond pulse.

# References

Bennett, M. J., & Weatherby, L. A. (1982). Newborn acoustic reflexes to noise and pure tone signals. *Journal of Speech and Hearing Research, 10,* 265–281.

Coats, A. C., & Martin, J. L. (1977). Human auditory nerve action potentials and brainstem evoked responses: Effects of audiogram shape and lesion location. *Archives of Otolaryngology, 103,* 605–622.

Djupesland, G. (1975). Advanced reflex considerations. In J. Jerger (Ed.), *Handbook of clinical impedance audiometry* (Chap. 5, pp. 85–126). Dobbs Ferry, NY: American Electromedics Corporation.

*Ear and Hearing.* (1984). Vol. 5 [Special issue: Middle ear measures.] Baltimore: Williams and Wilkins.

Feldman, A. S., & Wilber, L. A. (Eds.). (1976). *Acoustic impedance and admittance: The measurement of middle ear function.* Baltimore: Williams and Wilkins.

Givens, G. D., & Seidemann, M. F. (1984). Acoustic immittance testing of the Eustachian tube. *Ear and Hearing, 5,* 297–299.

Glattke, T. (1983). *Short-latency auditory evoked potentials.* Austin, TX: PRO-ED.

Goldstein, R., & Rodman, L. (1967). Early components of average evoked responses to rapidly repeating auditory stimuli. *Journal of Speech and Hearing Research, 10,* 697–705.

Hannley, M., Jerger, J., & Rivera, V. (1983). Relationships among auditory brainstem responses, masking level differences and the acoustic reflex in multiple sclerosis. *Audiology, 22,* 20–33.

Hayes, D., & Jerger, J. (1981). Patterns of acoustic reflex and auditory brainstem response abnormality. *Acta Otolaryngologica, 92,* 199–209.

Jacobson, J. T. (Ed.). (1985). *The auditory brainstem response.* San Diego: College-Hill Press.

Jerger, J. (Ed.). (1975). *Handbook of clinical impedance audiometry.* Dobbs Ferry, NY: American Electromedics Corporation.

Jerger, J. (Ed.). (1984). *Pediatric audiology.* San Diego: College-Hill Press.

Jerger, J., Anthony, L., Jerger, S., & Crump, B. (1974). Studies in impedance audiometry: III. Middle ear disorders. *Archives of Otolaryngology, 99,* 165–171.

Jerger, J., Burney, P., Mauldin, L., & Crump, B. (1974). Predicting hearing loss from the acoustic reflex. *Journal of Speech and Hearing Disorders, 39,* 11–22.

Jerger, J., Harford, E., Clemis, J., & Alford, B. (1974). The acoustic reflex in VIIIth nerve disorders. *Archives of Otolaryngology, 99,* 409–413.

Jerger, J., Oliver, T., & Stach, B. (1985). Auditory brainstem response testing strategies. In J. T. Jacobson (Ed.), *The auditory brainstem response.* San Diego: College-Hill Press.

Jewett, D., Romano, M., & Williston, J. (1970). Human auditory evoked potentials: Possible brainstem components detected on the scalp. *Science, 167,* 1517–1518.

Jewett, D., & Williston, J. (1971). Auditory evoked far fields averaged from the scalp of humans. *Brain, 94,* 681–696.

Kraus, N., Ozdamar, O., Heydemann, P. T., Stein, L., & Reed, N. (1984). Auditory brainstem responses in hydrocephalic patients. *Electroencephalography and Clinical Neurophysiology, 59,* 310–317.

Margolis, R. H., & Shanks, J. E. (1985). Tympanometry. In J. Katz (Ed.), *Handbook of clinical audiology* (3rd ed., Chap. 23, pp. 438–475). Baltimore: Williams and Wilkins.

Metz, O. (1946). The acoustic impedance measured on normal and pathological ears. *Acta Otolaryngologica* (Suppl. 63).

Northern, J., & Downs, M. (1984). *Hearing in children* (3rd ed.). Baltimore: Williams and Wilkins.

Ozdamar, O., & Kraus, N. (1983). Auditory middle-latency responses in humans. *Audiology, 22,* 34–49.

Picton, T. W., Woods, D. L., Baribeau-Braun, J., & Healey, T. M. G. (1977). Evoked potential audiometry. *Journal of Otolaryngology, 6,* 90–119.

Popelka, G. R. (Ed.). (1981). *Hearing assessment with the acoustic reflex.* New York: Grune and Stratton.

Popelka, G. R. (1984). Acoustic immittance measures: Terminology and instrumentation. *Ear and Hearing, 5,* 262–267.

Ruben, R. J., Knickerbocker, G. G., Sekula, J., Nager, G. T., & Bordley, J. E. (1959). Cochlear potentials in man. A preliminary report. *Laryngoscope, 69,* 665–671.

Schwartz, D. M., Larson, V. D., & DeChicchis, A. R. (1985). Spectral characteristics of air and bone conduction transducers used to record the auditory brainstem response. *Ear and Hearing, 6,* 274–277.

Shanks, J. E. (1984). Tympanometry. *Ear and Hearing, 5,* 268–280.

Silman, S. (Ed.). (1984). *The acoustic reflex: Basic principles and clinical application.* New York: Academic Press.

Sohmer, H., & Feinmesser, M. (1967). Cochlear action potentials recorded from the external ear in man. *Annals of Otology, Rhinology, and Laryngology, 76,* 427–435.

Sprague, B. H., Wiley, T. L., & Goldstein, R. (1985). Tympanometric and acoustic-reflex studies in neonates. *Journal of Speech and Hearing Research, 28,* 265–272.

Wright, P. F., McConnell, K. B., Thompson, J. M., Vaughn, W. K., & Sell, S. H. (1985). A longitudinal study of the detection of otitis media in the first two years of life. *International Journal of Pediatric Otorhinolaryngology, 10,* 245–252.

# 6

# Tests of Hearing—
# The Infant

## WILLIAM R. HODGSON

*T*he first purpose of an audiologist in dealing with children is to identify auditory disorder. If a hearing loss is found, its nature and magnitude must be determined. The audiologist must ask whether the disorder, as measured, is sufficient to explain observed behavior. The social, educational, and vocational implications of the disorder must be explored. Habilitative procedures must begin.

When working with infants, eliciting the information described above is not easy, but remarkable progress has been made in our ability to do so. Key elements in this progress are (1) the concept of evaluation as an ongoing process to assess disorders with greater precision over time and (2) the availability of a battery of audiologic tests, rather than a single procedure, so that children within a wide range of functional capacity can be accurately evaluated.

In this chapter I explain clinical and experimental procedures used to access auditory function in infants from birth to 2 years of age and discuss developmental norms and maturation of auditory behavior. I describe the variables that affect test responses and assess the validity of procedures used in infant audiometry. My major objective is to explain the techniques that have clinical utility in assessing the auditory sensitivity of infants.

# Infant Development and Response

To assess infants with auditory disorder, audiologists must know how normal infants behave and what the developmental norms for motor, auditory, language, and speech acquisition are. Audiologists should observe normal infants to become familiar with their appearance and behavior. The audiologist's training should include courses in child development, and he or she should have available for review and reference some books on child development, such as Mussen, Conger, and Kagan (1974) and Smart and Smart (1982). Audiologists must be sufficiently familiar with infants to feel at ease during testing, to know the capabilities of their patients, and to differentiate normal and abnormal behavior.

Some basic information about infant development is presented below. It must be remembered that developmental guidelines are averages and that a range of normal development reflects individual differences. Parents, too, should be reminded of this normal variability. Otherwise, they may react inappropriately to one child through comparison with the development of siblings.

## Neonates

The neonatal period is important to us because programs for early detection of auditory disorders concentrate on infants at this age. Almost all infants are in hospital nurseries at this time and are available for testing.

Determination of prematurity in neonates is important because this condition is correlated with such disorders found later on in life as increased behavioral and reading problems (Lubchenco et al., 1963) and hearing loss (Vernon, 1967). With considerable variability, the average weight of neonates is about 3,300 grams. If birth weight is less than 2,500 grams, infants are considered premature. Another criterion for prematurity is a gestation period of less than 37 weeks (Smart & Smart, 1982).

Although visual discrimination is reported to be poor (Held, 1979), the neonate can usually follow a slowly moving object directly in front of the face. Wolff (1966) found that 8 of 12 infants followed movement of a red ball within 2 hours of birth, and all responded within 24 hours. Control of motor activity in the neonate is limited. Visual responses may be slow, with jerky movements and poor coordination. Eye movement toward the source of sound (cochleo-oculogyric reflex) may be observed both independent of and in conjunction with head-turning responses. Motor behavior of the neonate that is useful for auditory testing is primarily limited to reflexive responses, and more of these responses are described below.

An eye blink in response to sound is called an auropalpebral reflex (APR) or cochleopalpebral reflex. This response is commonly observed in infants. The eyelid movement may be seen in waking or sleeping babies. Froding (1960) reported it to be the most reliable auditory response in neonates. Eisenberg, Coursin, and Rupp (1966) considered the APR a most useful response because it is common and resistant to extinction. That is, an infant may continue to respond with APRs even after repeated presentation of the stimulus. With both infants and adults, a relatively intense signal is required for elicitation of the APR. Wedenberg (1956) reported that SPLs of 105–115 dB were required for pure tones to result in APRs in neonates.

More recent information indicates that signal complexity plays an important role in determining whether or not the infant will respond. Babies respond more reliably and at lower levels to broad-band signals than to pure tones or other narrow-band signals (Gerber, 1985). Northern and Downs (1984) indicated that APRs can be reliably elicited, in a quiet room, with broad-band signals (noisemakers) at 50–70 dB SPL. They also indicated that APRs occur for speech signals at about 55–75 dB SPL. Broad-band signals with substantial energy across a wide frequency range, while they are more likely to elicit a response, are not good stimuli for detecting all hearing losses. Many individuals with handicapping high-frequency sensorineural loss have normal or near normal low-frequency sensitivity and can respond to a broad-band signal that has low-frequency components.

In addition to the APR, a startle response to auditory and other stimuli is frequently observed in neonates. Hardy, Dougherty, and Hardy (1959) observed startle responses in neonates from a noisemaker at a reported 64 dB as measured via the B-weighting network of a sound-level meter. Northern and Downs (1984) reported expected startle responses in infants to speech at a level of about 65 dB HL.

Other arousal or orientation responses may be observed. The sucking reflex may occur—and is probably more likely when the infant is hungry—on presentation of auditory stimuli. On the other hand, an infant already engaged in sucking may stop or diminish this activity when an auditory signal is presented, although Kaye and Levin (1963) did not demonstrate significant differences between experimental and control groups in this respect.

Changes in respiratory pattern can sometimes be seen on presentation of an auditory signal. In addition to the visually observable chest or abdominal movements, more sensitive graphic recordings of respiratory patterns during auditory stimulation as well as cardiac rate measurement (cardiotachometry) and impedance audiometry have been found useful. This latter has been particularly helpful in corroborating information about auditory response and indicating the status of the peripheral auditory mechanism. Evoked response audiometry and electrocochleography are also useful techniques.

Other factors that influence responses to acoustic signals are postconceptual age, the activity state of the neonate, and the ambient noise level. Gerber (1985) determined that a group of premature infants responded to stimuli on 28% of the trials while a group of full-term infants responded to the same stimuli on only 19% of the trials. Perhaps the difference is attributable to the less mature neuromuscular system of the preterm infant and reduced ability to inhibit responses to auditory stimuli.

Activity state contributes not only to whether the neonate responds but also to the type of response. This state may be described in terms of level of activity: deep sleep, light sleep, awake and quiet, or awake and active. Classifications and descriptions of activity states vary. Deep sleep, however, is characterized by little body movement except for sporadic startle responses, little or no eye movement, and rhythmic respiration. In light sleep there is considerable body and eye movement, with occasional flutter of the eyelids. Respiration is less regular than in deep sleep. Awake and quiet is characterized by open eyes and some movement of the head and limbs. Infants in the awake and active stage engage in generalized body movement, breathe irregularly, and vocalize. Northern and Downs (1984) suggested that deep and light sleep may be differentiated by flicking the eyelashes or touching the infant's eyelid lightly. The deeply sleeping infant does not respond, but the lightly sleeping infant responds with eye and other small body movements.

The type of response made by the infant not only varies according to state but also seems to follow the law of initial value (Bench, 1970). That is, the quieter the prestimulus state, the greater the increase in activity upon stimulation; the more active the prestimulus state, the greater the decrease in activity. Thus, a startle or body movement is a more likely response from quietly sleeping infants; reduction or cessation of movement is more probable from an active infant.

There is evidence suggesting that, especially for neonates, light sleep may be the best state for auditory assessment. False positive responses are likely to be reduced, and more responses may be observable than at other activity levels. Eisenberg, Griffin, Coursin, and Hunter (1964) observed a higher percentage of responses to noisemakers from neonates in light sleep or less than full wakefulness than from those either deeply asleep or fully awake. Bench and Mentz (1975) reported a similar finding when neonates, 6-week-old infants, and 6-month-old infants were stimulated with broad-band noise at 90 dB SPL. However, they found some interesting interactions between signal intensity, activity state, and age. That is, the neonates responded to the 90 dB SPL signal better when sleeping than when awake, but they responded better to a 60 dB signal when awake. An increase in signal complexity enhanced response. All groups responded better to broad-band than narrow-band signals. There was a relatively better response to a speech signal from infants in the 6-month-old group than from the younger subjects.

The probability of response increases in a quiet environment. For this reason, Northern and Downs (1984) recommended that auditory screening not be done in a room where the noise level exceeds 60 dB SPL.

## Older Infants

Growth and motor development are extensive during the first year; by the end of a year the infant may weigh about 24 pounds. Important motor development milestones are the ability to hold the head erect while sitting (3–4 months), to sit alone (6–7 months), and to walk alone (soon after the first birthday).

Several new responses that are useful in auditory evaluation develop during the first year. The developing ability to locate the source of sound is probably the most useful. Orienting responses in the first weeks of life may show crude localization attempts but are more commonly and noticeably manifested by reduction in general motor activity. Localization efforts mature with motor development and experience in hearing.

In normal infants localization efforts—searching for the source of sound—can be expected to begin by 3 months. By then motor control is sufficient for the baby to hold the head erect and make controlled if wobbly head movements to the right and left. Murphy (1969) reported maturation of localization as shown in Figure 6.1. By about 3 months (A), infants may localize on a horizontal plane, but do not look below or above eye level for the source of sounds unless an additional visual component directs them there. By 5 months (B), a horizontal localization effort may terminate in a vertical head movement toward a sound source originating below eye level. This inefficient movement may progress to an arc by 6 months (C) and to efficient direct localization by 7½ months (D). Quick and accurate localization of sound requires both motor coordination and listening experience. Therefore, usefulness of this orienting response is limited in infants either with motor retardation or with hearing loss, which reduces their auditory experience.

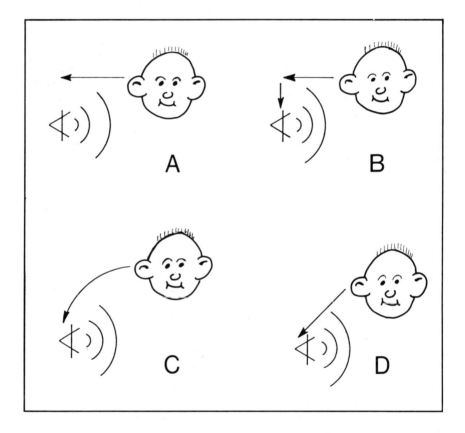

**Figure 6.1.** Stages in the development of auditory localization. A, 3 months: head movement along horizontal plane, generally toward sound source. B, 5 months: inefficient horizontal, then vertical orientation toward sound source. C, 6 months: improvement in moving head toward sound source. D, 7½ months: direct and efficient localization of a sound source. Based on Murphy (1969).

Experimenters have long demonstrated that neonates and other infants under 1 year can be conditioned to respond to auditory signals by classical or instrumental conditioning procedures. For example, Aldrich (1928) paired presentation of an acoustic signal and a pinscratch on the foot of a 3-month-old infant. After 15 trials the infant withdrew its foot on presentation of the acoustic signal only. Marquis (1931) successfully conditioned 7 out of 8 infants from 1 to 10 days of age to respond by sucking when they heard a signal that had been previously presented along with the infants' bottles. Fulton, Gorzycki, and Hull (1975) attempted to establish auditory stimulus-response control for pure-tone audiometry in 12 children 9–25 months of age, with a median age of 12 months (mean = 13.8 months). Edible reinforcers were used, and subjects responded by pressing a bar. The investigators successfully conditioned 7 of the 12 subjects to respond to low-level signals near expected normal threshold or at screening levels of 15 dB HL. Those successfully conditioned ranged in age from 12 to 25 months, with a median age of 14 months (mean = 16.4 months). The number of training sessions averaged 11.4, with a mean time of 11.5 minutes per session.

To summarize, numerous investigators have established responses from normal hearing infants under 12 months of age using classical or instrumental conditioning procedures under laboratory conditions. Use of reinforcement principles to strengthen and maintain auditory behavior already present in infants has shown clinical utility.

In addition to measures of auditory sensitivity, some information about auditory discrimination ability in infants also exists. Bronstein and Petrova (1967) demonstrated frequency discrimination in neonates. They obtained sucking responses on presentation of an auditory signal. Habituation occurred after repeated presentation, and the responses stopped. When the frequency of the signal was changed, the responses reoccurred. Butterfield and Hodgson (1969) demonstrated different sucking behavior in neonates when presentation of music was contingent on the infants sucking or not sucking.

Reduction of response through habituation must also be considered a form of auditory discrimination. Eisenberg, Marmarou, and Giovachino (1974a) found cardiac deceleration in neonates at least 70% of the time on presentation of the vowel /a/ at 68 dB SPL. In a companion article (Eisenberg, Marmarou, & Giovachino, 1974b), these authors reported differences in habituation rate between normal and high-risk infants. They believe this phenomenon may be useful in detecting infants in whom subtle auditory problems may later become evident. Eilers, Wilson, and Moore (1977) used visual reinforcement to establish that many infants 6 to 14 months of age could differentiate speech sounds. Continued study of infants' discrimination abilities and the development of age-related norms may lead to clinically useful tests of the auditory discrimination ability of hearing-impaired infants.

# Auditory Assessment

Now that we have had a brief look at infant development and the responses that babies are capable of, let's turn our attention to some actual test procedures and philosophies. We will begin by looking at the question of identification of hearing loss in neonates through programs that try to detect hearing loss in newborn infants.

There is no question that the neonate can hear. In fact, the presence of even prenatal response to sound is well established (Bench, 1968; Elliot & Elliot, 1964). However, the clinician must be alert to the possibility that anesthetics given to the mother may reduce auditory and visual responses of the neonate for several hours after birth.

According to Jaffe (1972), the external ear canal of the neonate can be expected to contain blood and vernix caseosum, the waxy substance that coats the skin of the newborn. However, Jaffe continued, these materials dehydrate in a few hours. Keith (1976) obtained tympanograms on 60 neonates. He had the vernix removed from the canals of 20 infants between 2½ and 20 hours of age, but did not clear the canals of the older neonates. Results were similar to normal tympanograms in older children, with maximum compliance near atmospheric pressure. Fourteen infants had tympanograms with a notch-shaped curve and two points of maximum compliance near atmospheric pressure. Keith concluded that the results ". . . are virtually incompatible with an ear full of fluid or mucous and the normal tympanogram indicates that middle-ear mobility is normal almost from birth. The findings of normal compliance measurements and well-aerated middle ears . . . would contradict statements in the literature that the middle ear is filled with a mucous cushion or mesenchymal tissue at birth" (p. 73). Bennett (1975) successfully obtained tympanograms from all 98 of his subjects between 5 and 218 hours of age. The tympanograms generally indicated normal middle ear pressure, although a fairly large number showed a notched tympanogram similar to that described in the study by Keith. Bennett felt that this notch was associated with the hypermobile neonatal tympanic membrane and that it disappears with maturation.

To repeat, there is no question that the neonate can hear. The questions needing answers are these: What are the least intense sounds that are audible? How useful is neonatal hearing? And, most important for our purposes, how can we detect those newborn infants who do not hear well? Possible answers to this last question are discussed below.

## Neonatal Hearing Screening Programs

Northern and Downs (1984) estimated that 1 in 750 neonates will be hearing-impaired. The occurrence of deafness among infants in the neonatal intensive care unit (NICU) is expected to be much higher. McFarland, Simmons, and Jones (1980) found hearing impairment in 1 in 954 babies in a well-baby nursery but in 1 in 56 in an intensive care nursery. It is most important that hearing loss be detected early to reduce the possible effects of sensory deprivation, to maximize use of remaining hearing to help the child learn language and speech, and to afford the parents an opportunity to learn the many things they need to know to cope with a hearing-impaired child.

In the 1960s large-scale efforts to detect hearing loss through neonatal audiometric screening got underway (Downs & Sterritt, 1964). As experience was gained in neonatal screening, two tracks developed. One consisted of identification audiometry. In most programs, a moderately intense high-frequency signal was delivered to the infant in the hospital nursery while one or more observers looked for a motor response. However, more sophisticated procedures, such as brainstem evoked response audiometry (BERA), have been utilized (Despland & Galambos, 1980). The other is use of a high-risk register, a list of conditions in the neonate with which a high incidence of hearing loss is known to be associated. Use of such a register alerts nursing personnel to infants who have an increased probability of hearing loss.

An example of a large-scale program of identification audiometry and follow-up was reported by Feinmesser et al. (1982). They screened 18,000 newborn infants and saw these babies again in well-baby clinics at the age of 5 to 7 months. On the basis of this experience, they concluded that the newborn screening program was too costly and impractical and changed their emphasis to use of a high-risk register at birth and a universal screening program when babies are 7 to 9 months old. After 40,000 infants had gone through this program and 69 had been detected with hearing impairment, it was determined that 35 of the infants would have been identified by use of a high-risk register alone. The other 34 were

not at risk, and therefore hearing impairment was detectable only by identification and audiometry procedures.

Herein lies the dilemma of the individual who attempts to detect hearing loss in infants: audiometric screening of all neonates has a high incidence of false positive and false negative results (Northern & Downs, 1984)
and is an expensive proposition. However, limiting our attention to infants
who appear on a high-risk register results in missing a significant number
of hearing losses.

In 1982 the Joint Committee on Infant Hearing Screening (1982)
published its current recommendations regarding detection of hearing
loss in infants. The committee recommended identification of hearing-
impaired infants by means of five risk criteria and suggested that follow-up
evaluation of infants at risk continue until accurate assessment of hearing is accomplished. The risk criteria are as follows:

1. A family history of childhood hearing impairment

2. Congenital perinatal infection such as cytomegalovirus, rubella, herpes,
   toxoplasmosis, or syphillis

3. Anatomic malformations involving the head or neck, such as dysmorphic appearance including syndromal and nonsyndromal abnormalities, overt or submucous cleft palate, or morphologic abnormalities
   of the pinna

4. Birth weight less than 1,500 grams

5. Hyperbilirubinemia at a level exceeding indications for exchange
   transfusion

6. Bacterial meningitis, especially *H. influenza*

7. Severe asphyxia, which may include infants with APGAR scores of
   0–3 who fail to institute spontaneous respiration within 10 minutes
   and those with hypotonia persisting to 2 hours of age.

For all infants in one or more of the above categories the committee
recommended audiometric screening under the supervision of an audiologist, preferably by 3 months and no later than 6 months of age.

Members of the Nova Scotia Conference on Early Identification of
Hearing Loss (Mencher, 1976) recommended that the high-risk register
may be supplemented by individual behavioral screening following a particular model. First, the ambient noise level at the time of the test should
be measured and reported. I believe that the conference members should
also have stipulated that the noise level not exceed 60 dB SPL, as recommended by Northern and Downs (1984). Second, the conference recommended that the infant be asleep prior to testing. One study indicated

that neonates sleep 80% of the time (Mussen et al., 1974). Therefore, although requiring a pretest state of sleep will obviously complicate the test procedure, it is not an impossible criterion. The evidence previously discussed justifies this requirement, and a state of light sleep, as defined earlier, is preferable. The conference members further recommended that the test stimulus be a predominately high-frequency complex signal with a sharp rise time, a maximum SPL of 90 dB, and a duration of ½ to 2 seconds, with an interstimulus interval of at least 5 seconds. The arousal response they stipulated can be any generalized body movement that involves more than one limb and that is accompanied by some form of eye movement. They suggested one of two scoring criteria: that the observer not know when a signal is presented or that two observers score the infant's response independently. Finally, they recommended that two or more responses out of eight stimuli be a passing score. Individual neonatal hearing screening should be done in addition to maintenance of a high-risk register if the procedures and criteria just presented can be met without equivocation. Particular attention to infants in the NICU is warranted. If not, the evidence suggests that the screening program will not be efficient or valid and that it would be better to rely on use of a high-risk register alone.

Objective automated devices for neonatal screening have been developed and are being assessed. One such unit was described by Altman, Shenhav, and Schaudinischky (1975, 1976). The device, called an Accelerometer Recording System, picks up movements of the infant's crib, and samples are recorded in association with stimulus presentations. Another device is the Crib-O-Gram (Simmons, 1976; Simmons & Russ, 1974). This device consists of a motion-sensitive transducer attached to a bassinet, a graphic recorder that records the measured motion, and timing and signal-generating equipment. Each test period consists of a 10-second prestimulus recording of bassinet activity, presentation of a 16-second test signal, and recording of activity during the subsequent 6 seconds. McFarland et al. (1980) reported that to that date over 12,000 neonates had been screened. Of this number, 10,497 were from well-baby nurseries and 1,576 were from NICUs. Eleven hearing-impaired babies had been detected from the well-baby nurseries and 28 from the NICUs. False positive results (babies with normal hearing who failed) and false negative results (infants with hearing loss who passed) were also given. Improved scoring criteria in effect since 1973 were reported to have reduced the false positive rate to an overall 9% and the false negative rate to 0.02%. However, Durieux-Smith, Picton, Edwards, Goodman, and MacMurray (1985) evaluated 306 infants in a NICU and reported a false positive rate with the Crib-O-Gram of about 33%. These results were obtained by comparing Crib-O-Gram results with those obtained by brainstem electric response audiometry (BERA). When the criterion for failing was 30 dB HL, compared to BERA results, the Crib-O-Gram test resulted in a false negative rate of about 52% for infants between 31 and 37 weeks of age and about 35% for infants between 38 and 54 weeks. While part of the disparity reported in the studies cited above is associated with the method used by the investigators to compute false positive and false negative rates (Ventry, 1982), the study by Durieux-Smith et al. suggests that the false positive rate with the Crib-O-Gram is disappointingly high. Moreover, 280 of the subjects were tested twice with the Crib-O-Gram, and 32% passed one and failed one Crib-O-Gram test. Test-retest reliability with BERA was not obtained. The investigators concluded that, for use in NICUs with populations similar to that tested, the Crib-O-Gram is unreliable, yields too many failures of infants with normal hearing sensitivity, and may miss babies with mild hearing losses that are detectable with BERA.

Automated procedures appear successful in detecting large hearing losses, but improvement is apparently needed in their ability to detect small hearing losses and in overall reliability. They are attractive in that they can be used with minimal disruption of nursery routine. Scoring of the infant's response is simplified. Validation of the procedures discussed above through field testing is still required. When these things are accomplished, automated procedures may come into routine use in neonatal screening programs.

In conclusion, high-risk registers have been shown to be reasonably effective in identifying infants who should be considered at risk for deafness. A register has been established for follow-up that strikes a fair compromise between the number of false positives and false negatives resulting from its use. Its use should be routine in all nurseries. However, if attention is limited to neonates at risk for deafness, some deaf babies will be missed. For this reason, hearing screening should also be conducted if a quality program can be maintained. Three final points should be kept in mind. First, authorities agree that current feasible procedures for screening neonates are sensitive only for severe to profound hearing losses (Mencher, 1976; Northern & Downs, 1984). Second, we know that at least some neonates with normal hearing at birth have progressive degenerative loss occurring early in childhood. Third, children are subject to developing and fluctuating conductive disorders. For these reasons, attention to hearing sensitivity must continue throughout childhood, and formal screening programs are a good idea whenever they can be instituted and done well (e.g., in well-baby clinics, nurseries and preschools, and regular schools).

## Behavioral Evaluation of Infants from Birth to 2 Years of Age

Clinical evaluation is required when infants at risk for hearing loss are isolated by a high-risk register, when infants fail hearing screening, or when auditory disorder is suspected for any reason. Screening procedures are often carried out by technicians or others trained for a nonprofessional role whereas clinical evaluation is the job of the audiologist. The successful pediatric audiologist is flexible, sees evaluation as an ongoing process, and is prepared to use a battery of procedures to adapt to the capacities of a particular infant. Table 6.1 shows response levels expected in normal hearing infants as a function of type of stimulus and age. A steady reduction occurs in the level needed to elicit a response, although simple signals (warble tones) continue to require a higher level.

During the last 30 years, great progress has been made in our ability to evaluate and habilitate hearing-impaired infants. Liden and Harford (1985) point out that the prevailing medical viewpoint in the early 1950s was that remediation with deaf children could not begin until they were 7 years of age and old enough to go to a school for the deaf. They note that the greatest contribution of pediatric audiology has been in emphasizing the importance of early education, speech, and language training and in changing the attitude of the medical community toward the management of hearing-impaired children. Unfortunately, traces of the regressive attitude remain. Not too long ago, Shah, Chandler, and Dale (1978) reported that a substantial delay often occurs between the first suspicion of hearing loss in young children and a firm diagnosis. Parents indicated

**TABLE 6.1**
**Minimum Response Levels as a Function of Stimulus and Age**

| Age | Noisemakers (Approx. dB SPL) | Warble Tones (dB HL) | Speech (dB HL) |
|---|---|---|---|
| 0–6 weeks | 50–70 | 78 | 40–60 |
| 6 weeks–4 months | 50–60 | 70 | 47 |
| 4–7 months | 40–50 | 51 | 21 |
| 7–9 months | 30–40 | 45 | 15 |
| 9–13 months | 25–35 | 38 | 8 |
| 13–16 months | 25–30 | 32 | 5 |
| 16–21 months | 25 | 25 | 5 |
| 21–24 months | 25 | 26 | 3 |

*Source:* Northern and Downs (1984, p. 135).

that a leading cause of the delay was the reluctance of the primary-care physician to believe parental concerns, to perform office screening tests, and to refer young children for audiologic evaluations.

Electrophysiological procedures—particularly brainstem evoked response audiometry and impedance measures—are helpful, as mentioned earlier. In conjunction with these tests, two other procedures with proven clinical utility for infants are discussed below.

One such procedure is behavioral observation audiometry. Testing infants up to 4 to 6 months of age generally involves stimuli similar to those used in screening neonates, and similar responses are sought. In other words, moderately intense stimuli are presented to elicit reflexive responses. The generalizations regarding activity state referred to earlier still obtain. The task may be more difficult than auditory screening because the audiologist is trying to get a more detailed measure of audition. Therefore, more auditory stimuli must be presented over a longer time, and adaption (habituation) as well as fatigue may affect responses.

In spite of these difficulties, procedures have been suggested to obtain differential information about auditory function for this age range. Wedenberg (1956) established that normal neonates were awakened by pure tones of 70–75 dB SPL, and APRs occurred at 105–115 dB SPL. Using this information, Wedenberg (1972) concluded that his procedure could be used to differentiate infants as follows. First, of course, if the infant awakens at signal intensities of 70 to 75 dB and gives APRs at 105–115 dB SPL, hearing is assumed normal. Second, a cochlear problem with recruitment may be present if an APR occurs at the expected signal intensity but the infant requires more than 75 dB to awaken. Third, a conductive or retrocochlear disorder may be present if no APR occurs at 105–115 dB and if the infant awakens in response to some level above 75 dB. Finally, deafness is indicated by no response. As is the case with most tests, the results of this procedure alone should not be considered definitive. Along with other tests, however, it may provide useful information.

I believe it is best to use electronically generated signals, even with children from 3 to 4 months of age. We are kidding ourselves when we attribute precise intensity and frequency measurements to most noise-makers. Bove and Flugrath (1973) analyzed 25 noisemakers and concluded that 20 had spectra too wide for clinical use. They found only 5 that had acceptable high-frequency characteristics. We may agonize over a signal that achieves an appropriate compromise between the frequency-restricted stimulus we would like to use to determine configuration of the hearing loss and a signal that is sufficiently complex to maximize auditory response in infants.

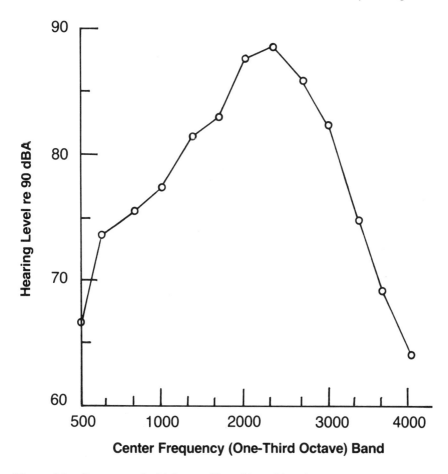

**Figure 6.2.** Spectrum of a high-pass filtered broad-band noise recommended for auditory evaluation of infants. Data from Mencher (1976).

Figure 6.2 shows the signal recommended by the Nova Scotia Conference on the Early Identification of Hearing Loss (Mencher, 1976). This predominantly high-frequency signal should be most sensitive to the high-frequency configuration that prevails in sensorineural disorders but still maintain enough broad-band energy to encourage responses in normal hearing infants.

Because infants at 3 or 4 months of age sleep much less than neonates, it may be difficult to find them quiet enough for testing. By letting them take a bottle, responses in the resultant relatively quiet state may be observed, and after eating they may fall asleep. Responses may include startle, APR, initiation or cessation of sucking, observable change in respiration pattern, or arousal. More than one observer should record responses independently. Responses should not be accepted unless they can be repeated.

A second useful procedure for infants is visual reinforcement audiometry (VRA). From 3 to 4 months of age, as motor control develops, the orientation response mentioned earlier may develop. This response lends itself to auditory testing in a sound field. The stimuli generally used are warble tones or narrow bands of noise. Some infants, especially younger ones, may respond only to speech. As mentioned earlier, the disadvantage of a broad-band signal is that infants with normal sensitivity across any part of the signal's spectrum may respond; as a consequence, high-frequency losses are missed or their severity underestimated. I have had some success with filtering the speech spectrum to supply a more useful signal. I prefer to do this with live voice, using variable-frequency filters in the audiometer circuit for the additional flexibility afforded. Use of a tape-recorded signal is awkward when working with infants and younger children, since constraints associated with selecting and cuing desired signals add another variable to an already complex situation.

Proposals to divide speech into several frequency bands may have clinical utility to provide estimates of hearing sensitivity (Franklin, 1980). However, we must remember that the results may be influenced by irregular audiometric configurations. That is, when signals other than pure tones are used, there is always the possibility that the patient is responding to energy that is remote from the central frequency that we think is being tested (Koval & Stelmachowicz, 1983). The result, in patients with high-frequency loss, may be underestimation of hearing deficit; the broader the band of the signal, the greater the error may be.

A convenient sound-field audiometry setup is shown in Figure 6.3. The infant is placed between two loudspeakers, either supported in an infant seat or seated in a highchair. The head should be free to turn. It may be better for the parent not to hold the child because of distraction or inadvertent clues. However, infants who will remain quiet only when held should sit on the parent's lap, facing forward, with no more support of the head and upper trunk than is necessary.

It is a good idea to have an assistant in the test room to keep the infant's attention minimally directed toward the front between signals and otherwise to help keep the test situation under control.

Attractive animated toys adjacent to the loudspeakers may provide reinforcement and reduce habituation, although they may not be very effective for 3- to 5-month-old infants. Moore, Wilson, and Thompson (1977) reported that use of an animated toy reinforced responses in infants

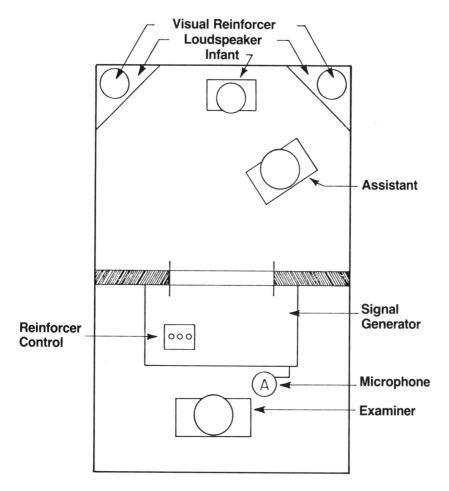

**Figure 6.3.** Setup for localization audiometry.

between 5 and 11 months of age. However, their study showed no statistically significant differences in responses of a group of 4-month-old infants compared with a control group who received no such reinforcement.

Various stimuli have been used as reinforcers in addition to the animated toys just mentioned. These have included flashing lights and lighted pictures. Moore, Thompson, and Thompson (1975) reported stronger reinforcement from the complex visual image of an animated, lighted toy than from a reinforcer consisting of only a flashing light. However, a few infants, especially younger ones, may be frightened by an animated toy. Therefore, it is probably better to have available both an animated toy for its superior reinforcing strength and a simpler flashing light or lighted picture for the few babies who may react with fear to the complex reinforcer.

In VRA the signal is presented, and, if the child looks toward the loudspeaker, the reinforcer is activated briefly. If there is no response, the assistant may direct the child's attention toward the loudspeaker, physically moving the head if necessary. If a reliable stimulus-response pattern can be established, with accurate localization, both loudspeakers can be used. Slavish alternation between loudspeakers should be avoided to prevent anticipatory false responses. After each response, the assistant should bring the infant's attention back to midline.

It may help to do initial conditioning and testing with a broad-band signal to optimize probability of response. The initial presentation level should depend on a pretest observation of the child's responses to environmental sounds. To minimize the overall number of stimulus presentations, an ideal level would be one that is obviously audible but not a great deal above apparent threshold. After sufficient conditioning trials to establish a consistent head-turning response, search for threshold begins. Thompson and Wilson (1984) recommended a "down 20, up 10" procedure in which the level is reduced 20 dB after each response and then increased in 10 dB steps until the child again responds. In this manner the minimum response level is determined. Testing can then continue with signals that are more frequency-selective.

Presumably because of reduced auditory experience, infants with severe or profound hearing loss may not respond consistently to sounds above their auditory threshold. If they do attempt to respond, they may not be able to localize accurately. When I see such confusion in localization attempts, I use only one loudspeaker for all signal generations. Then, if the animated toy does in fact serve as a reinforcer, the infant has only one source toward which to look for reinforcement.

The biggest limitations of sound-field localization audiometry lies in two areas. First, infants—especially those under 1 year of age—who have a severe or profound loss may not respond at all in this situation. Of course, even this eventuality provides helpful information, indicating the probability of a hearing loss of considerable magnitude. Additional confirming information may be available through some of the procedures described above or through techniques such as auditory brainstem response and impedance measures. Second, as is true with all sound-field audiometry, the information obtained is almost exclusively associated with the infant's better ear. A unilateral hearing loss will probably not be identifiable. Nevertheless, an estimate of the infant's functional auditory status can be obtained.

One marked advantage of sound-field localization audiometry is that it provides a quick and easy method of substantiating functionally normal hearing sensitivity in situations where an infant's hearing is suspect for one reason or another. If the orientation response has developed, the infant will respond to low-intensity test signals without lengthy training sessions or much specialized equipment beyond that routinely present in an audiometric test unit.

Let us review some experimental results obtained with localization audiometry. Suzuki and Ogiba (1961) reported on a procedure they called conditioned orientation reflex (COR) audiometry. In their procedure two loudspeakers are placed some distance apart, and near each is a semi-transparent doll with a light behind it. A signal is presented, and a second later the light behind the doll is lighted. The visual stimulus, if not the auditory, causes the child to look toward the source. The hope is to condition the child to respond to the auditory signal. If the conditioning is successful, the doll is subsequently lighted only after response to the auditory stimulus occurs—in the hope that this procedure will be reinforcing and maintain response. In this event, intensity and frequency of test signals are varied until the desired information is obtained. Suzuki and Ogiba reported that COR audiometry required an average of 5 minutes for infants under 1 year of age and was successful in 44.8% of their test sample. The success rate for older children was much higher.

Liden and Kankkunen (1969), who coined the term visual reinforcement audiometry (VRA), placed loudspeakers near and on either side of the infant's head. Associated with the loudspeakers on either side were frosted glass windows on which slides of attractive pictures could be projected. They presented the test signal and visual stimuli using the same procedure described by Suzuki and Ogiba. In addition to orientation response, Liden and Kankkunen accepted any visible response. They reported VRA could reliably evaluate infants from about 6 to 8 months of age. By plugging the ear that was not being tested and observing responses, they were able to obtain information from each ear separately when differences between ears did not exceed the attenuation characteristics of the plug plus the magnitude of the head shadow. In a group of normal infants between 3 and 11 months of age, they reported mean monaural thresholds for warble tones at octave intervals from 250 through 4000 Hz at about 30 dB HL.

Haug, Baccaro, and Guilford (1967) also reported on a modification of the localization procedure that permits evaluation of each ear separately.

They called their procedure the PIWI technique, which stands for ''puppet in the window illuminated,'' a description of the reinforcer they used. After testing in sound field with a procedure similar to that of Suzuki and Ogiba, they placed earphones on their subjects and continued the stimuli, hoping that the previously conditioned response would generalize to the new situation. Of eight subjects between 5 and 12 months of age, most of whom had a hearing loss, the authors reported 100% success in the initial sound-field segment of the test. On six of the eight subjects, they reported success in obtaining complete pure-tone air- and bone-conduction audiograms. That is, the response that generalized to earphone testing was also maintained when the test signals were delivered by the bone-conduction vibrator.

Close agreement has been reported between minimal response levels obtained from localization audiometry and air-conduction thresholds obtained with earphones. Matkin (1973) compared better-ear results so obtained in a group of 26 children between 1–3 and 4–5 years of age. For 1000 Hz, 3 of the children showed no difference in the thresholds obtained by two methods, 3 of the children showed a 5 dB difference, 4 showed a 10 dB difference, 3 showed a 15 dB difference, and 2 showed a difference greater than 15 dB.

As children reach the age where some language may develop, the audiologist should be alert to the possibility of exploiting this modality as a means of evaluation. Patients nearing 2 years of age may have enough receptive language to point to body parts (nose, tummy, feet), clothing (shirt, shoes), or familiar objects (ball, toy airplane, toy car). If three or four stimulus words can be established and reliable responses obtained, speech thresholds can be established. As always, speech stimuli only determine overall hearing sensitivity and may not detect the presence of a high-frequency loss or other irregular audiometric configuration. Nevertheless, this test can sometimes give valuable information that cannot otherwise be obtained. It may be helpful to confirm other results. Because it can be performed with earphones, it may provide critical information about the relative function of each ear. Bone-conduction speech thresholds are occasionally useful in conjunction with impedance measures to differentiate conductive and sensorineural loss.

While a response to sound means that the child can hear, it is important to realize that failure to respond may not indicate a hearing loss. Some variables that reduce the probability of a response have already been discussed—state of the infant, nature of the stimulus, and presence of environmental noise. Other factors, such as delay in intellectual, emotional, and motor development, may reduce responsiveness to sound. Information about these attributes may be gathered by scales such as the

*Denver Developmental Screening Test* (Frankenburg & Dodds, 1967) and the *Minnesota Child Developmental Inventory Profile* (Ireton & Thwing, 1980). Both give norms over an age range from 1 month to 6 years. If a child is uniformly low in function on the variables measured by these scales and does not respond to sound, the probability of a disorder other than or in addition to hearing loss is greater than for the nonresponding child who measures high on these scales. Additionally it should be noted that both scales have a language subsection. It provides information about the language delay associated with hearing loss in a child known to be hearing-impaired. This subsection also helps in a diagnostic sense. That is, failure to respond to sound and reduced scores on the language subtest in the presence of normal scores in other areas is evidence to suggest a hearing loss.

# Case History

The following case history demonstrates most of the techniques I have discussed. In this instance, we did some things well and some things poorly, and we were able to get an aid on the child at an early age. To our gratification he is now progressing well and using his hearing, I believe, to maximum benefit.

I first saw Gregory when he was 8 weeks old. Since 2 weeks of age, his mother had been concerned about his hearing. Normal pregnancy and birth were reported, and the otologic examination was negative. There was no familial history of hearing loss, and the child was not at high risk for hearing disorder for any other reason. The only unusual report was periodic nasal congestion. The mother's impression was that Gregory did not respond to sound at all during the first few weeks of his life, but was currently responding to sound directed to the right ear. Consistent APRs were obtained when pure tones were directed to the right ear at hearing levels of 90 to 110 dB. Responses were obtained at octave intervals from 500 to 8000 Hz. No response of this sort could be obtained on the left ear. Attempts at impedance testing were unsuccessful because I could not maintain a seal on either ear.

The infant's responses together with the mother's observation suggested the possibility of resolving conductive hearing loss. I concluded that hearing was functional—and perhaps functionally normal—on the right ear, with a probable loss on the left. I was not sufficiently convinced of the probability of permanent or handicapping hearing loss to recommend more extensive immediate testing. With the referring physician concurring, I recommended a retest in 2 months.

I next saw Gregory when he was 20 weeks old. The clinical picture had changed. Efforts at localization audiometry using narrow bands of noise and warble tones were unsuccessful, although the baby responded to speech in sound field at 70 dB HL. APRs still resulted from pure-tone stimulation at 100 to 110 dB (500 to 4000 Hz) on the right ear only. Tympanograms were Type C bilaterally, and there were no acoustic reflexes. It seemed likely that my earlier impression of possible near-normal hearing in the right ear was probably in error. Current test results suggested a moderate loss in the right ear and a severe or profound loss in the left, with the possibility of a conductive component being present.

We enrolled Gregory for a period of diagnostic observation and therapy, seeing him three times each week. Our goals were to learn more about his hearing loss, to find an appropriate hearing aid, to stimulate awareness of sound, and to help his parents understand problems and solutions associated with hearing loss.

Over a period of 2 months we sometimes obtained Type C and occasionally Type B tympanograms. APRs could not always be elicited on stimulating the right ear, and never on the left ear. Concurrent ear, nose, and throat examinations were normal except for the observation that tympanic membrane movements were sluggish. The suspicion of bilateral secretory otitis media was established, and a decongestant medication was initiated.

During this same period we began trying various moderately powerful body-type hearing aids. The child consistently responded to conversational-level speech with the aid on the right ear but never with it on the left ear. No tolerance problems were noted. When Gregory was 26 weeks old, a body-type aid was recommended for the right ear, and the aid was purchased. The aid had an HAIC maximum gain of 55 dB, maximum power output of 126 dB, and a frequency range of 380 to 4000 Hz. With this aid, speech awareness responses at 30 to 35 dB could be obtained. I did not recommend an aid with extended low-frequency response because of Gregory's demonstrated hearing across all of the speech range and my concern about possible masking of speech sounds by amplified low-frequency noise.

We began a period of hearing-aid orientation for Gregory and his parents. It was fortunate that he had enough residual hearing to be aware already of the utility of sound. He must have quickly recognized the advantages of amplification, because he soon objected to removal of the hearing aid. We taught the parents how to put the aid on, adjust the controls, replace the batteries, and take care of the aid. We gradually increased the gain setting until consistent responses were seen for low-level speech, and we also increased daily use of the aid. By 34 weeks of age, Gregory was wearing the aid full time.

When Gregory was 10 months old we instituted a home training program, teaching the parents effective methods of visual and auditory stimulation during everyday activity. We concentrated on achieving good speech-to-noise ratios. The child's vocalizations increased at an encouraging rate. At 14 months he would wave bye-bye in response to the verbal stimulus and would look for the family pet when its name was spoken.

When Gregory was 16 months of age, the primary responsibility for his training was shifted to a local preschool center for the hearing-impaired. At the same time, working with the preschool, we began efforts to condition him to respond to pure tones with earphones via play audiometry. By 22 months of age thresholds were tentatively established as shown in Figure 6.4.

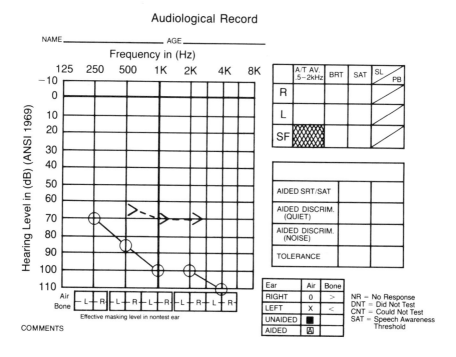

**Figure 6.4.** Tentative thresholds established for Gregory by 22 months of age. (There was no response to air-conducted signals in the left ear or to 8000 Hz in the right ear. Bone-conduction responses were unmasked.)

Because of continuing evidence of a possible conductive component, manifested in otologic examinations by sporadically abnormal tympanograms and air-bone gaps, ventilating tubes were inserted through the tympanic membranes when Gregory was 24 months old. Their presence was maintained for about 6 months.

At the age of 3½ years, Gregory's unaided SRT, obtained with spondee picture cards, was 70 dB. A crude discrimination check revealed that, aided with 50 dB HL presentation, the child could discriminate 8 of 10 monosyllabic words. At the time of this evaluation he achieved a receptive vocabulary age of 2 years and 2 months on the *Peabody Picture Vocabulary Test*.

In preschool Gregory made very good progress in language and speech development. He was originally enrolled in a Total Communication program, but his excellent development of verbal language prompted his teacher to move to an exclusively oral-aural model. His spontaneous speech at this time consisted of two- and three-word sentences. His voice quality was good and his rate and accent pattern quite good. He routinely produced vowels correctly but omitted many consonants.

I should also mention that, during the time described above, Gregory went through three hearing aids of the same model. A strong and active child, he simply demolished the aids.

We were fortunate to recommend from the beginning a hearing aid that was quite appropriate. In many cases, revision of hearing-aid recommendations is necessary as a child matures and we learn more about his or her hearing. We sometimes first recommend a Y-cord amplification arrangement if we cannot determine the ear best suited to amplification. Sometimes we realize the initial recommendation needs changing to achieve more or less gain. Because of this fact, flexible body aids with internal adjustments were useful. If both ears are eventually found to be appropriate for amplification, binaural aids may be recommended. I knew I would probably eventually recommend an at-the-ear aid for Gregory, but at this age, when optimum amplification is critical, a body-type aid seemed best. Gregory learned to adjust and care for his aid himself, and this learning was probably facilitated by use of a body aid.

Gregory is now 12 years old and in the sixth grade. He is in public school, where he spends much of his time in a resource room and attends some regular classes. His latest audiogram is shown in Figure 6.5. There has been little change in his right ear thresholds over the years, and eventually we obtained some response on the left ear but with a fragmented audiogram and responses limited to the low frequencies. Tympanograms have been normal bilaterally for several years, the fluctuating middle ear problem experienced in early childhood having cleared up. The figure shows aided warble-tone thresholds. Gregory has worn a behind-the-ear aid on his right ear since he was about 4 years old. Given today's hearing aids and my current outlook, I would have probably recommended an ear-level aid at an earlier age. In the classroom Gregory uses an FM radio-frequency receiver to receive a signal from the transmitter worn by his teacher.

Consistent with the magnitude of his loss, his auditory discrimination remains poor, about 40% for an open-set test. He uses his hearing and vision together effectively. Recent administration of the Craig Lipreading Inventory resulted in a score of 54% without voice and 79% with voice. Recent results from the *Test of Auditory Comprehension* are shown in Figure 6.6. Gregory passed all sections of the screening task (subtests I through V), and testing began with subtest VI. He passed subtests VII through VIII and failed IX. His performance on subtests VI through IX was at least one standard deviation above the average for children his age with his amount of hearing loss. When Gregory's

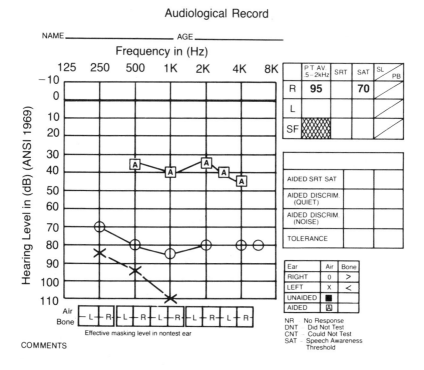

**Figure 6.5.** Gregory's audiogram at age 11. (No response to air-conducted or bone-conducted signals except as shown.)

chronological age was 11-0, his Receptive Language Age was 9-5 as measured by the *Peabody Picture Vocabulary Test*. In retrospect, I am pleased with my contribution to Gregory's development.

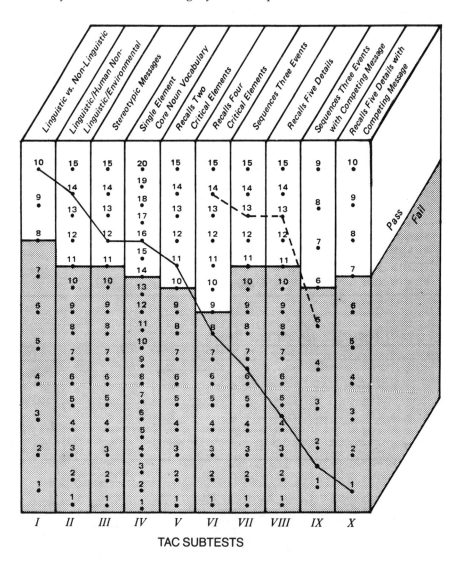

**Figure 6.6.** Results from *Test of Auditory Comprehension*. Solid line shows average scores for subjects who are the same age and have the same magnitude of hearing loss as Gregory. Broken line shows Gregory's scores.

To summarize, the probability of a severe hearing loss was established when Gregory was 20 weeks old. This early identification facilitated enrollment in a program of diagnostic therapy and permitted his parents to begin the counseling and orientation training that is important to help parents understand, accept, and effectively work with the problem of hearing impairment. Early use of appropriate amplification helped Gregory to develop successfully in an aural-oral program. Good preschool training helped him to participate successfully in an aural oral school curriculum, an undertaking which is often not possible for a child with the amount of hearing loss that Gregory has. Today he can communicate successfully with his family and other normal hearing individuals.

# Needs

Further validation is needed of tests and procedures in clinical use. More effective and efficient screening procedures are needed—ones that result in fewer false positives and false negatives and that can be universally applied with reasonable expense. Because of progressive and postnatally acquired loss, we should investigate development of a system that incorporates screening procedures between birth and school age to supplement existing neonatal and school screening.

We need better diagnostic procedures for assessment of infants who fail screening tests as well as tests that give more sensitive measurement of auditory threshold for each ear separately and are applicable at an earlier age. Recent progress has demonstrated that infants can respond at levels lower than previously thought. We must continue to look for methodology that will elicit even better responses. Assessment of compatible test batteries is required. The usefulness of BERA in neonatal screening requires further evaluation (Downs, 1982). Clinically feasible methods are needed for assessing auditory discrimination ability of hearing-impaired infants.

Coordination of diagnostic and habilitation programs and cooperation between professionals who operate these programs have at times been lacking, and ways to reduce this problem should be explored. Family doctors must have been trained in recognizing the warning signs for hearing loss by the end of medical school or residency (Gibson, 1985). Research to improve effectiveness of amplification and of training in its use is still needed, although substantial improvement in the quality of amplification is occurring.

# Summary

To summarize, the following constitutes a battery of tests or procedures that should be useful in evaluating auditory sensitivity of infants. The greater the number of tests applied to an individual infant, the greater the confidence that can be placed in the results.

1. Noisemakers may give useful preliminary and supplementary information. They are simple and easy to use, and sometimes may give information where more complex procedures fail. Electroacoustically obtained estimates of frequency and intensity characteristics should be available. Those who use noisemakers should remember that such measures are indeed estimates and that these soundmakers cannot be calibrated with the precision of electronic generators. They are useful in obtaining reflexive, arousal, and orientation responses in infants.

2. Localization procedures may give useful information about the better ear in infants from 3 or 4 months to 1 year and older. Speech (possibly filtered), narrow-band noise, and warble tones are good stimuli. By covering one ear or by delivering signals through earphones, a previously conditioned response may generalize to give information about each ear separately or about bone-conduction sensitivity. Bone-conducted speech stimuli are useful for a quick estimate of cochlear levels.

3. Impedance audiometry is very helpful, giving sensitive information about the status of the conductive mechanism and corroborative evidence about auditory sensitivity and sensorineural levels.

4. Evoked-response audiometry, electrocochleography, and other electrophysiologic procedures may give additional information. These more complex procedures may not be necessary if good behavioral audiometry is done. In any case, behavioral and electrophysiologic tests should be used together to supplement and corroborate each other.

Future progress in detecting hearing loss in infants must be directed toward a reliable, accurate, and inexpensive screening procedure as well as an accurate method for detecting small hearing losses. As an example of the need for the latter, Shurin, Pelton, and Klein (1976) caution that middle ear effusion (fluid) associated with infection or eustachian tube dysfunction is more common in the infant than has been suspected. Balkany, Berman, Simmons, and Jafek (1978) reported suppurative middle ear effusions in 30% of a sample of NICU infants, and Kitajiri, Sando, Hashida, and Doyle (1985) found middle ear fluid in 16 of 20 infants with palatal abnormalities. Fria, Cautekin, and Eichler (1985) established that middle ear effusion was associated with an average speech awareness of 24.6 dB HL in 222 infants 7 to 24 months of age. An older group of children with the same problem had a loss of similar magnitude, with best sensitivity at 2000 Hz consistent with mass and stiffness influences of this disorder. Bess (1985) reviewed evidence that children with middle ear disease with effusion, unilateral hearing loss, and mild bilateral (around 25 dB) sensorineural loss have more educational and communicative difficulty than previously supposed. This finding is an argument for early detection and for sharpening our diagnostic skills to detect small hearing losses early.

# References

Aldrich, C. (1928). A new test for hearing in the newborn: The conditioned reflex. *American Journal of Diseases of Children, 35,* 36–37.

Altman, M., Shenhav, R., & Schaudinischky, L. (1975). Semi-objective method for auditory mass screening of neonates. *Acta Otolaryngologica, 79,* 46–50.

Altman, M., Shenhav, R., & Schaudinischky, L. (1976). Semi-objective method for auditory mass screening of neonates. In G. Mencher (Ed.), *Proceedings of the Nova Scotia Conference of Early Identification of Hearing Loss* (pp. 181–189). Basel: S. Karger.

Balkany, T. J., Berman, S. A., Simmons, M. A., & Jafek, B. W. (1978). Middle ear effusions in neonates. *Laryngoscope, 88,* 398–405.

Bench, J. (1970). The law of initial value: A neglected source of variance in infant audiometry. *International Audiology, 9,* 314–322.

Bench, J., & Mentz, L. (1975). Stimulus complexity, state and infants' auditory behavioral responses. *British Journal of Disorders of Communication, 10,* 52–60.

Bench, R. (1968). Sound transmission in the human fetus through the maternal abdominal wall. *Journal of Genetic Psychology, 113,* 85–87.

Bennett, M. (1975). Acoustic impedance bridge measurements with the neonate. *British Journal of Audiology, 9,* 117–124.

Bess, F. H. (1985). The minimally hearing-impaired child. *Ear and Hearing, 6,* 43–47.

Bove, C., & Flugrath, J. (1973). Frequency components of noisemakers for use in pediatric audiological evaluations. *Volta Review, 75,* 551–556.

Bronstein, A., & Petrova, E. (1967). The auditory analyzer in young infants. In Y. Brackbill & G. Thompson (Eds.), *Behavior in infancy and early childhood* (pp. 163–172). New York: Free Press.

Butterfield, E., & Hodgson, W. (1969, November). *Tools for the audiologic study of neonates.* Scientific exhibit at the meeting of the American Speech and Hearing Association, Chicago.

Despland, P., & Galambos, R. (1980). The auditory brainstem response (ABR) is a useful diagnostic tool in the intensive care nursery. *Pediatric Research, 14,* 154–158.

Downs, D. W. (1982). Auditory brainstem response testing in the neonatal intensive care unit: A cautious perspective. *Asha, 24,* 1009–1015.

Downs, M., & Sterritt, G. (1964). Identification audiometry with neonates: A preliminary report. *Journal of Auditory Research, 4,* 69–80.

Durieux-Smith, A., Picton, T., Edwards, C., Goodman, J. T., & MacMurray, B. (1985). The Crib-O-Gram in the NICU: An evaluation based on brain stem electric response audiometry. *Ear and Hearing, 6,* 20–24.

Eilers, R. E., Wilson, W. R., & Moore, J. M. (1977). Developmental changes in speech discrimination in infants. *Journal of Speech and Hearing Research, 20,* 766–780.

Eisenberg, R., Coursin, D., & Rupp, N. (1966). Habituation to an acoustic pattern as an index of differences among human neonates. *Journal of Auditory Research, 6,* 239–248.

Eisenberg, R., Griffin, E., Coursin, D., & Hunter, M. (1964). Auditory behavior in the human neonate: A preliminary report. *Journal of Speech and Hearing Research, 7,* 245–269.

Eisenberg, R., Marmarou, A., & Giovachino, P. (1974a). Heart rate changes to a synthetic vowel. *Journal of Auditory Research, 14,* 21–28.

Eisenberg, R., Marmarou, A., & Giovachino, P. (1974b). Heart rate changes to a synthetic vowel as an index of individual differences. *Journal of Auditory Research, 14,* 45–50.

Elliot, G., & Elliot, K. (1964). Some pathological, radiological and clinical implications of the precocious development of the human ear. *Laryngoscope, 74,* 1160–1171.

Feinmesser, M., Tell, L., & Levi, H. (1982). Follow-up of 40,000 infants screened for hearing defect. *Audiology, 21,* 197–203.

Frankenburg, W. K., & Dodds, J. B. (1967). The Denver Developmental Screening Test. *Journal of Pediatrics, 71,* 181–191.

Franklin, B. (1980). *Speech-band audiometry manual.* San Francisco: San Francisco State University.

Fria, T., Cantekin, E., & Eichler, J. (1985). Hearing acuity of children with otitis media with effusion. *Archives of Otolaryngology, 111,* 10–16.

Froding, C. (1960). Acoustic investigation of newborn infants. *Acta Otolaryngologica, 52,* 31–40.

Fulton, R., Gorzycki, P., & Hull, W. (1975). Hearing assessment with young children. *Journal of Speech and Hearing Disorders, 40,* 397–404.

Gerber, S. E. (1985). Stimulus, response, and state variables in the testing of neonates. *Ear and Hearing, 6,* 15–19.

Gibson, G. C. (1985). The role of the family physician—A front line view. *Ear and Hearing, 6,* 59–63.

Hardy, J., Dougherty, A., & Hardy, W. (1959). Hearing responses and audiologic screening in infants. *Journal of Pediatrics, 55,* 382–390.

Haug, O., Baccaro, P., & Guilford, F. (1967). A pure-tone audiogram on the infant: The PIWI technique. *Archives of Otolaryngology, 86,* 435–440.

Held, R. (1979). Development of visual resolution. *Canadian Journal of Psychology, 33,* 213–221.

Ireton, H. R., & Thwing, E. J. (1980). *Minnesota Infant Development Inventory.* Minneapolis: Behavior Sciences Systems.

Jaffe, B. (1972). Heredity and congenital factors affecting newborn conductive hearing. *Conference on Newborn Hearing Screening* (pp. 87–101). Washington, DC: Alexander Graham Bell Association for the Deaf.

Joint Committee on Infant Hearing Screening. (1982). Position statement. *Asha, 24,* 1017–1018.

Kaye, H., & Levin, R. (1963). Two attempts to demonstrate tonal suppression of non-nutritive sucking in neonates. *Perceptual Motor Skills, 17,* 521–522.

Keith, R. (1976). *The use of impedance measurements in infant hearing programs.* In G. Mencher (Ed.), *Proceedings of the Nova Scotia Conference of Early Identification of Hearing Loss* (pp. 68–75). Basel: S. Karger.

Kitajiri, M., Sando, I., Hashida, Y., & Doyle, W. (1985). Histopathology of otitis media in infants with cleft and high-arched palates. *Annals of Otology, Rhinology, and Laryngology, 94,* 44–50.

Koval, C., & Stelmachowicz, P. (1983). Clinical validity of "speech-band" audiometry. *Journal of Speech and Hearing Disorders, 48,* 328–329.

Liden, G., & Harford, E. R., (1985). The pediatric audiologist: From magician to clinician. *Ear and Hearing, 6,* 6–9.

Liden, G., & Kankkunen, A. (1969). Visual reinforcement audiometry in the management of young deaf children. *International Audiology, 8,* 99–106.

Lubchenco, L., Horner, F., Reed, L., Hix, I., Jr., Metcalf, D., Cohig, R., Elliott, H., & Bourg, M. (1963). Sequelae of premature birth. *American Journal of Diseases of Children, 106,* 101–115.

McFarland, W. H., Simmons, F. B., & Jones, F. R. (1980). An automated hearing screening technique for newborns. *Journal of Speech and Hearing Disorders, 45,* 495–503.

Marquis, D. (1931). Can conditioned response be established in the newborn infant? *Journal of Genetic Psychology, 39,* 479–492.

Matkin, N. (1973). Some essential features of a pediatric audiologic evaluation. In *Evaluation of Hearing Handicapped Children* (Chap. 5). Denmark: Fifth Danavox Symposium.

Mencher, G. (Ed.). (1976). *Proceedings of the Nova Scotia Conference on Early Identification of Hearing Loss.* Basel: S. Karger.

Moore, J., Thompson, G., & Thompson, M. (1975). Auditory localization of infants as a function of reinforcement conditions. *Journal of Speech and Hearing Disorders, 40,* 29–34.

Moore, J., Wilson, W., & Thompson, G. (1977). Visual reinforcement of head-turn responses in infants under twelve months of age. *Journal of Speech and Hearing Disorders, 42,* 328–334.

Murphy, K. (1969). The psychophysiological maturation of auditory function. *International Audiology, 8,* 46–51.

Mussen, P., Conger, J., & Kagan, J. (1974). *Child development and personality* (4th ed.). New York: Harper & Row.

Northern, J., & Downs, M. (1984). *Hearing in children* (3rd ed.). Baltimore: Williams and Wilkins.

Shah, C. P., Chandler, D., & Dale, R. (1978). Delay in referral of children with impaired hearing. *Volta Review, 80,* 206–215.

Shurin, P. A., Pelton, S. I., & Klein, J. O. (1976). Otitis media in the newborn infant. *Annals of Otology, Rhinology, and Laryngology, 85* (Suppl. 25), 216–222.

Simmons, F. (1976). Automated hearing screening test for newborns: The Crib-O-Gram. In G. Mencher (Ed.), *Proceedings of the Nova Scotia Conference on Early Identification of Hearing Loss* (pp. 171–180). Basel: S. Karger.

Simmons, F., & Russ, F. (1974). Automated newborn hearing screening: Crib-O-Gram. *Archives of Otolaryngology, 100,* 1–7.

Smart, M., & Smart, R. (1982). *Children: Development and relationships* (4th ed.). New York: Macmillan.

Suzuki, T., & Ogiba, Y. (1961). Conditioned orientation reflex audiometry. *Archives of Otolaryngology, 74,* 192–198.

Thompson, G., & Wilson, W. (1984). Clinical application of visual reinforcement. *Seminars in Hearing, 5,* 85–99.

Ventry, I. (1982). Computing false positive and false negative rates for the Crib-O-Gram. *Journal of Speech and Hearing Disorders, 47,* 109–110.

Vernon, M. (1967). Prematurity and deafness: The magnitude and nature of the problem among deaf children. *Exceptional Children, 33,* 289–298.

Wedenberg, E. (1956). Auditory tests on newborn infants. *Acta Otolaryngologica, 46,* 446–461.

Wedenberg, E. (1972). Auditory tests on newborn infants. In G. Cunningham (Ed.), *Conference on Newborn Hearing Screening* (pp. 126–131). Washington, DC: Alexander Graham Bell Association for the Deaf.

Wolff, P. (1966). The causes, controls and organization of behavior in the neonate. *Psychological Issues, 5,* 1–99.

# Pure-Tone Tests with Preschool Children

## ROSS J. ROESER
## WENDE YELLIN

$T$he importance of auditory function in the acquisition and development of language, speech, and cognitive skills cannot be stressed enough. Almost from birth an infant begins the process of learning language, which forms the basis for other aspects of development. The infant with adequate hearing will learn language skills primarily through the auditory channel. Vocabulary is learned by hearing words that are associated with objects, events, and experiences. By hearing combinations of words, meaningful phrases and sentences are developed. Moreover, the acquisition of reading and writing depends on the knowledge of spoken language. Since hearing is so essential to the natural learning of language, it follows that a hearing impairment early in life, at birth or in the years before linguistic skills are learned, will interfere significantly with most areas of language and academic development. Therefore, to minimize its handicapping effects (physiological, educational, psychological, and social), hearing loss in children must be identified as early as possible.

This chapter covers the procedures that are employed in screening and evaluating hearing in the preschool child. An emphasis is placed on using pure tones, but many of the evaluation procedures discussed can be used with, and indeed can be more successful with, other types of stimuli, including narrow bands, filtered noises, and speech. Before we begin our discussion of screening and evaluation procedures, the question of the prevalence of hearing loss in the preschool population is addressed.

# The Prevalence of Hearing Loss in the Preschool Population

Statistics estimating the prevalence of hearing loss in young children vary from survey to survey. With regard to profound congenital hearing loss, Frasier (1971) and Stewart (1974) have estimated the incidence as 1 in 1,000 live births, while the American Academy of Pediatrics Committee on Children with Handicaps (1973) estimates 1 in 1,500 live births. Estimates of hearing impairment among school children range from 2% to 20% (Connor, 1961). These wide variations can be illustrated by two reports: the National Health Examination Survey found that 1% of 7,417 children had losses of 25 dB or more (Leske, 1981); the National Academy of Science found that 18.9% of the 1,639 children tested had hearing loss (Kempe, Silver, & O'Brien, 1984). The differences between studies may be due to testing conditions or the ages of the populations or, more significantly, to differences in the definition of hearing loss.

The criterion used for defining hearing loss typically has been hearing thresholds of 25 dB or greater. This standard, obtained by computing the average of thresholds at 500 Hz, 1000 Hz, 2000 Hz, and 3000 Hz, was established by the American Academy of Otolaryngology Committee on Hearing and Equilibrium and the American Council of Otolaryngology Committee on the Medical Aspects of Noise (1979). As will be discussed later in this chapter, hearing screening programs generally employ pure tones at hearing levels between 20 and 30 dB HL. However, evidence is mounting that even 20 dB may be an inappropriate cutoff to define normal hearing for children. As discussed by Northern and Downs (1984), a loss of 20 dB may interfere with the normal acquisition and development of speech and language. They feel that 15 dB HL should be the upper limit of normal hearing for children.

Using this stricter criterion, Northern and Downs estimate that hearing impairment occurs in 13% of the children in the 2- to 3-year-old age group, 12% of the children in the 3- to 4-year-old age group, and 9.2% of the children in the 4- to 5-year-old age group. This approximate incidence figure of 1 out of 10 preschool children stresses the importance of early identification of hearing loss through audiometric screening and evaluation procedures, which are discussed throughout this chapter.

# Considerations for Preschool Hearing Screening

General considerations for any hearing screening program, whether it be designed for preschool or school-aged children or even adults, include the test environment, equipment, personnel supervising and administering the testing (examiner criteria), equipment, test procedures, and follow-up. With the preschool population, special provisions for dealing with the child who is difficult to test should also be made in planning the program.

### Test Environment

The test environment in which one chooses to perform audiometric screening should be well lighted, adequate in size to accommodate the tester and equipment, well ventilated, and free of high ambient noise levels. The most critical requirement of the test environment is an acceptable ambient noise level, because serious problems can occur in hearing screening if the background noise levels are too high. The most desirable space for hearing screening is located as far away as possible from noise sources such as heating units, air conditioners, and other mechanical equipment. The best areas for hearing screening include quiet offices and library areas; generally good areas are auditorium stages with the curtains drawn, a nurse's office, or the teachers' lounge if these areas are available in the preschool building. However, the exact location depends entirely on the building itself and the schedule of daily activities.

The problem with testing in environments having high ambient noise levels is that the noise in the environment has the potential to mask or block out the test stimuli. High ambient noise levels have a limiting effect on the frequencies and intensity at which hearing screening can be performed and are the reason for imposing many of the recommended guidelines for hearing screening. The main energy of most noise is concentrated in the frequencies below 1000 Hz. This one factor is the primary reason why hearing screening programs have recommended testing at 1000 Hz and above, even though some important data can be obtained at 500 Hz and 250 Hz (American Speech and Hearing Association [ASHA] Committee on Audiometric Evaluation, 1975). Moreover, screening tests performed at intensities of 10–15 dB HL can be severely affected by noise, even though these intensities are more sensitive to certain types of hearing loss.

It has been reasoned by some that if background noise levels are too high, simply increasing the intensity level of the test stimuli will solve the problem. However, this solution is not acceptable, because by increasing the intensity level, the sensitivity of the screening test is reduced and those children who have significant hearing loss at the screening level initially chosen may pass at the higher level. In no case should the levels of the test stimuli be increased above those specified by the screening program; an alternate test site should be selected if the ambient noise levels are too high.

The problem of ambient noise can be solved by the use of sound-isolating rooms. Such enclosures were recommended by the National Conference on Identification Audiometry (Darley, 1961). Small, portable sound-isolating rooms are commercially available, and studies have shown them to provide significant benefit to hearing screening programs in schools (Fisher, 1976). However, they are expensive, and most preschool hearing screening programs will not have them available. Furthermore, since the smaller test chambers will not allow both the child and the examiner into the room at the same time, these units would be limited to older, cooperative preschoolers who would give voluntary responses to the test signals and would not be anxious in a small enclosure by themselves.

Another possible solution for eliminating unwanted background noise is the use of noise-excluding earphone enclosures. These devices contain large cups that surround the ear and help to increase attenuation of the background noise. It has been found that certain types of these enclosures are more effective in reducing background noise than standard (supra-aural) headsets. Musket and Roeser (1977) compared thresholds using four types of noise-excluding headsets to those obtained with a standard (MX-41/AR) cushion in quiet and in the presence of wide-band noise. Testing was done at 60 dB SL with children aged 8 to 12 years. They found that only one of the four noise-excluding headsets provided significant benefit with this population of children in the presence of background noise. Clinicians choosing to use a particular type of noise-excluding system should be aware of the data that support their use.

Noise-excluding headsets also present inherent problems, particularly the placement of earphones on the head. They are larger than the standard headset, and they can be misplaced easily—especially on children, whose heads are smaller than those of adults—making them more apt to move around. Noise-excluding earphones should be utilized only by highly experienced examiners who are aware of the difficulties that may occur with their use. The ASHA Committee on Audiometric Evaluation (1975) did not endorse or encourage the use of noise-excluding earphones; this conservative approach is most likely due to the possible problems that might occur with their use.

There are two methods for checking whether the ambient noise level of the test environment is acceptable. The first is to use a sound level meter with an octave band filter. Table 7.1 provides the allowable noise levels for screening at 20–25 dB HL. The tester would simply measure the test environment to determine whether the noise levels of the room fall below these values. If sound-measuring equipment is not available, and typically it is not, the second procedure would be to use a biological check. The biological check is performed by screening one or preferably two subjects with proven normal hearing sensitivity, possibly including the tester. If these individuals fail to perceive one or more of the test stimuli, the environment most likely is not satisfactory, provided that the equipment is in proper calibration. The biological check should be performed routinely at the beginning of each test session, even if sound-measuring equipment is available, to ensure acceptable noise levels and proper equipment function.

## Equipment

*The Audiometer.* There are various types of audiometers presently available from a number of different manufacturers and suppliers that are suitable for preschool hearing screening. The types of audiometers commercially available vary from basic screening models to very complex clinical instruments, and the signals generated range from simple pure tones to the more complex stimuli used in comprehensive testing. However, for preschool hearing screening programs a simple pure-tone air-conduction audiometer is needed. The audiometer should be capable of generating pure tones at least at these frequencies: 250, 500, 1000, 2000, 3000, 4000, 6000, and 8000 Hz. There is no need for the audiometer to have bone-conduction or speech audiometry capabilities. Simple pure-tone air-conduction instruments are available for about $600 to $700.

**TABLE 7.1**
**Octave Band Levels Allowable for**
**Screening at 20–25 dB Level Recommended by the ASHA Committee**
**on Audiometric Evaluation (dB SPL)**

| Test Frequency | 500 | 1000 | 2000 | 4000 |
|---|---|---|---|---|
| Octave Band Cutoff | 300 | 600 | 1200 | 2400 |
| Frequencies | 600 | 1200 | 2400 | 4800 |
| Allowable ambient noise for threshold at 0 HL (ANSI 1969) | 26 | 30 | 38 | 51 |
| Plus ASHA screening level (ANSI 1969) | 20 | 20 | 20 | 25 |
| Resultant maximum ambient noise allowable for ASHA screening | 56 | 50 | 58 | 76 |

*Source:* Based on ASHA (1975).

Other specific considerations in the purchase of equipment for preschool hearing screening include the following: (1) the equipment should have an AC voltage line (battery-operated instruments are not stable); (2) the equipment should include two standard earphones and cushions; and (3) the instrument should have been calibrated to ANSI 1969 specifications for audiometers.

*Calibration.* All audiometers, whether they are used for screening or diagnostic purposes, must meet minimum requirements set by the American National Standards Institute. (The standard can be obtained for a small fee by writing to the American National Standards Institute at 1430 Broadway, New York, NY 10018, or the Acoustical Society of America at 335 East 45th St., New York, NY 10017.) While it is not mandatory to have the standard, it may be helpful if the basic equipment necessary for calibration is available.

Studies have documented the unfortunate finding that audiometers used for hearing screening often tend to go out of calibration (Walton

& Wilson, 1972). Thus it is important that calibration procedures be used routinely with all audiometers, including those used in preschool hearing screening programs.

There are four types of calibration schedules. These include a daily listening check, a monthly biological check, a periodic check (yearly), and an exhaustive check (every 5 years).

*Daily listening check.* Each morning following an appropriate warm-up time (10 minutes) the tester should listen to the signal emitted from the audiometer for transient clicks or distortions of the signal at various intensities at all frequencies. The tester should also determine that the signal is in the correct earphone. It is far better to discover a malfunction in the equipment than to face inappropriate referrals.

*Biological calibration.* Each month that the audiometer is in use, a biological calibration check is required on at least one subject whose hearing threshold is known. The procedure involves obtaining baseline threshold measurements on three to five normal hearing individuals who will be available for comparison testing throughout the year. If on the monthly check a threshold difference greater than 5 dB is found for one of the individuals at any test frequency between 500 Hz and 6000 Hz, then the other subjects should be checked. If a shift greater than 5 dB in the same direction is confirmed by the additional biological checks, an electronic calibration of the audiometer is required. The results from each monthly biological calibration check should be recorded on a form that is kept in a calibration file maintained for each audiometer.

*Periodic (yearly) calibration.* At least once a year, every audiometer should have an electronic calibration to ensure that it meets the minimum standards defined by ANSI. This service is provided by electronic or acoustic firms using specialized electronic equipment. If it is necessary to ship the audiometer to another location for calibration, it should be packed carefully so that the instrument will be protected from damage in transit. As soon as the audiometer is returned from calibration or repair, the user should perform a biological check in order to reestablish new baseline threshold records on subjects as described above.

*Exhaustive calibration.* Every 5 years each audiometer must have an exhaustive electronic calibration. This calibration is more comprehensive than the periodic electronic calibration and includes the testing of all settings on the frequency and intensity (HL/HTL) dials as well as replacing switches, cords, earphones, and cushions.

**Care of Audiometers.** Audiometric equipment should not be handled roughly or dropped at any time. This equipment is delicate and expensive, and should be protected from extremes in temperature and humidity.

The life of an audiometer is much shorter in coastal cities if the audiometer is not properly cared for due to high humidity and temperature variations.

When transporting instruments in a car, keep them in the passenger compartment, protected from freezing or hot temperatures and abusive handling. On hot days never allow them to remain in a closed, unventilated vehicle for long periods of time. Summer temperatures in a closed car may well reach over 100°F within a few minutes.

When not in use, instruments should be stored off the floor under a protective cover in an area of relatively even temperature. Dusty and salty conditions may rapidly affect the calibration and operation of the equipment. The storage compartment, available on most equipment, should be reserved for storing that instrument's earphones and cords. Never interchange earphones between machines.

The earphones are the most delicate part of the equipment and are the most likely component to go out of calibration as a result of being dropped or some other form of misuse. The cushions may be cleaned with a mild solution of soap and water. It is advisable to never use alcohol on the cushions, as it tends to dry them out and make them hard, resulting in frequent replacement. The receiver inside the cushion should be protected from getting wet, and the diaphragms of the earphones should be protected from liquids and sharp objects that can enter the perforations in the grids protecting them.

Earphone cushions should never be pressed down on a flat surface or packed cushion-to-cushion without a separating pad, such as foam rubber, which helps keep a vacuum from forming and prevents damage from percussion blows. The earphone cords should not be twisted or knotted and should be packed loosely in the storage compartment. If plugs or cords do not have to be regularly removed from the earphone jacks, a corrosive film may form between the plug and the jack. This film can be loosened by periodically pulling the plugs in and out several times. However, care should be taken to replace plugs in their proper output jacks and see that they are pushed in all the way.

## Examiner Criteria

Two levels of personnel may be utilized in preschool hearing screening programs, one supervisory and one technical (ASHA, 1975; Darley, 1961). The supervisor of the program should be an audiologist holding the Certificate of Clinical Competence from the American Speech-Language-Hearing Association. As supervisor of the program, the audiologist is responsible for selecting the screening procedures to be used, training and monitoring the support staff, ensuring proper equipment calibration, attempting to screen the difficult-to-test preschoolers who are not testable by the technical staff, referring failures for comprehensive audiological testing, discussing test results with medical personnel, and generally carrying out the higher administrative functions of the program.

The support personnel perform the actual screening tests and carry out the day-to-day activities of the program, such as performing daily calibration checks and filling out statistical reports. Many preschool screening programs use nurses or speech-language pathologists in this role. Because of their training, such professionals are effective, but they still should be provided with in-service training to reacquaint them with the general area of hearing, hearing disorders, and audiometric testing.

When paraprofessionals or professionals with no training in hearing screening are used as support staff, additional training is mandatory. The National Conference on Identification Audiometry recommended that for such persons the training course be conducted over a 2- to 6-week period, with at least one half of the time devoted to supervised practice in testing (Darley, 1961). Since the success of the entire hearing program can rest on the support personnel, the need for adequate training of these individuals cannot be stressed enough. The absolute minimum training period for paraprofessionals should be no less than 5 days, with one half of the time spent in supervised practicum. Topics that should be included in the training program are as follows:

1. Basic physical principles of sound

2. Anatomy and physiology of the auditory system

3. Disorders of the ear and types of hearing loss

4. Use, care, maintenance, and calibration of audiometers

5. Screening procedures

6. Threshold measurement and referral procedures

7. Record keeping

## Screening Test Procedures

The screening test is conducted in two parts: the otoscopic inspection and the audiometric screening.

## Otoscopic Inspection

Otoscopy is the process by which the ear canal and tympanic membrane are inspected by an examiner, using an instrument called an otoscope (see Figure 7.1). The purpose of the inspection is to assess the overall condition of the outer ear and tympanic membrane.

Should the ear canal be inspected as part of a preschool hearing screening program? There are those who feel that this procedure is not necessary because any significant abnormality such as wax impaction will show up on the screening test results; if it does not, then the condition should not be considered significant in screening for hearing loss. But some conditions, such as a foreign object in the ear canal, partial occlusion of the ear canal by wax, and the early stages of otitis media, will not be detected by the hearing screening measures. Thus, there are good reasons to support otoscopic inspection of the external auditory canal as part of the screening test battery. Ginsberg and White (1978) support this notion by stating that all audiologists should have an otoscope at hand and should check each patient before testing. When immittance tests are used as part of the screening, otoscopy is even more important, since the presence of cerumen can give misleading information regarding the

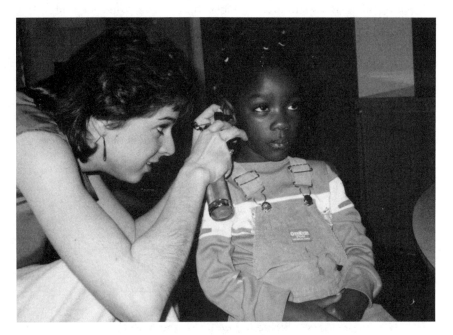

Figure 7.1.   Otoscopic inspection of the external ear.

condition of the middle ear. Moreover, the presence of a foreign object may cause damage to the ear if a probe is inserted into the ear canal, forcing the object against the eardrum and possibly causing a perforation.

What if an examiner finds a foreign object in the ear canal, suspects a medical abnormality, or feels that an abnormal amount of cerumen is present in the ear canal in the pretest otoscopic inspection? In the case of a foreign object or suspected medical abnormality, it is clear that medical referral is necessary. However, there is no simple answer to the question of what to do when excessive earwax is encountered.

The incidence of impacted cerumen in the preschool population is not known. However, in 2,959 school-aged children who failed hearing screening tests, Watkins, Moore, and Phillips (1984) found that 137 (4.9%) had impacted cerumen. Bricco (1985) screened 349 Native American children less than 7 years of age and found that 35 (10%) failed due to impacted cerumen. These statistics represent a high incidence and make it clear that procedures should be developed to deal with the condition. If there is an extreme amount of cerumen present, it is advisable to make a referral to the family physician to have it removed. If there is simply an abnormal amount, this finding should be brought to the attention of the parents so that it can be checked by the managing physician during a routine health examination. Under no circumstances should the examiner remove cerumen or any other material from the ear canal unless under the direct supervision and with the approval of a physician.

Watkins, Moore, and Phillips (1984) described an innovative program whereby the audiologists and nurses in a school hearing conservation program, under the direction of a physician, hold cerumen-removal clinics. One hundred thirteen children who failed screening tests before irrigation successfully passed after irrigation. There were no complications following the irrigation.

With preschool children the otoscopic examination might be frightening, especially if they have had a medical examination of their ears previously. Musket and Dworaczyk (1980) describe a modification of an otoscope in which it is disguised as a puppet so it will be more acceptable to younger children. Figure 7.2 shows this innovative modification. Following the otoscopic inspection, if no major contraindications are found, the examiner proceeds to the audiometric portion of the screening test.

## Audiometric Screening

*Speech vs. Pure Tones.* Two choices of test stimuli are available for screening hearing: speech and pure tones. Speech has the advantage of being less abstract than pure tones, so tests using speech can generally be administered more successfully to younger preschool children. Based on this one principle, several procedures using speech stimuli were developed and perhaps are still in use today in some preschool and school screening programs. However, those using speech stimuli for hearing screening must realize its severe limitations in identifying high-frequency and frequency-specific hearing loss.

*The Individual Pure-Tone Sweep-Check Test.*   The most widely preferred pure-tone test is the sweep-check screening test (Fay, Hochberg, Smith, Rees, & Halpern, 1972) originally described by Newhart (1948). The pure-tone sweep-check test is the screening procedure recommended by the ASHA Committee on Audiometric Evaluation (ASHA, 1975).

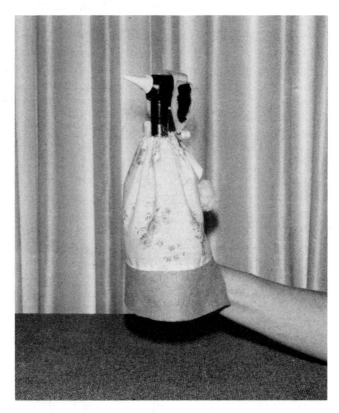

**Figure 7.2.**   Disguising the otoscope as a puppet may reduce apprehension in preschool children.

In this procedure, stimuli are presented at predetermined frequencies and fixed intensity levels, and the child is instructed to respond by raising a hand or finger. Earphones are placed over both ears of the child, and a practice tone is presented at a level above the test tone (i.e., 40 dB HL) to acquaint the child with the type of signal to be heard. All of the test stimuli are first presented to one ear and then the other, and a record is made as to the presence or absence of a response at each frequency; no attempt is made to alter the attenuator dial from the specified level to determine threshold when the child fails to respond. The sweep-check procedure can be successfully administered to a fully cooperative preschool child in about 2 to 4 minutes.

*Frequencies and Intensities.* Controversy exists over the specific frequencies and intensities to test in the individual pure-tone sweep-check test. In general, the frequencies recommended have been in the 500–6000 Hz range. Tones below 500 Hz typically are not recommended because they are more easily masked by ambient noise and do not provide significant information in the testing procedure. These two problems also occur at 500 Hz, and most recent guidelines do not recommend using this frequency (ASHA, 1975). The use of 6000 Hz in screening has also been questioned due to its variability (Hood & Lamb, 1974).

At one time it was believed that limiting the test signals to one or two frequencies would significantly reduce the time required for the individual sweep-check test without affecting the overall test results. Some have suggested screening only with one (4000 Hz) tone (House & Glorig, 1957) whereas others perform screening with two tones, using 2000 and 4000 Hz (Norton & Lux, 1961); 500 and 4000 Hz (Siegenthaler & Sommers, 1959); and 1000 and 4000 Hz (Maxwell & Davidson, 1961).

Although studies are available to support limited-frequency screening, conclusive data indicate that limited-frequency screening procedures are not as effective as the pure-tone sweep-check test. Siegenthaler and Sommers (1959) evaluated the audiometric test results of more than 19,500 children and estimated that 35% of those failing the sweep-check test did not demonstrate losses at 4000 Hz. Stevens and Davidson (1959) report similar observations on 1,784 audiograms. These findings suggest that limiting the screening to a single frequency, or even to two frequencies, significantly reduces the sensitivity of hearing screening, at least in school children. In light of these reports, it is apparent that screening should be performed at three or four frequencies.

The recommended intensity or intensities at which screening should occur has generally varied between 20 and 30 dB HL (American National

Standards Institute [ANSI], 1969). In selecting screening level, two factors should be considered: the effect of the background noise and the sensitivity of the test in detecting even slight hearing loss. Background noise was discussed previously in this chapter. Needless to say, as the screening level decreases, the ambient noise will have a greater effect on the test signal. This one factor has prevented schools from screening at and below 15–20 dB HL.

By decreasing the level at which the test is performed, the sensitivity of the test can be increased, and children with even slight hearing loss can be identified. Since audiologists feel that even slight hearing losses affect the development of speech and language, the goal of many programs is to reduce the screening level to identify these children. However, we are forced into accepting screening levels of 20–25 dB HL because of the conditions under which most screening is performed. Unfortunately, reduction of the screening level to 10 or 15 dB HL would significantly increase the number of unnecessary referrals because of false positive identification due to background noise.

*Pass/Fail Criteria.* The specific pass/fail criteria used in the program will depend entirely on the frequencies and intensities at which the screening is performed. However, results from several studies make it quite clear that referral should be based on failure of two screening tests given several hours apart on the same day or several days apart. In this procedure, children are referred for follow-up only if they fail the second screening test. The reason for requiring the second test is that temporary factors, such as noise in the test environment, the child's nervousness, and transient conductive hearing loss can be allowed to abate, thus reducing the number of unnecessary referrals.

There are no extensive data from preschool populations on how the second screening affects the referral rate. However, data from the elementary grades highly support the use of follow-up screening prior to referral. Melnick, Eagles, and Levine (1964) found that the inclusion of a second screening reduced the number of unnecessary referrals by 23%. Wilson and Walton (1974) rescreened 411 children in grades K–5 who failed an initial screening test and found that slightly more than 50% passed the second screening test. Results from these two studies on school-aged children certainly support the need for rescreening preschoolers before referral.

Table 7.2 summarizes six widely used recommended procedures. These protocols in no way exhaust the possible screening guidelines that have been suggested. They represent the wide range of screening pro-

**TABLE 7.2**

**Comparison of Recommended Test Frequencies, Intensity Levels, and Pass/Fail Criteria for School Hearing Screening**

| Source | Test Frequencies | Intensity Levels (ANSI 1969) | Pass/Fail Criteria |
|--------|------------------|------------------------------|--------------------|
| National Conference on Identification Audiometry | 1000, 2000, 4000, and 6000 Hz | 20 dB at 1000, 2000, and 6000 Hz 30 dB at 4000 Hz | Failure to hear any signals at these levels in either ear |
| State of Illinois Department of Public Health | 500, 1000, 2000, and 4000 Hz | 25 or 35 dB | Failure to respond to one tone at 35 dB in either ear or to any two tones at 25 dB in the same ear |
| American Speech-Language-Hearing Association Committee on Identification Audiometry | 1000, 2000, and 4000 Hz | 20 dB at 1000 and 2000 Hz 25 dB at 4000 Hz | Failure to respond at any frequency in either ear |
| Northern and Downs (1984) | 1000, 2000, and/or 4000 and 6000 Hz | 25 dB | Failure to respond to one tone at 1000 or 2000 Hz or failure to respond to two out of three tones at 3000, 4000, and 6000 Hz |
| Anderson (1978) | 1000, 2000, and 4000 Hz | 20 dB | Failure to respond to any one signal in any ear |
| Downs (1978) | 1000, 2000, 4000, and 6000 or 8000 Hz | 15 dB | Failure to respond to either 1000 Hz or to both 4000 and 6000–8000 Hz in either ear |

cedures employed in the schools. We support the guidelines proposed by the American Speech-Language-Hearing Association (ASHA, 1975) because they represent the most acceptable screening procedures available to date.

It should be recognized that although the ASHA procedures will detect those children with educationally significant hearing loss, these guidelines are not exclusive in identifying only educationally significant hearing loss. Specifically, those who fail at 4000 Hz only will not experience significant auditory problems in the classroom unless the loss is in the severe range and also affects responses at 3000 Hz. This is because 4000 Hz falls outside of the critical speech range. However, those children with hearing loss at 4000 Hz need to be identified so that comprehensive audiological testing can be performed and appropriate action (medical follow-up or counseling) initiated to prevent any further decrease in hearing. Moreover, the ASHA guidelines do not detect minimal hearing loss. Thus, these screening guidelines should be used with immittance measures, since minimal hearing loss is frequently associated with middle ear disorders.

*The Difficult-to-Test Child.*   The standard pure-tone sweep-check test can be administered successfully to most preschool children 30 months of age and older (Watkins, Moore, & Phillips, 1984), but some difficulty will often be experienced with younger children and ''immature'' children.

With younger and immature children, special techniques must be used in the hearing screening program. Two of the techniques that can be used with the difficult-to-test child are play conditioning and test training. These two procedures are typically used by audiologists for threshold testing and are described in detail later in this chapter. However, they can be adapted for screening and are successful for many children who initially will not provide a voluntary response by raising a hand or finger.

It is important to point out that to complete an accurate screening test successfully on the difficult-to-test child requires special skills. In the hands of an evaluator unskilled with preschool children errors can be made. To avoid false positive or, even worse, false negative outcomes, preschool children who fall into the difficult-to-test category should be evaluated by the audiologist supervising the program whenever possible. If this is not possible, these children should be referred to evaluators who have had comprehensive training in working with the difficult-to-test child, and to avoid making errors the results should be reviewed by the audiology consultant.

# Follow-Up

Once the preschool child has failed the hearing screening tests, appropriate follow-up needs to be carried out. Follow-up considerations should be made for audiological, medical, and educational involvement.

*Audiological Follow-Up.*   In traditional preschool hearing screening programs, all children who fail are immediately referred for medical follow-up. Such referral is important to identify significant medical problems but might be considered premature in the sequence for some failures. The hearing screening tests administered to the preschool child must be considered only as a preliminary indication of the presence of hearing loss. Before the exact nature and extent of the loss can be determined, additional audiological testing should be performed by an audiologist under acceptable testing conditions. This testing would minimally include pure-tone air- and bone-conduction audiometry, speech audiometry, and immittance testing.

It would be ideal for all failures to be referred to a clinic where both medical and audiological facilities are available. In that way the physician and audiologist could work together in assessing the nature and extent of the problem and providing appropriate follow-up. Many of the larger metropolitan areas have such facilities. However, where such facilities are not available, follow-up audiological threshold testing should be performed prior to the medical referral. In this way the referral physician will have the necessary audiological data available in order to make a valid diagnosis and begin proper treatment if indicated.

The current guidelines of the American Speech-Language-Hearing Association (ASHA, 1975) support the need for audiological follow-up before medical referral. In addition, the guidelines indicate that completed diagnostic audiological evaluation for those children failing the hearing screening is especially important for the following categories, listed in order of priority:

1. Binaural loss in both ears at all frequencies tested

2. Binaural loss at 1000 and 2000 Hz only

3. Binaural loss at 1000 or 2000 Hz only

4. Monaural loss at all frequencies

5. Monaural loss at 1000 and 2000 Hz only

6. Binaural or monaural loss at 4000 Hz only

Thus, any preschool child falling into one of these categories should receive a complete audiological evaluation, preferrably before the medical referral.

*Medical Follow-Up.*   One of the dilemmas regarding medical follow-up for preschool children failing the screening test is the choice of the physician to whom to send the child. Traditional medical ethics dictate that the child be referred to the family physician. Typically, the family physician is a general practitioner or pediatrician. The general medical practitioner plays a very important role in the overall management of the family's medical needs but often does not have the expertise required in the diagnosis and management of otological problems. For this reason those children failing the screening program may be best served if referred directly to an ear specialist (otologist). In most cases, for the overall well-being of the child, referral to an otologist, with proper notification and approval from the managing physician, is most appropriate when auditory disorders are found.

Whenever referral is made for medical follow-up, the parents must be contacted. Initially contact can be made by phone, but written recommendations should also be made. In addition, feedback from the physician should be requested and records kept on all medical referrals. An example of an effective form letter that can be used to inform parents is provided in Figure 7.3

*Educational Follow-Up.*   When significant hearing loss is found in preschool children, the school system must be notified so that special provisions can be made for educational follow-up. In many cases, the hearing loss will be transient; the extent and duration of the impairment will depend on the nature of the abnormal condition. In other cases, the loss will be permanent. However, for both transient and permanent losses concern exists regarding their effect on speech and language development and educational achievement. Preschool children who fail hearing screening tests and who show any sign of delayed psychoeducational development should be referred for developmental testing. Many school systems have programs to conduct psychoeducational testing for children 3 years of age and older.

If the child is enrolled in a regular preschool program, the teacher must be made aware of the hearing loss. It is important to offer the teacher

HEARING REFERRAL FORM REGARDING _____
(name of child)

Dear Parent:

Your child was recently screened for hearing problems on _____,
and was retested on _____.

Results of this screening indicate that your child may have difficulty
hearing, and you are urged to take him/her to your doctor for further hearing
evaluation.

Please take this form with you when your child is examined and ask the doctor
to complete the bottom half.

-------------------------------------------------------------------------------

Dear Doctor:

See the attached screening audiogram.

Please complete the following checklist and return this form at your earliest
convenience
to: _____

_____

I have examined _____ on _____ and find:
(date)
( ) a fully treatable problem
( ) a partially treatable problem
( ) a nontreatable problem

Hearing problem was found to be one of the:

( ) outer ear  ( ) middle ear  ( ) inner ear  ( ) other (please specify)
_____

I expect that on completion of treatment there will be:

( ) no significant hearing handicap that may interfere with learning
( ) a handicap that may interfere with learning

Special recommendations: _____

_____

_____

I feel that this referral was: ( ) valid  ( ) invalid.

Signed: _____

**Figure 7.3.** Sample letter to inform parents of hearing loss.

suggestions in managing the hearing-impaired child, whether the loss is transient or permanent, so that learning takes place in a positive environment without alienation. Preferential seating is a must to assure the child's attention. A buddy system can help bring the child into group activities. Visual aids can assist not only in educational instruction but also class routines. Figure 7.4 provides a letter we have found to be useful in notifying teachers of the presence of hearing loss.

*The Child with Unilateral Hearing Loss.* The problems manifested by children with unilateral hearing loss have been ignored because of the assumption that performance in psycho/social/educational environments will not be affected by the loss. Typically, audiologists recommend preferential classroom seating, hearing protection from loud noise, and aggressive action for middle ear disorders. Avoidance of ototoxic drugs should also be considered, and the child's hearing should be monitored on a regular basis, especially to assess threshold sensitivity of the better ear. In these children speech and language most often develop normally, and they do not display the apparent handicaps typical of the hearing-impaired child.

Despite these early clinical impressions, evidence is mounting that unilateral listeners do experience communication difficulties. Giolas and Wark (1967) interviewed adults with unilateral losses and found that they had extreme difficulty understanding speech in noisy situations. Problems were also noted when listening to a speaker from a distance, even in quiet situations. Several recent studies have documented the problems encountered by children with unilateral hearing loss. Recently, Bess and Tharpe (1984) reported that children with unilateral hearing impairment exhibit more negative behaviors, failed one or more grades at a higher percentage, and had lower verbal IQ scores than their normal hearing counterparts. Even more recently, Bess and Tharpe (1986) reviewed case history information on 60 unilaterally hearing-impaired children and found that approximately one half exhibited delays in the educational process; 35% had failed at least one grade, and an additional 13% needed special resource assistance. Certainly these data strongly urge educators to give special consideration to the child with unilateral hearing loss. These children should be monitored carefully for learning problems at home and at school, and resource help should be made available. The use of wireless amplification systems is a consideration with these children, as they provide an improved message-to-competition ratio, meaning that the child would be less distracted by background noise and classroom instruction would be more intelligible (Bess, Tharpe, & Gibler, 1986).

Student's Name: _____

Dear _____ :

The above-named child, who is enrolled in your class, was tested and found to have a hearing impairment. With the parent's permission we are sending you this letter providing you with suggestions for helping a hearing-impaired child succeed in a class with normally hearing children.

1. Preferential seating. Seat the child close to where you usually stand to give instructions. Check to make sure that lighting is such that the child can see your face while you are talking. It is also helpful if you do not give important instructions while you are walking about the room or when your back is toward the child. When other children recite, allow the child to turn around so that he or she can see the child reciting. The child's face should be toward the speaker.

2. Talking to the child. Secure the child's attention before you begin to speak. Then talk naturally in your normal tone of voice. Shouting is not helpful. If the child does not understand something, repeat what you just said. If he or she still seems uncertain, then rephrase what you said using different words.

3. Special hints. If the child has trouble during spelling tests, try using the words in a sentence. Many words look alike to the lipreader. When the child makes other mistakes, make sure he or she has understood the question or direction (by having the child repeat) before you correct the error. When giving homework assignments or important directions, have the child write the assignment so you can make sure he or she understands what to do.

   Children with a hearing loss who need to see the speaker's face often cannot take notes and listen at the same time. You may wish to allow a "buddy" to take notes for the child using a carbon paper. Special assignments requiring the child to watch a television program may also be difficult, as the child cannot always see the speaker's face. Providing notes for the child to study at home would be helpful in this situation. During reading class you should make sure that the child knows the meaning of the words and does not simply "call" words that he or she does not understand. In a reading circle these children will have difficulty keeping their places because they cannot see and understand the other children as well as they do the teacher. Another problem area for some hearing-impaired children is hearing the various bells used to signal the end of class, fire drills, etc. Assign these children a "buddy" to tap them on the shoulder to alert them to the bell.

4. Parents can be helpful. Because children with a hearing loss can follow instructions better if they are already prepared for the vocabulary in the new lesson, it is often most helpful if teachers allow interested parents to bring the child's textbooks home. Using the teacher's recommendations, the parent can individually introduce the child to the vocabulary in the next lesson.

5. The hearing aid. Even if the child wears a hearing aid, he or she still needs to watch the face of the speaker to understand what is being said. A child with a hearing aid should wear it constantly while at school except for swimming class. Encourage the parents to provide the child with an extra battery so that the battery can be replaced if it goes out while the child is in school. We have enclosed additional information regarding hearing aid use and maintenance that you may wish to refer to for further assistance.

Your understanding of this child can be an important contribution to his or her success in school. If you have questions or comments concerning this letter, please feel free to call me.

Yours very truly,

_____ , MS, CCC/A
Clinical Audiologist

**Figure 7.4.** Sample letter to inform teachers of hearing loss.

# Evaluation Procedures

Much research has been carried out to determine the most efficient method for obtaining comprehensive audiological tests on preschool children. Table 7.3 provides a summary of the major test procedures that are available to the audiologist; these procedures are described in detail below. Before discussing the actual evaluation procedures we should review two preevaluation considerations: test stimuli and the role of the parent during the evaluation.

## Test Stimuli

With each of these procedures, a variety of test stimuli can be employed for evaluation, including pure tones, filtered noise, white noise, environmental sounds, filtered speech, and speech. Generally, for behavioral observation audiometry, conditioned orientation reflex audiometry, and visual reinforcement audiometry, pure tones produce the lowest percentage of response and are not as effective a signal when compared with other types of stimuli, especially speech. However, pure tones provide frequency-specific information that is helpful in identifying high-frequency hearing loss, and they must be employed routinely as part of the evaluation process to rule out high-frequency or frequency-specific hearing loss.

Precaution is needed in interpreting test results obtained with narrow-band noise. Many clinicians assume that narrow-band noise generated by clinical audiometers is frequency-specific. That is, the energy produced is limited to a narrow band of frequencies centered at the test frequency. Figure 7.5 shows the results of spectral analysis on narrow-band noise signals generated by a microprocessor-based diagnostic audiometer. The fact that the audiometer incorporates a microprocessor indicates that it was designed using updated technology. As shown in this figure, the narrow-band signals are reasonably frequency-specific. The rejection rate is at least 40 to 50 dB per octave for all stimuli. With this audiometer, results obtained with the narrow-band stimuli can be considered frequency-specific. The maximum possible error when testing a cooperative patient would be 40 to 50 dB at one octave frequency when a precipitous, frequency-specific hearing loss is present. While this audiometer does produce narrow-band noise that is frequency-specific, other audiometers, especially the older versions based on earlier technology, may not. For this reason, it is imperative that spectral analysis be performed in order to make frequency-specific clinical judgments if narrow-band signals are used with preschool children and other difficult-to-test populations.

**TABLE 7.3**
**Summary of Preschool Audiological Evaluation Procedures**

| Name of Test | Explanation of Technique | Indications for Use | Advantages/Disadvantages |
|---|---|---|---|
| Behavioral Observation Audiometry (BOA) | *Conditioning:* None<br><br>A variety of test signals are presented through loudspeaker(s). Minimal intensity is determined where behavioral changes are observed (e.g., alerting, scanning, cessation of activity, or change in sucking during testing).<br><br>*Reinforcement:* None | Infants under 6 months and older youngsters with severe developmental delays.<br><br>*Alternative:* Auditory evoked responses (particularly if test findings suggest a significant hearing loss). | *Advantages:* Can be used with unconditionable children.<br><br>*Disadvantages:* 1. Rapid habituation of unconditioned behavior.<br><br>2. Unilateral losses may be missed.<br><br>3. Can only rule out severe and profound losses since relatively high intensities are required to elicit unconditioned responses even in normal hearing infants. |

**Table 7.3.** continued

| | | |
|---|---|---|
| Conditioned Orientation Reflex Audiometry (COR) | *Conditioning*: Establish bond between auditory signal and flashing lighted toy. | Toddlers from 6 to 24 months and many older children with developmental delays. |
| Visual Reinforcement Audiometry (VRA) | *Reinforcement*: Lighted toy as well as social praise during test phase. | *Alternative*: Auditory evoked responses. |

*Advantages:*
1. Stimuli can be presented by earphones, bone conduction, or loudspeaker.
2. Does not require voluntary response.
3. Capitalizes on heightened visual alertness of hearing-impaired children.

*Disadvantages:*
1. Approximately 35% of infants under 12 months of age cannot be conditioned.
2. Many toddlers will not accept earphones initially.
3. If stimuli are presented in the sound field, a unilateral hearing loss may be missed.

**Table 7.3.** continued

| | | |
|---|---|---|
| Tangible Reinforcement Operant Conditioning Audiometry (TROCA) | *Conditioning*: Connection is established between auditory stimuli and "button-pressing."<br><br>*Reinforcement*: A tangible reinforcement (such as cereal) that is automatically dispensed following a correct response. | Preschoolers, especially those with short attention spans and those who work best with structure. Also many older mentally retarded children.<br><br>*Alternative*: VRA (auditory evoked responses). |

*Advantages*: 1. Stimuli can be presented by earphones, bone conduction, or loudspeakers.

2. Can be used in conjunction with frequency-specific measures.

*Disadvantages*: 1. Time-consuming and requires repeated sessions to establish conditioning.

2. Children will often insist upon eating the reinforcer between trials, thus increasing the length of the test session substantially.

**Table 7.3.** continued

| | | |
|---|---|---|
| Play Condi-<br>tioning<br>Audiometry<br>(PCA) | *Conditioning:* Connection is established between auditory stimuli and play activity.<br><br>*Reinforcement:* Play activity and social reinforcement during conditioning and testing. May also use visual reinforcement. | Preschoolers, 30 months to 4 years, and older children with mild developmental delays.<br><br>*Alternatives:* TROCA or VRA (auditory evoked responses). | *Advantages:* Can be used in conjunction with any frequency-specific measures.<br><br>*Disadvantages:* A variety of activities are needed to maintain interest in the activity; otherwise, response behavior habituates. |

*Source:* Adapted from Brookhouser, Worthington, Stelmachowicz, Cyr, and Gorga (1985). Reprinted by permission.

## The Role of the Parent

Flexibility and adaptability are two important examiner requirements for testing preschool children. Also important for successful testing is the establishment of cooperation and trust. When initially meeting the child, the audiologist should greet both the child and the parent and suggest that they all go to another room to "play some games." Never ask children whether they want to come—a typical 3-year-old will answer "no!"

The role of the parent when testing the preschool child should be determined on an individual basis. Some children may be cooperative when separated from the parent, performing well in the structured test environment. Others may feel threatened sitting with a stranger in an enclosed room. Still others may feel comfortable with the parent outside the test room watching through a window. For many children, though, the parent must be in the test room. The parent may sit quietly and watch, or actually participate by helping the audiologist. In either case, what the

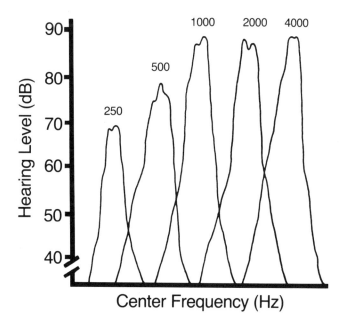

**Figure 7.5.** Spectral analysis of narrow-band noise signals at octave frequencies of 250–4000 Hz produced by a microprocessor-based diagnostic audiometer through sound-field speakers.

parent observes during testing can be beneficial during counseling. The parent who has first-hand observation will better understand the limitations of testing children. If sound-field tests are conducted with the parent inside the sound suite, the parent will hear the levels at which the child responds and better understand the degree of loss, if one is found. However, one word of caution is needed. If sound-field stimuli are used at high intensities (above about 65 dB HL), all observers in the sound room must be given hearing protectors to prevent possible legal suits from exposure to loud noise. Generally parents should be welcomed to observe the testing if they desire, and be treated warmly to help establish cooperation and trust from the preschool child. Now that these two preevaluation considerations have been covered, specific audiological evaluation procedures will be presented.

## Behavioral Observation Audiometry (BOA)

This procedure often provides only minimal information concerning threshold sensitivity, but it may be the only successful behavioral test method with difficult-to-test preschool children and special populations. This form of testing is passive in that the child is not conditioned to respond, and as a result it is nonthreatening to the young child. Typically, testing takes place in the sound field (see Figure 7.6) because many times the child will not accept earphones. However, if the child will accept earphones the testing can be done with the earphones worn. A stimulus is presented, and a behavioral response is observed. Ideally, two evaluators should be available for the testing, one directly observing the child within the test room and one observing the child outside the test room while presenting the test stimuli. During the test the two evaluators can compare their interpretations of a child's activity as a way of validating true responses to the auditory stimuli.

The procedure is carried out as follows:

1. The child is seated between two speakers. The stimulus intensity at this spot has been calibrated. If children will not separate from their parent(s), they may sit on either parent's lap, but the parent must not prompt the child. If a child will sit alone, a small chair or high chair is useful to restrict excessive movement.

2. The test room must be quiet, with conversation and ambient noise at a minimum. The child is distracted by looking at pictures or playing with quiet toys. The examiner with the child should direct the activity (Figure 7.6A).

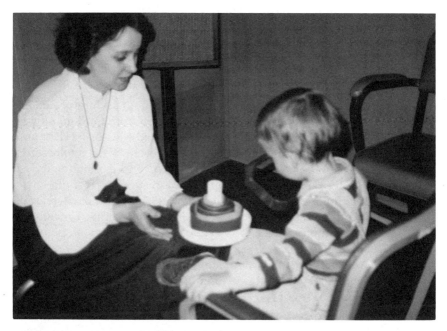

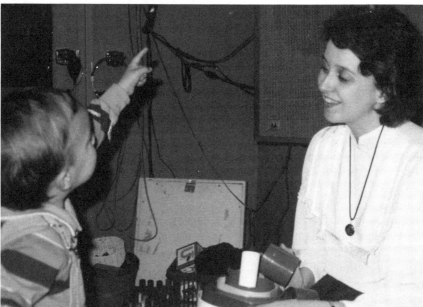

**Figure 7.6.** Behavioral observation audiometry in sound field.

3. A warble tone or narrow-band noise stimulus is presented at 0 dB HL, and the intensity is increased in 10 dB steps until a response is observed. The procedure is repeated until three reliable responses are observed. Stimuli should be presented first at 500 Hz and 2000 Hz, and if the child does not fatigue, 1000 Hz and 4000 Hz are tested.

4. A behavioral change following stimulus presentation is interpreted as a response, but often it can be difficult to discern from random movement. The most recognizable response is a head turn or localization reponse. If the child appropriately looks at each speaker following stimulus presentation, a response is accepted and ear symmetry is assumed (Figure 7.6B). Other behavioral responses include eye-widening or blinking, cessation of play activity, increased or decreased sucking, increased respiration, verbalization, or searching. Time intervals between stimulus presentation should be varied to avoid patterning. The child needs to be observed between stimuli to determine how often the behavior occurs without stimulus presentation. If the examiner is not sure that the child is responding, the intensity is increased; a more pronounced behavior should occur if the child was responding to the sound.

5. Testing must proceed quickly, as the child may fatigue, lose interest, or become restless. If no response is observed to low-intensity stimuli, an intense stimulus should be presented to cause a startle response.

While BOA is often successful, results should be interpreted as minimum response levels as opposed to true thresholds. Downs and Sterritt (1967) and Thompson and Weber (1974) found that responses follow a sequential pattern as the child matures, reaching threshold levels by 2 years of age. The Index of Auditory Behaviors (Northern & Downs, 1984), shown in Table 7.4, describes the expected response levels by chronological age. However, several variables can affect these expected ranges of results. Children from special populations may not follow normal response patterns at their chronological age. Dahle and McCollister (1983) point out that auditory behavior should be correlated to developmental age rather than chronological age for mentally retarded children. The normally developing child may not respond as expected due to boredom with the task. Thompson and Weber (1974) found that lower (better) thresholds were obtained using play audiometry than BOA with children able to perform play audiometry. The audiologist must be aware of the developmental level of each child tested to incorporate the best test procedure and correctly interpret the results.

**TABLE 7.4**

**Auditory Behavior Index for Infants: Stimulus and Level of Response***

| Age | Noisemakers (Approx. SPL) | Warbled Pure Tones (dB HL) | Speech (dB HL) | Expected Response | Startle to Speech (dB HL) |
|---|---|---|---|---|---|
| 0–6 weeks | 50–70 dB | 78 dB | 40–60 dB | Eye widening, eye-blink, stirring or arousal from sleep, startle | 65 dB |
| 6 weeks– 4 months | 50–60 dB | 70 dB | 47 dB | Eye-widening, eye-shift, eye-blinking, quieting; beginning rudimentary head turn by 4 months | 65 dB |
| 4–7 months | 40–50 dB | 51 dB | 21 dB | Head turn on lateral plane toward sound; listening attitude | 65 dB |
| 7–9 months | 30–40 dB | 45 dB | 15 dB | Direct localization of sounds to side, indirectly below ear level | 65 dB |
| 9–13 months | 25–35 dB | 38 dB | 8 dB | Direct localization of sounds to side, directly below ear level, indirectly above ear level | 65 dB |
| 13–16 months | 25–30 dB | 32 dB | 5 dB | Direct localization of sound on side, above, and below | 65 dB |
| 16–21 months | 25 dB | 25 dB | 5 dB | Direct localization of sound on side, above, and below | 65 dB |
| 21–24 months | 25 dB | 26 dB | 3 dB | Direct localization of sound on side, above, and below | 65 dB |

*Testing done in a sound room.

*Source:* Northern and Downs (1984, p. 135). Reprinted by permission.

Thompson and Wilson (1984) reviewed data collected using BOA on children aged 3–59 months and provide the following summary statements regarding this technique:

1. The potential for observer bias in judging responses complicates the task.

2. The obtained thresholds improve substantially as a function of age.

3. The obtained thresholds vary substantially as a function of signal used—pure tones are not an effective signal.

4. Infants and young children habituate to the test stimulus, which results in large intrasubject variability in a substantial number of cases.

5. A substantial variability in threshold estimates occurs across infants—this variability makes it difficult to establish "norms" using the BOA procedure.

Despite these limitations, BOA is useful and should be incorporated into testing the preschool child at least as a screening technique when other procedures are unsuccessful. Significant hearing loss can be ruled out, and conditioning levels for other behavioral test procedures can be determined. However, results should be interpreted cautiously, as these responses tend to be elevated and only represent sensitivity in the better ear.

## Conditioned Orientation Reflex (COR) and Visual Reinforcement Audiometry (VRA)

Before describing the specific procedures used with COR and VRA, the theories of behavioral conditioning should be addressed. Many audiological test methods have their roots in classical or operant conditioning procedures.

Classical conditioning involves the presentation of a stimulus or creation of an event to elicit a response or a change of behavior in some way. The two response modes that make up classical conditioning are unconditioned and conditioned reflexes or responses. An unconditioned response occurs when a stimulus elicits a specific response without prior conditioning or learning. An example of an unconditioned response would be the startle reflex to intense acoustic stimuli. A conditioned reflex or response occurs when the unconditioned reflex is transferred to a neutral event. The neutral event then controls the response and will elicit the desired response. In audiological testing, COR and VRA are based on the principles of classical conditioning.

In operant conditioning, the response to the stimulus is controlled by the consequences of the response. When the response to a stimulus is followed by an event that strengthens or reinforces the response, the event is called a positive reinforcement. Examples of positive reinforcements are providing candy, tokens, money, or praise after a correct response occurs. When the response is followed by an event that weakens the response through punishment, the event is called a negative reinforcement. Examples of negative reinforcements are shocks and withdrawing positive reinforcement. Although negative reinforcement can be effective in some learning situations, the use of positive reinforcment is much more successful in audiometric testing. Two examples of the use of operant conditioning in audiometry are Tangible Reinforcement Operant Conditioning Audiometry (TROCA) and Play Conditioning Audiometry (PCA).

Dix and Hallpike (1947) provided one of the early visual conditioning test procedures successful with children under 6 years of age based on the principles of conditioning. In this procedure, named the Peep Show, the child initially is presented with an auditory stimulus and simultaneously a light is illuminated. By pressing a button, a darkened box with a picture inside was designed to light up, reinforcing the child. After conditioning the child to the auditory and visual stimuli, the auditory stimulus alone is presented. Through the conditioning technique, the meaningless sound of the auditory stimuli has been made interesting, thus keeping the child's interest. Complex instructions are also avoided, because an instructor can demonstrate the child's role. Dix and Hallpike (1947) reported this technique to be successful with the otherwise untestable preschool child.

Pressing the button for reinforcement proved too difficult a motor task for some children. To overcome this weakness, Conditioned Orientation Reflex (COR) audiometry was developed (Suzuki & Ogiba, 1961). The COR procedure expands upon the orientation reflex. When a light stimulus is presented, a young child will turn reflexively toward the light source (see Figure 7.7). By pairing an auditory stimulus with the light stimulus, the child can be conditioned to orient to the light when the sound stimuli alone are perceived. Suzuki and Ogiba (1961) reported success in testing over 80% of their children in the 1- to 3-year-old age range with the COR technique.

The procedure for using COR is as follows:

1. A sound-field test room is set up with a darkened box placed upon each speaker. Animated toys (dolls) are hidden in these boxes. The tester can illuminate the box to reveal the doll by activating a switch.

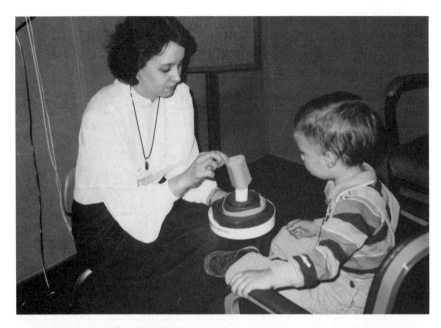

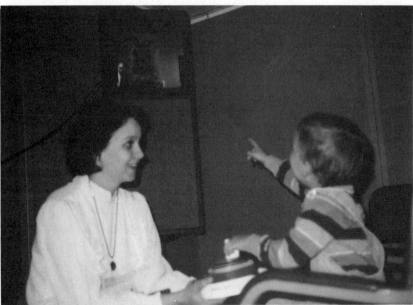

**Figure 7.7.** Conditioned Orientation Reflex (COR) audiometry being applied to a preschool child.

2. The child is seated alone or on a parent's lap or in a high chair between two speakers. The child should be quietly distracted, looking at pictures or a toy (Figure 7.7).

3. An auditory stimulus is presented at approximately 70 dB above the child's expected threshold and the doll box illuminated (Figure 7.7). This conditioning is alternated between the speakers, with the auditory and visual stimuli presented for 3 or 4 seconds as the child watches.

4. The auditory stimuli are next presented alone, with the box lighting up as a reward after the child (without visual reinforcement) looks toward the speaker. This procedure is continued, decreasing the intensity until the child does not respond and the minimal response level is obtained.

The COR technique is a quick and efficient procedure. It does not require the child to perform a motor task, which makes it especially helpful when evaluating children under 3 years of age. The main disadvantage of COR is that thresholds are obtained in sound field. Thus, the information obtained only reflects hearing sensitivity of the better ear, so unilateral impairment may be missed. The success rate of the test and the information it provides, however, does make it a valuable and useful clinical tool.

The Puppet in the Window Illuminated (PIWI) test is a form of COR audiometry developed by Haug, Baccaro, and Guilford (1967). Successful with children unable to perform fine motor tasks, PIWI accepts the eye orientation reflex, cessation of activity, startle, or searching as response behaviors.

The PIWI procedure is as follows:

1. An auditory stimulus is presented through a sound-field speaker. A darkened box containing a puppet is located above the speaker.

2. When a response is observed, the puppet box is illuminated.

3. Stimulus intensity is decreased until threshold is reached, with responses reinforced by the illuminated puppet. An interesting aspect of PIWI is that the child's interest may be maintained by changing puppets.

4. Earphone and bone-conduction testing is next carried out if the child will cooperate.

Although COR is useful in obtaining thresholds on normal hearing children, children with hearing impairment often find this procedure too difficult. Liden and Kankkunen (1969) expanded upon COR by changing the test technique and modifying the response criteria. Their technique is called Visual Response Audiometry (VRA).

VRA accepts several behaviors as responses instead of limiting positive responses to localization or the eye orientating reflex. Infants may display a reflexive behavior, such as widening of their eyes, wrinkling of their forehead, or changing their facial expression. An investigatory response is accepted when a child is conditioned to associate an auditory stimulus with a visual reinforcement. An orientation response occurs when the child quickly learns that an auditory stimulus is followed by a visual stimulus and is not surprised by the pattern. A spontaneous response occurs if children report they hear the auditory stimulus by vocalizing, raising their hands, or any other response mode. Acceptance of these four behavioral patterns gives the audiologist more freedom when testing young children.

VRA protocol follows one of two methods, the 60 dB procedure and the 30 dB procedure. Both of these procedures are described below.

## 60 dB Procedure

1. An auditory stimulus is presented initially at 60 dB HL and paired with a visual stimulus. This simultaneous presentation is repeated to condition the child.

2. Once the child is conditioned, stimulus intensity is decreased in 20 dB steps. When no response is observed, the intensity is increased in 10 dB steps.

3. Threshold or the minimum response level is determined when the child responds to three out of six presentations at the lowest intensity level.

## 30 dB Procedure

1. An auditory stimulus is presented initially at 30 dB HL.

2. If no response is observed, the intensity is increased and the 60 dB procedure is followed.

3. If a response is observed, a visual reinforcement is presented.

4. The procedure is repeated. The intensity is then decreased in 20 dB steps. When no response is observed, the intensity is increased in 10 dB steps.

5. Threshold or the minimum response level is the lowest intensity at which the child gives two consecutive responses.

Thompson and Folsom (1984) found no significant difference between the 30 dB and 60 dB procedures. The 30 dB procedure may be more time-efficient for the normal hearing child, but the 60 dB procedure may provide a better starting intensity for the hearing-impaired child.

VRA has proven to be a successful technique for assessing hearing sensitivity of children under 3 years of age. Because it accepts many different response patterns, hearing-impaired children who have difficulty localizing sound or responding consistently to sound will be identified (Hodgson, 1978). Thompson and Wilson (1984) reported success with children as young as 5 months of age when reinforcers were made interesting with different colors, movements, and contours. Thompson and Wilson (1984) also studied VRA using earphones. Although responses were observed, thresholds appeared elevated. They related this to either earphone leakage or to play techniques used to distract the infants. Further study is needed in this area.

## Tangible Reinforcement Operant Conditioning Audiometry

Tangible Reinforcement Operant Conditioning Audiometry (TROCA) is a procedure that uses an object to reinforce a child's response to an auditory stimulus. Originally developed by Lloyd, Spradlin, and Reid (1968) for use with mentally retarded children, this procedure has been adapted for many difficult-to-test populations. The technique requires the use of specially designed equipment that will dispense a tangible reinforcer to the child upon activating a switch. The procedure is generally performed as follows:

1. A tangible reinforcer is selected. This reinforcer may be food, such as candy or cereal; a drink, such as juice or soda; a small trinket or toy; or a reinforcer that the child is accustomed to using. The reinforcers may be placed in a cup or bag as the child receives them for later use, or may be immediately given to the child. The reinforcement must be viewed positively by the child, but it must not detract from the task.

2. To begin testing, a 500 Hz auditory signal is presented at 50 dB HL, and a reinforcement button is lit. The audiologist presses the button, the reinforcement is obtained and given to the child, and both stimuli stop. This procedure is repeated twice, or until the child becomes aware of the task.

3. On the third trial, the audiologist guides the child's hand to press the lighted button and receive the reinforcement. As the trials continue,

the audiologist gradually stops guiding the child through the task in the hope that the child will perform the behavior independently.

4. Once the child is able to respond to the auditory stimulus and lighted button without assistance, the light is gradually removed (faded) until only the auditory stimuli cue the child's response. The response should be generalized across frequencies, and thresholds often can be obtained.

Difficult-to-test children will require several training sessions to obtain reliable results. The training may require the child to return for five or six sessions, or possibly more, with the sessions lasting no longer than about 15 minutes. A parent, teacher, or speech-language pathologist may include test training with TROCA in daily activities.

## Play Conditioning Audiometry

Play Conditioning Audiometry (PCA) provides the most reliable threshold information when successfully used with the preschool child. Although a young child may respond to conventional testing (hand-raising or button-pressing), the task is boring and interest is quickly lost. PCA makes testing a game. A block is dropped in a bucket, a ring placed on a stack, a bead snapped to another bead, or some other reinforcing behavior is carried out when the child hears the stimulus. The gross motor movement, accompanied by verbal praise, becomes reinforcing, and the child becomes involved in an enjoyable activity. Play audiometry is successful with children as young as 30 months of age, but may be needed with difficult-to-test children as old as 10 or more, or even adults.

To use PCA the child must be conditioned to perform the response task before proceeding to threshold testing. Conditioning is carried out by presenting a suprathreshold stimulus and guiding the child through the response mode. When responses occur without the evaluator's urging or guidance, the intensity is decreased until threshold is obtained. If a child does not condition to an auditory stimulus, it is helpful to switch to another sensory modality in order to differentiate inability to perform the task from inability to perceive the stimulus. One helpful procedure, suggested by Thorne (1962), incorporates the tactile mode and proceeds as follows (see Figure 7.8):

1. The child holds the bone vibrator from the audiometer in one hand and a block in the other hand, so that the two objects are touching (Figure 7.8A).

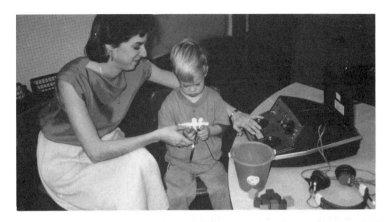

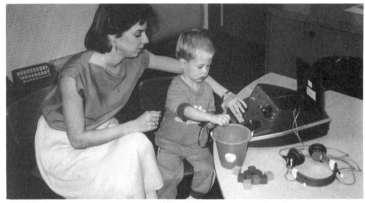

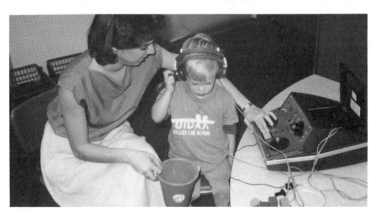

**Figure 7.8.** Tactile stimulation using the bone-conduction oscillator can assist in play conditioning audiometry.

2. A 500 Hz stimulus is presented at equipment limits (usually 60–65 dB HL), causing a tactile sensation in the child's hand.

3. As the child feels the vibratory stimulus, his or her hands are shaken together. The block is guided by the examiner and dropped in a bucket, and the stimulus is stopped. The child is rewarded by clapping and praise. This procedure is continued until the child can perform the task alone (Figure 7.8B) or until it is determined that the child will not condition to the tactile stimulus.

4. The bone vibrator is next placed on the mastoid. If severe hearing impairment is suspected, conditioning is attempted with a 500 Hz tactile stimulus. If hearing impairment is not suspected, a 500 Hz signal at 40 dB HL is presented. Conditioned thresholds should be obtained at 500 Hz and 2000 Hz. The task is then transferred to earphones (Figure 7.8C).

Using a tactile stimulus assures the audiologist that the child can be conditioned for PCA. The bone vibrator may also appear less threatening to a child who will not accept earphones.

Roeser and Northern (1981) describe a simple play conditioning technique named Play Audiometry Reinforcement using a Flashlight (PARF). PARF is carried out in the following way (see Figure 7.9):

1. The examiner holds a flashlight, and the child holds the object used to respond (block, ring, etc.) under the flashlight. The light from an otoscope can be used if a flashlight is not available (Figure 7.9A).

2. The light is turned on for 1 or 2 seconds, and the child's hand is guided to make the appropriate response (put block in box, stack the ring, etc.). This procedure is repeated until the child is conditioned or until it is determined that the child will not condition.

3. If the child can be conditioned to the light, the audiologist sets the earphones on the table next to the audiometer close to the child. The intensity is set to a high level (90–100 dB HL) and the frequency at 1000 Hz. The child is given the response object to hold to the cheek, and a 2- or 3-second tone is presented. The child's hand is guided to make an appropriate response. Usually the child will condition within three to five trials, at which point the audiologist proceeds to Step 4. However, even if the child does not condition, Step 4 is tried because it might be possible that the child did not perceive the stimulus.

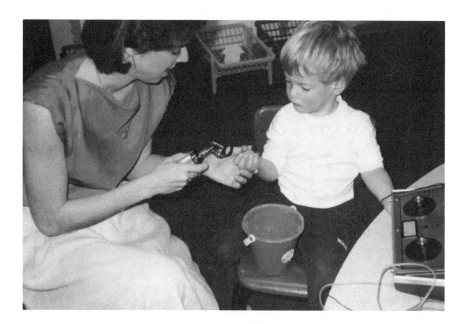

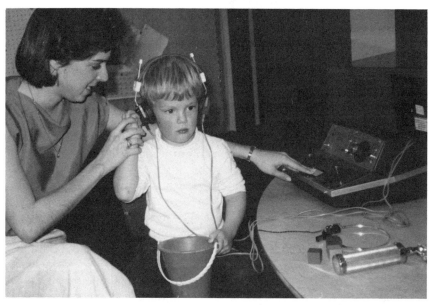

**Figure 7.9.** Example of Play Audiometry Reinforcement using a Flashlight (PARF). In this example the clinician is substituting the light from an otoscope for the flashlight.

4. Earphones are then placed on the child, and the child holds the response object to the earphone or the cheek (Figure 7.9B). A 1000 Hz stimulus at 50 dB HL is presented, and the examiner guides the child's hand to make the response. If the child does not appear to respond, the intensity is increased.

5. Once the child is conditioned, thresholds are obtained.

Using a visual stimulus adds some "magic" to the test procedure. Most children can transfer visual conditioning to an auditory signal without difficulty. Clinical experience with PARF has shown that the child who cannot be conditioned to the visual stimulus used in this procedure will not condition to an auditory stimulus. Thus, these children should be considered for BOA, VRA, COR, or even auditory brainstem response audiometry.

# Masking

As a result of the high prevalence of middle ear disorders in the preschool population, the majority of hearing losses are conductive in nature. Furthermore, it is usually during the preschool years when unilateral sensorineural hearing loss is first discovered. Both of these conditions require the use of masking for accurate testing. Otherwise, spurious results will be obtained. Figure 7.10 is a typical example of erroneous results that are found when masking is not used. This figure illustrates unmasked pure-tone findings from a 3½-year-old child who was known to have normal right-ear hearing sensitivity and a profound left-ear sensorineural hearing impairment. Yet, due to the lack of masking, the audiogram indicates only a moderate degree of left-ear loss, which is shown to be conductive rather than sensorineural.

The introduction of masking noise can be disruptive to some children. Many cannot discriminate between the pure tones and the masking noise, and stop responding. Others respond only to suprathreshold stimuli, increasing the intensity level at which they respond as the masking level is increased. This linear shift may appear to be a plateau effect when it is actually only the child's response pattern to the masking noise. Because of these problems, results obtained with masking must be interpreted carefully, and the importance of a test battery approach and the utilization of the cross-check principle (described below) becomes more evident.

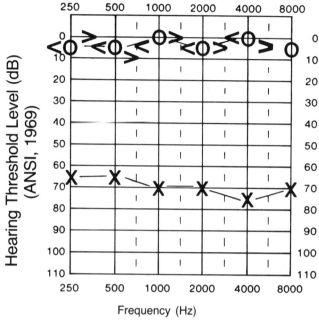

O = RIGHT EAR AIR     < = RIGHT EAR BONE

X = LEFT EAR AIR     > = LEFT EAR BONE

**Figure 7.10.** Classical example of unmasked pure-tone findings for a child known to have normal right-ear hearing sensitivity and a profound left-ear sensorineural hearing loss. Without masking, the audiogram erroneously shows a moderate conductive hearing loss due to crossover.

If masking is attempted, standard masking formulae should be employed (Martin, 1986), with some added explanation. Children should be told that a rain noise or "Mr. Wind" will blow in their ears, and that they need to ignore that noise but keep listening for the "ticklebug." Introducing the noise gradually will help reduce the effects of the noise by not frightening the child and will interfere less with the established criteria for responding.

A new development is the introduction of insert earphones for clinical audiometry. These devices fit directly into the external auditory canal, rather than fitting over the pinna, and provide significantly more interaural attentuation. Killion, Wilber, and Gudmundsen (1985) have shown that as much as 40 dB extra interaural attenuation can be gained from the insert earphone compared with a standard earphone. The added interaural attenuation will eliminate or greatly reduce the need for masking and can be highly beneficial for valid audiological testing of preschoolers.

# The Cross-Check Principle

A basic tenet of all diagnostic testing is that the results from only one procedure should not be considered in isolation when formulating the clinical diagnosis, especially when other procedures are available; results from a battery of tests should be used. The cross-check principle formally elaborates this very important concept. First described by Jerger and Hayes (1976), the basic hypothesis of the cross-check principle is that often other handicaps, such as mental retardation, cerebral palsy, blindness, and autism, interfere with a child's ability to cooperate for pure-tone testing and that true thresholds cannot be obtained on one test only.

Behavioral testing is compromised by ambiguous response modes, nonrepeatable responses, and suprathreshold responses. The cross-check principle employs a battery approach so that pure-tone tests are verified by independent measures. In this way, threshold sensitivity can be reported more validly. When acoustic immittance measures are included, the effects of middle ear disorders can be considered. Sensitivity Prediction from the Acoustic Reflex (Jerger, Burney, Mauldin, & Crump, 1974) provides a means of classifying degree of loss, and results can be compared to behavioral findings. If results from these two measures are noncontributory or contradictory, auditory brainstem response (ABR) audiometry will predict hearing sensitivity in the 1000–4000 Hz region. Although low-frequency and frequency-specific information is compromised by ABR, recommendations for educational placement and amplification oftentimes can be made with better confidence through the use of this technique.

By employing the cross-check principle, more accurate results can be reported, and critical errors and misdiagnoses can be avoided. Thus, it is critical that the cross-check principle be applied to testing the preschool child, especially the difficult-to-test preschool child. All children failing the diagnostic audiological test battery must be scheduled for additional testing, including immittance tests and ABR testing. These diagnostic procedures are covered elsewhere in this text.

# Summary

Early identification of hearing loss is a critical factor in preventing possible language and educational handicaps. Throughout this chapter we have presented procedures to be used in screening hearing and a variety of audiological diagnostic procedures to obtain the most information possible from a preschool child. Emphasized is the need for flexibility. If one procedure fails, the astute clinician will try something else; if the child is successful at one task and is still attentive, clinicians should proceed to the next step to add more information. A complete pure-tone audiogram may not be obtained from every preschool child, but even partial information can help establish appropriate educational settings, preliminary hearing-aid fittings, the need for psychoeducational testing, or neurological referral. With patience and perseverance, preschool children can be evaluated successfully and given the opportunity to develop to their full potential.

# References

American Academy of Otolaryngology Committee on Hearing and Equilibrium and the American Council of Otolaryngology Committee on the Medical Aspects of Noise. (1979). Guide for the evaluation of hearing handicap. *Journal of the American Medical Association, 19,* 2055–2059.

American Academy of Pediatrics Committee on Children with Handicaps. (1973). The physician and the deaf child. *Pediatrics, 51,* 1100.

American National Standards Institute (ANSI). (1970). *American National Standard specifications for audiometers, ANSI S3.6-1969.* New York: American National Standards Institute.

American Speech and Hearing Association (ASHA), Committee on Audiometric Evaluation. (1975). Guidelines for identification audiometry. *Asha, 17,* 94–99.

Anderson, C. (1978). Hearing screening for children. In J. Katz (Ed.), *Handbook of clinical audiology* (pp. 48–60). Baltimore: Williams and Wilkins.

Bess, F. N., & Tharpe, M. A. (1986). Case history data on unilaterally hearing-impaired children. *Ear and Hearing, 7,* 14–19.

Bess, F. N., & Tharpe, M. A. (1984). Unilateral hearing impairment in children. *Pediatrics, 74,* 206–216.

Bess, F. N., Tharpe, M. A., & Gibler, A. M. (1986). Auditory performance of children with unilateral sensorineural hearing loss. *Ear and Hearing, 7,* 20–26.

Bricco, E. (1985). Impacted cerumen as a reason for failure in hearing conservation programs. *Journal of School Health, 55,* 240–241.

Brookhouser, P., Worthington, D., Stelmachowicz, P., Cyr, G., & Gorga, M. (1985). *Evaluation of hearing and vestibular function in the child: Methods and pitfalls.* Short course presented at the annual meeting of the American Academy of Otolaryngology—Head and Neck Surgery, Atlanta.

Connor, L. (1961). Determining the prevalence of hearing-impaired children. *Exceptional Children, 28,* 337–344.

Dahle, A., & McCollister, F. (1983). Considerations for evaluating hearing. In G. Mencher & S. Gerber (Eds.), *The multiply handicapped hearing-impaired child* (pp. 171–206). New York: Grune and Stratton.

Darley, F. L. (1961). Identification audiometry for school-age children: Basic procedures. *Journal of Speech and Hearing Disorders,* Monograph Supplement 9, 26–34.

Dix, M. R., & Hallpike, C. S. (1947). The peep-show: New technique for pure-tone audiometry in young children. *British Medical Journal, 2,* 717–723.

Downs, M. (1978). Auditory screening. *Otolaryngology Clinics of North America, 11,* 611–629.

Downs, M. P., & Sterritt, G. M. (1967). A guide to newborn and infant hearing screening programs. *Archives of Otolaryngology, 85,* 37–44.

Fay, T. H., Hochberg, I., Smith, C. R., Rees, N., & Halpern, H. (1972). Audiologic and otologic screening of disadvantaged children. In A. Glorig & K. Gerwin (Eds.), *Otitis media* (pp. 163–170). Springfield, IL: Charles C. Thomas.

Fisher, L. I. (1976). Efficiency and effectiveness of using a portable audiometric booth in school hearing conservation programs. *Language, Speech, and Hearing Services in Schools, 7,* 242–249.

Frasier, G. R. (1971). The genetics of congenital deafness. *Otolaryngology Clinics of North America, 4,* 227–247.

Ginsberg, A., & White, T. P. (1978). Otological considerations in audiology. In J. Katz (Ed.), *Handbook of clinical audiology* (2nd ed., pp. 8–22). Baltimore: Williams and Wilkins.

Giolas, T. G., & Wark, D. J. (1967). Communication problems associated with unilateral hearing loss. *Journal of Speech and Hearing Disorders, 32,* 336–343.

Haug, O., Baccaro, P., & Guilford, F. (1967). A pure-tone audiogram on the infant: The PIWI technique. *Archives of Otolaryngology, 86,* 435–440.

Hodgson, W. (1978). Testing infants and young children. In J. Katz (Ed.), *Handbook of clinical audiology* (2nd ed., pp. 397–409). Baltimore: Williams and Wilkins.

Hood, B., & Lamb, L. E. (1974). Identification audiometry. In K. S. Gerwin & A. Glorig (Eds.), *Detection of hearing loss and ear disease in children* (pp. 14–39). Springfield, IL: Charles C. Thomas.

House, H. P., & Glorig, A. (1957). A new concept in auditory screening. *Laryngoscope, 67,* 661–668.

Jerger, J., & Hayes, D. (1976). The cross-check principle in pediatric audiometry. *Archives of Otolaryngology, 102,* 614–620.

Jerger, J., Burney, P., Mauldin, L., & Crump, B. (1974). Predicting hearing loss from the acoustic reflex. *Journal of Speech and Hearing Disorders, 39,* 11–22.

Kempe, C. H., Silver, H. K., & O'Brien, D. (1984). Current pediatric diagnosis and treatment. *Lange Medical Publications*, 309–310.

Killion, M. C., Wilber, L. A., & Gudmundsen, G. I. (1985). Insert earphones for more interaural attenuation. *Hearing Instruments, 36,* 34–36.

Leske, M. C. (1981). Prevalence estimates of communicative disorders in the U.S. language, hearing and vestibular disorders. *Asha, 23,* 229–236.

Liden, G., & Kankkunen, A. (1969). Visual reinforcement audiometry. *Acta Otolaryngologica, 67,* 281–292.

Lloyd, L. L., Spradlin, J. E., & Reid, M. J. (1968). An operant audiometric procedure for difficult-to-test patients. *Journal of Speech and Hearing Disorders, 33,* 236–245.

McConnell, F., & Ward, P. H. (1967). *Deafness in childhood.* Nashville, TN: Vanderbilt University Press.

Martin, F. N. (1986). *Introduction to audiology.* Englewood Cliffs, NJ: Prentice-Hall.

Maxwell, W. R., & Davidson, G. D. (1961). Limited frequency screening and ear pathology. *Journal of Speech and Hearing Disorders, 26,* 122–125.

Melnick, W., Eagles, E. L., & Levine, H. S. (1964). Evaluation of a recommended program of identification audiometry with school-age children. *Journal of Speech and Hearing Disorders, 29,* 3–13.

Musket, C. H., & Dworaczyk, R. D. (1980). Using an otoscope with preschoolers in acoustic immittance screening programs. *Language, Speech, and Hearing Services in Schools, 11,* 109–111.

Musket, C. H., & Roeser, R. J. (1977). Using circumaural enclosures with children. *Journal of Speech and Hearing Research, 20,* 325–333.

Newhart, H. A. (1948). A pure-tone audiometer for school use. *Archives of Otolaryngology, 28,* 777–779.

Northern, J. L., & Downs, M. P. (1984). *Hearing in children.* Baltimore: Williams and Wilkins.

Norton, M. C., & Lux, E. (1961). Double-frequency auditory screening in public schools. *Journal of Speech and Hearing Disorders, 26,* 293–299.

Roeser, R. J., & Northern, J. L. (1981). Screening for hearing loss and middle ear disorders. In R. J. Roeser & M. Downs (Eds.), *Auditory disorders in school children* (pp. 120–150). New York: Thieme Stratton.

Siegenthaler, B. M., & Sommers, R. K. (1959). Abbreviated sweep-check procedures for school hearing testing. *Journal of Speech and Hearing Disorders, 24,* 249–257.

Smith, C. (1976). Pediatric audiology. *Maico Audiology Library Series, 9,* 29–32.

Stevens, D. A., & Davidson, G. D. (1959). Screening test of hearing. *Journal of Speech and Hearing Disorders, 24,* 258–261.

Stewart, J. (1974). *HRS screening.* Paper presented at the annual meeting of the Western Society for Pediatric Research, Carmel, CA.

Suzuki, T., & Ogiba, U. (1961). Conditioned orientation reflex audiometry. *Archives of Otolaryngology, 74,* 192–198.

Thompson, G., & Folsom, R. C. (1984). A comparison of two conditioning procedures in the use of visual reinforcement audiometry (VRA). *Journal of Speech and Hearing Disorders, 49,* 241–245.

Thompson, G., & Weber, B. A. (1974). Responses of infants and young children to Behavior Observation Audiometry (BOA). *Journal of Speech and Hearing Disorders, 39,* 140–147.

Thompson, G., & Wilson, W. (1984). Clinical application of visual reinforcement audiometry. *Seminars in Hearing, 1,* 85–98.

Thompson, G., Wilson, W., & Moore, J. (1979). Application of visual reinforcement audiometry (VRA) to low-functioning children. *Journal of Speech and Hearing Disorders, 44,* 80–90.

Thompson, M., & Thompson, G. (1972). Response of infants and young children as a function of auditory stimuli and test methods. *Journal of Speech and Hearing Research, 15,* 699–707.

Thorne, B. (1967). Conditioning children for pure-tone testing. *Journal of Speech and Hearing Disorders, 27,* 84–85.

Walton, W. K., & Wilson, W. R. (1972). Stability of routinely serviced portable audiometers. *Language, Speech, and Hearing Services in Schools, 3,* 36–43.

Watkins, S., Moore, T., & Phillips, J. (1984). Clearing impacted ears. *American Journal of Nursing, 9,* 1107.

Wilson, W. R., & Walton, W. K. (1974). Identification audiometry accuracy: Evaluation of a recommended program for school-age children. *Language, Speech, and Hearing Services in Schools, 5,* 132–142.

# 8

# Speech Tests with Preschool Children

## FREDERICK N. MARTIN

*I*n the complete audiological evaluation of the adult patient, speech audiometry serves a number of useful and valuable functions. Determination can be made of the extent to which a hearing handicap affects the ability to hear, discriminate, and tolerate speech. Through the use of speech audiometry, diagnosis can be made regarding the type of hearing disorder and the general site of pathology, including auditory processing difficulties. Speech audiometry is also an aid in determining the type of rehabilitative measures needed and their prognoses. In addition, it is an aid in verifying the reliability of pure-tone test results.

All of the above advantages of speech audiometry for adults can be applied to children. However, in many audiological settings, speech audiometry is absent in the testing of small children, often because facilities do not allow for the additional time and equipment required. Often speech tests with children require two clinicians, or an audiologist and a trained assistant, a price judged too dear to pay in some centers.

Most of the speech tests require two-room settings with excellent sound isolation between the test and control rooms, an environment not always available. At times speech audiometric procedures are not attempted because of an a priori decision that they will not work with a given child or that the results to be obtained do not justify the efforts involved.

Speech signals are obvious selections as stimuli for the assessment of hearing sensitivity in children. There is evidence that speech items were in use as early as 1883 (Meyerson, 1956) to determine hearing thresholds. It was pointed out over a half century ago (Bunch, 1934) that an important reason for performing speech audiometry with children is that speech items have higher face validity than do nonspeech items. This fact increases the probability of accurate responses from those children whose language skills allow the use of speech as test stimuli, since children pay closer attention to verbal than to nonverbal stimuli (Hardy & Bordley, 1951). Clawson (1966) points out that mentally retarded children show an arousal to speech stimuli at significantly lower intensities than they do to pure tones, resulting in a poorer correlation between these two measures than is normally seen in children with normal intelligence. He feels that speech tests, in addition to confirming pure-tone results, reveal insights into the difficulties that retarded children have in paying attention to sound.

While there is no doubt that in many cases speech audiometry with children may be arduous, the practical value obtained from these tests makes the efforts worthwhile. Many children find speech audiometry easier and less abstract that pure-tone tests and are willing participants in such procedures. Often the results of speech tests serve to verify or deny the clinical impressions of hearing disorders gleaned from subjective impressions or from other tests. There are times, in fact, when speech audiometry is the only procedure that can be successfully completed on a child. In such cases, the child must, of course, be returned for further audiometric study, but a valuable beginning will have been made.

To be sure, there are children who, because of their deficits in language skills, maturity, or intelligence, cannot be tested using speech audiometry. The skilled examiner often recognizes this problem early in the evaluation. In any case, where speech test results are obtainable, they should be pursued.

Measurements made during speech audiometry include tests for speech detection, speech reception, and speech discrimination as well as most comfortable and uncomfortable loudness levels. Test results aid the clinician in such matters as aural (re)habilitation, referral for medical treatment, educational placement, and, very importantly, the selection of appropriate hearing aids. The more formal the test is, the easier the interpretation of results and subsequent disposition of the case. Nevertheless, audiologists working with small children must often sacrifice this kind of reliability in favor of more informal and subjectively scored examinations.

# Speech Detection Threshold

The speech detection threshold (SDT) may be defined as the lowest level at which a listener can detect the presence of an ongoing speech signal and identify it as speech. While it is not known how frequently the SDT is used as a measurement of hearing in children, it is probably safe to assume that it is used with some regularity. It seems important to discuss the reason why the SDT should be obtained.

The usual rationale for obtaining the SDT is that it may be the only speech test obtainable from some children and that, while its usefulness is limited, there may be some predictability from the SDT to the speech *reception* threshold (SRT), since studies have shown that the intensity generally required to obtain the SRT is about 10 to 12 dB greater than that for the SDT (Egan, 1948). Hirsh (1952, p. 127) correctly points out that the SDT provides about as much information as the threshold for a buzzer, a combination of pure tones, or a number of different kinds of sounds. Since speech is a broad-band signal, it is impossible to predict audiometric configuration from the SDT (Giolas, 1975, p. 41). If patients are properly conditioned to respond to a signal when presented with a broad band of frequencies, they will indicate a response when any portion of that spectrum becomes audible. Since the spectrum of speech contains peaks and valleys and since most of the energy is concentrated in the lower frequencies, a child with a high-frequency hearing loss will respond to the low-frequency components of the signal, perhaps without discriminating the entire word(s) at all. Frisina (1962) found the SDT to be +/−5 dB of the 500 Hz threshold in cases of flat audiograms, or those which fall slightly or precipitously in the higher frequencies. When the audiometric curve rises in the higher frequencies, as it does in some cases of conductive hearing loss or some congenital sensorineural losses (Ross & Matkin, 1967), the SDT will be +/−5 dB of the pure-tone threshold revealing the best hearing sensitivity on the audiogram.

It must be remembered that some variability is to be expected when measuring the SDT, especially in children. Giolas (1975) points out that the data collected on a set of subjects under specific conditions of recording may not be the same with a different speaker or another set of variables. Giolas recommends finding the SDT by giving a child a set of instructions such as ''Put the ring on the peg.'' The child is encouraged to perform this act, and once the concept is grasped, the intensity is lowered until the child can no longer follow the instruction. It would seem to me that the level at which obedience to commands ceases may be above the SDT by several decibels in some cases and may, in fact, correlate highly with the threshold of intelligibility for sentence material.

Obviously the pure-tone audiogram may be a reasonably good predictor of the SDT, but the reverse is not the case. In fact, if the audiometric configuration is irregular across the frequency range, the SDT may considerably underestimate the SRT, suggesting that it is lower than it truly is. Agreeing that the audiometric contour is not indicated by the SDT, Giolas (1975) nevertheless feels the procedure has advantages, especially in the sound field. In light of the preceding discussion the spectrum of the speech signal must always be kept in mind.

Certainly opinions vary on the relative values of different audiometric procedures. The SDT is a measurement I make only as a last resort, when all attempts at pure-tone and speech reception thresholds have failed. Since the SDT can be very misleading, especially in the often-seen cases of high-frequency hearing loss, these results must be interpreted with the greatest care.

In one of the larger sound suites at the University of Texas we have set up a special output from our diagnostic audiometer so that speech, pure tones, or a variety of noises can be directed to any one of six loudspeakers that are mounted near the ceiling in the child's room. A small console contains six buttons, labeled to correspond to the speakers (right front, right mid, right rear, etc.). Since most children above 6 months of age can localize sound unless they have unilateral losses or central disorders, we use a variety of speech signals, such as calling the child's name or asking ''Where's mommy?'' We are able to observe startle responses at times when the level is above threshold, but if the child can be kept interested in the game, we can also approximate the sound-field SDT.

## Procedure for Obtaining the SDT with Children

Before testing can be undertaken, the child must be made as comfortable and unafraid as possible. It is common that when the SDT is the test of choice, the child is either very young or otherwise too uncooperative to take more advanced and definitive tests. It is frequently a mistake to attempt to separate children from their parents or other adults who may have brought them to the clinic lest they become fretful.

If the child will accept earphones, this situation is ideal. If not, the sound-field system may be the only alternative. The clinician or other person assisting the audiologist should seat the child in the chair, which has been placed in a calibrated position, and should assure that no objects or bodies are placed between the child and loudspeaker. The child should be occupied with objects or small toys that make as little noise as possible. It is important that these objects not have too much fascination, or they will take the place of the auditory stimulus in occupying the child's attention. Often it is possible to request that the persons who accompany the child to the audiology clinic bring such objects from home.

The clinician at the controls of the audiometer may present a series of stimuli, perhaps alternating them between or among several speakers in the test room. These signals may be delivered by monitored live voice or prerecorded on tape. Looking for a response to such things as the child's name, "Mama," or the names of toys is useful. Asking the child to point to body parts is sometimes effective as well as giving the child a set of simple instructions, if a previous interview suggests that these may be followed, such as "Put the ball on the table." Once the child gives any form of response, the intensity of the signal may be lowered until the SDT is estimated.

If measurements through the audiometer prove difficult or impossible, estimates of the SDT may be attempted by having a clinician give the kinds of instructions or other verbal stimuli from within the same room where the child is otherwise occupied. In this way, of course, only the most gross estimation of signal intensity can be made.

## Using the SDT with Children

There may be times in the clinical evaluation of small children when the SDT is the only measurement obtained on a given day. The experienced audiologist recognizes the limitation of this finding and should view it as the threshold for a broad-band signal, recalling always the spectrum of speech. If the SDT is felt to be reliable and a hearing loss is indicated, the examiner is encouraged to test further and to begin to consider remediation for the child. In such cases the extent of the hearing loss may be underestimated, but proper follow-up will have begun and the error should eventually be corrected. If the SDT suggests normal hearing or "hearing adequate for speech acquisition" (an expression commonly seen in the files of small children with language disorders) and no further audiometry is pursued, a tragic misdiagnosis may occur. The hearing loss may not be discovered until much later in the child's life when valuable therapy time will have been lost.

# Speech Reception Threshold

Hirsh (1952, p. 127) points out that in proceeding from the concept of speech detectability to that of speech intelligibility, we must ask what the required level is for speech to be just intelligible to a listener and, given a particular sample of speech, how intelligible that speech is. The definition for "just intelligible speech" is not entirely agreed upon, but we will say that the speech reception (intelligibility) threshold is the lowest hearing level at which *at least* 50% of a list of spondaic words can be correctly identified.

Words alleged to be spondees are usually found to have at least slightly greater stress on one syllable than the other. Most two-syllable words are either iambic (greater stress on the first syllable) or trochaic (greater stress on the second syllable). Hudgins, Hawkins, Karlin, and Stevens (1947) found that two-syllable words uttered with spondaic stress are more uniform in their audibility than one-syllable words or two-syllable words uttered with iambic or trochaic stress. The increased homogeneity of spondees would seem to allow for measurement of the SRT with a lesser number of test words. Nevertheless, spondaic stress in English is unnatural and may be difficult for some small children to understand.

On the subject of stress in spondaic words when testing children, Northern and Downs (1984, p. 149) state, "It is more important that the child knows and enjoys the toy than that it conforms to equal-stress-on-each-syllable principle." Martin and Mussell (1981) found that the six stimulus words recommended by Frank (1980) and commonly used in testing small children (*airplane, baseball, cowboy, cupcake, hotdog, popcorn*) showed no differences in spondee thresholds for young normal-hearing children whether uttered with spondaic or trochaic (natural) stress. They noted informally that response time seemed to be slightly longer for spondaic stress than for trochaic stress. Martin and Checkles (1983) repeated the above study, comparing speech thresholds for spondees and trochees on normal-hearing children and those with conductive and sensorineural hearing loss, and again found no significant differences. The obvious conclusion that can be drawn from these studies is that trochaic stress may be substituted for the more traditional spondaic stress when measuring the speech thresholds of young children if this is deemed to be clinically advantageous.

Most audiologists today appear to prefer SRT testing with monitored live voice over the use of prerecorded stimuli. This allows the freedom to substitute or eliminate words according to the apparent needs of the child being tested, to alter the speed of the test, and generally to tailor the procedure to the patient. While there is no doubt that stimulus control is usually better with recorded material, the flexibility of monitored live voice generally makes it preferable for small children.

In recent years the literature has shown a tendency toward standardization in SRT test procedures. The historic 50% criterion allowed for a good deal of variability in technique, with consequent potential for significant differences in the SRT according to the procedure used. I feel that precise methods for obtaining the SRT that allow the least subjective interpretation of results (ASHA, 1979; Martin & Stauffer, 1975; Tillman & Olsen, 1973; Wilson, Morgan, & Dirks, 1973) are preferable for adults, especially when the SRT is obtained without prior knowledge of the audiogram, thus objectifying the test even further. For children, the use of such precision may prevent completion of the test if it takes too long. Precision is directed toward the clinician's desires, not those of the child, a fact that must be borne in mind since without patient cooperation speech audiometry is impossible. Monitored live voice testing using steps of 5 dB or sometimes even 10 dB often yields rapid and acceptable results.

While many children give reliable test results on pure-tone tests (Eagles & Wishik, 1961; Frisina, 1973, p. 160), in many cases test results with pure-tone stimuli are quite poor. In such cases the SRT lends valuable assistance in determining the extent of a hearing deficit. Children are likely to react more positively to more familiar speech sounds than to abstract pure-tone stimuli—in the absence, of course, of any confounding linguistic deficits. Speech tests take considerably less time than do pure-tone tests, an important factor considering the generally shorter attention span of young children.

The highly positive correlation between the SRT and the pure-tone average (PTA) has encouraged some authorities (Davis, 1970, p. 208; Hirsh, 1962; Silverman & Hirsh, 1955) to argue that the determination of SRT is actually unnecessary. While it is true that the SRT does not provide the estimation of social efficiency for hearing that was once hoped for, the finding of a discrepancy between SRT and PTA is an important one in determining the accuracy of both tests. The SRT, therefore, seems to be an indispensable test, especially with children.

Many clinicians feel that the SRT is a reliable measurement on children with normal intelligence and even on some difficult-to-test children like the mentally retarded (Lloyd & Reid, 1966). While some children give reliable results on speech tests as young as 3 years or even younger (Martin & Coombes, 1976), many people feel that the SRT is an inconsistent measurement below the age of 4 years (Meyerson, 1956; Siegenthaler, Pearson, & Lezak, 1954). Generally the success rate in testing children is greater for speech than for pure tones (Hodgson, 1978).

While familiarization with the test items has the effect of lowering the SRT for most subjects (Tillman & Jerger, 1959), only 55% of audiologists actually do this, according to a recent national survey (Martin & Sides, 1985). With respect to testing adult SRTs with spondaic words, Beattie, Svihovec, and Edgerton (1975) found that using 18 of the 36 spondees from CID Auditory Test W-1 gave greater precision and accuracy to the SRT procedure. Conn, Dancer, and Ventry (1975) found that by using 18 selected spondees, prior familiarization is unnecessary. Since three of those words fell outside the recorded range of $+/-4$ dB acceptable by most clinicians, a final list of 15 words was recommended. No such lists have been designed for children, and pretest conditioning is generally required to familiarize children, especially low-level retardates, with the words (DeWachter-Schaerlaekins, 1969).

Many children who have sufficient language and intelligible speech can take the SRT test rather easily, simply by repeating the words presented to them through an earphone or loudspeaker. While special forms of encouragement and reward may be used, the procedure is essentially the same as for adults. Other children are simply not sufficiently motivated to go along with this kind of exercise, and the SRT procedure must be modified into a form of game. Children often actually enjoy pointing to pictures or objects representing the stimulus word.

A number of point-to-the picture tests have been described in the literature. Keaster (1947) used pictures of 25 nouns taken from a kindergarten-level word test. Commands were given to the child, such as ''Put the rabbit on the floor.'' The level of the commands was progressively lowered until threshold was approximated. This test appeared to have appeal to the children and required no verbal response, although the child was required to remember and understand not only the stimulus word but the entire command. Lloyd, Reid, and McManis (1967) used pictures of standard spondaic words. They found these pictures easy to obtain and the results generally quite good, despite the fact that they were working with retarded children. Other procedures utilizing colored pictures have resulted in frequently reliable results with children (Frank, 1980; MacFarlan, 1940; Siegenthaler & Haspiel, 1966; Siegenthaler et al., 1954).

To measure speech thresholds of non-English-speaking children whose primary language was Spanish, Martin and Hart (1978) developed a picture-pointing test. Pictured items were recorded in Spanish on one channel of a stereo tape with the English translation on the other channel. In essence, the child listened to the Spanish version while the audiologist listened to the English version to monitor the responses. Each tape channel fed a different channel of a speech audiometer. Instructions were recorded directly on the Spanish channel and were augmented by gestures and pantomime. Accurate picture-pointing was socially reinforced by a second clinician seated with the child as intensity was varied on the audiometer in the control room. Very good PTA-SRT agreement was evinced in children aged 3 to 6. Using this technique, one can tape any combination of two languages to determine speech thresholds of children whose language is not spoken by the clinician. It is essential in developing such tests that vocabulary level and pronunciation be appropriate to the children to be tested.

Toys have been used as inducements to get SRTs from young children who are unwilling or unable to give verbal responses. Sortini and Flake (1953) used toys with two-syllable names, uttering the words with spondaic stress. Using different commands, they obtained results with children as young as 26 months. Northern and Downs (1984, p. 150) suggest the use of toys in obtaining the SRT. They feel that the carrier phrase is important and recommend a procedure whereby the phrase "Show me . . ." is uttered and then the hearing level dropped quickly by 10 to 15 dB. Northern and Downs urge that the carrier phrase be audible when the words themselves are at or slightly below threshold. While research on adults should often not be generalized to children, Martin and Weller (1975) found that the presence of a carrier phrase, or its sensation level with reference to the spondaic word, has no effect on the SRT. Using their procedure, Northern and Downs suggest speed in testing, even at the sacrifice of some accuracy. Since working with small children usually means that a limited number of spondee pictures may be used (often only three or four), the SRT thus measured may actually be closer to the SDT than many clinicians realize (Hodgson, 1972, p. 512).

Agreeing with other authors that SRTs are frequently unreliable in children below 4 years of age, Griffing, Simonton, and Hedgecock (1967) developed a screening speech audiometric procedure for preschool children. The *Verbal Auditory Screening for Preschool Children* (VASC) test utilizes a board with pictures representing 12 spondaic words. Griffing et al. found that the procedure worked particularly well with 4- and 5-year-olds. Mencher and McCulloch (1970) tested kindergarten children with the VASC and compared the results to an audiometric screening with pure tones at 20 dB (ANSI 1969) and concluded that the test may miss children in the mild hearing loss range of 30 to 40 dB. Ritchie and Merklein (1972) also found the VASC procedure to have less than desired efficiency in identifying hearing loss in children, being less accurate than pure-tone tests. Hasegawa, Yoshida, Ohashi, Manage, and Itami (1974) did not find the VASC useful in the auditory screening of a group of 2,564 children aged 3 through 6 years. Identifying pictures, particularly spondee pictures, can be accomplished with hearing sensitivity up to 1000 Hz, considering that the task requires a closed-set response.

Accurate determination of SRTs on children presents a number of problems that have not changed in the nearly four decades since they were outlined by Keaster (1947):

1. The test must have sufficient appeal to maintain the child's attention long enough for threshold to be determined.

2. Most young children have a brief attention span, requiring a rapid procedure.

3. Since verbal comprehension is more highly developed than verbal production in small children, nonverbal responses are preferred.

4. Children's short attention spans must not be exceeded nor their abilities to understand the task.

5. Test words must be within the child's vocabulary.

While varieties of reinforcers have been used to encourage responses from children to pure-tone stimuli, in the case of speech tests the reinforcement has been mostly social. Social reinforcement, such as a smile, pat on the head, nod, or word of praise, is sufficient with many young children, while others find such intangibles insufficiently motivating to continue repeating words or pointing to pictures or objects. With this in mind Martin and Coombes (1976) developed a procedure for immediate tangible reinforcement of appropriate responses to speech items. The child is instructed to touch a part of a brightly colored clown (see Figure 8.1). If the response is correct, the child is immediately rewarded with a small piece of candy that falls into a cup held in the clown's hand. Parts of the clown are wired in series with a programming unit in the control room of a two-room audiometric suite. More than one response or an incorrect response locks out a possible reward. The procedure was found to be extremely rapid and accurate with children down to the age of 2½ years with normal hearing. As a matter of fact, the children so enjoyed the procedure that it seemed to place them in a good humor so that other tests, such as immittance measures, could be completed with less difficulty than

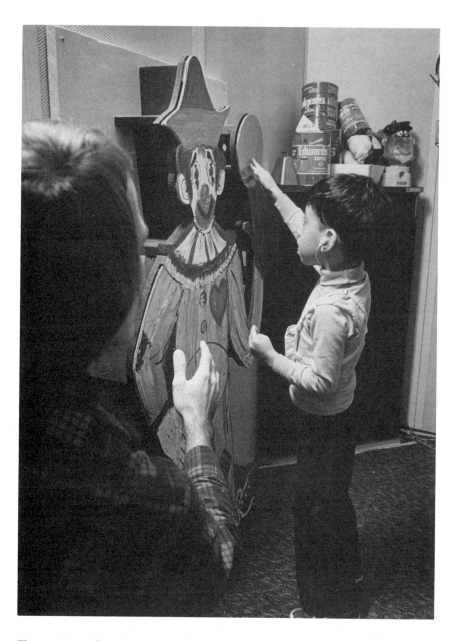

**Figure 8.1.** A hearing-impaired child being tested in the sound field for speech thresholds using a tangible reward (candy pellets). From Martin (1986, p. 374). Reprinted by permission.

is normally found. The procedure has subsequently proven useful in the determination of speech thresholds in mentally retarded children (Weaver, Wardell, & Martin, 1979) and mentally retarded adults (Martin, Durbon, & Maddock, 1984; Martin, Maddock, & Durbon, 1984).

Most modern diagnostic audiometers are capable of delivering speech stimuli to a bone-conduction vibrator. While manufacturers provide no standards for normal hearing for speech by bone conduction, most clinicians find that a correction factor of 5 to 30 dB is necessary, since the speech circuit is designed in most cases to drive the small diaphragm in the earphone and not the plastic case of the bone vibrator. There is at least one new audiometer for which no correction factor is necessary when testing speech thresholds by bone conduction. Speech can be routed to the bone-conduction vibrator, which can be placed on the mastoid or forehead of the child. A comparison of SRTs obtained by bone conduction with those obtained by air conduction reveals the presence of a conductive component. Goetzinger and Proud (1955) and Merrell, Wolfe, and McLemore (1973) found high correlations between the average bone-conduction thresholds at 500, 1000, and 2000 Hz and the bone-conduction SRT.

Regardless of the procedure used, the SRT is only as useful as the pediatric audiologist makes it. The SRT is never a goal in itself. Recognizing the possibility of missing high-frequency hearing losses, Meyerson (1956) used high-pass filters with spondaic words. This idea has great merit, but the extent to which it is practiced today is not known. Several research projects along these lines are underway at the University of Texas.

## Procedure for Obtaining the SRT with Children

The child should first be seated comfortably in the patient room of a two-room audiometric suite, close to the talkback microphone. A parent or other accompanying adult should be seated quietly nearby within the room if this is deemed appropriate. Before a formal SRT procedure is attempted, the clinician should speak with the child, however briefly, to get an estimate of the severity of any problem. If the child answers questions posed in a normal conversational voice, the SRT should not show more than a mild hearing loss, at least in the better ear, assuming that the clinician has been careful to avoid lipreading cues. From observation of the child the audiologist determines the formality of the tests to be used. Furthermore, the investment of a few minutes in talking with the child prior to testing may be invaluable in getting the child to cooperate. Unfortunately many audiologists begin testing before the child has had an opportunity to become comfortable with them. Talking *with* children and not *to* them may greatly facilitate testing.

In the case of an older child with adequate speech and language, a traditional SRT procedure may be used. The child may be instructed to repeat words into a microphone. The suggestion that this is an "airplane game," with the child the pilot, often makes the procedure more fun for the child. The clinician should initially set the talkback gain at a low level since many children will feel compelled to shout their responses. This is especially true if the clinician is wearing a headset, which is often a good idea since children often enjoy having these accoutrements in common with their older game partners.

While earphone SRTs are preferable, the child may fear these or find them uncomfortable. In some cases the clinician may successfully insist that the test continue under earphones, while in others it may be better to go to a less accurate but more feasible procedure. One clever innovation was developed by Harris (1980), who modified a bright yellow telephone by substituting an audiometer earphone and talkback microphone for the receiver and microphone of the telephone. Speech thresholds obtained with this device closely approximated those under earphones. Harris found this approach extremely useful in obtaining both speech and pure-tone thresholds.

Testing in the sound field accomplishes the objective of determining the level at which the child is receiving speech, at least in the better-hearing ear. The child should be encouraged to look toward the loudspeaker, which often requires an assistant to direct the child's attention. While a child's movement about the room compromises sound-field calibration, at times this is unavoidable with active children, but this behavior should be prominently noted in audiological reports. A small table, at which the child is seated, can hold toys and other test and play items, keeping the child close to a calibrated place in the room.

If a child will repeat test words, this procedure is best. If spondees are not usable, then pointing to body parts, items of clothing or furniture, or other persons in the room may be used. The simple instruction "Show me the . . ." is often useful. The child may be encouraged to engage in conversation and to answer questions with the hope that through either verbal or nonverbal indications the words have been heard and discriminated at a given hearing level.

A good hearing level at which to begin testing is 50 dB. This is loud enough to elicit responses from children with mild losses without being alarmingly loud for those with normal hearing. If no reaction is observed at this level, it may be increased in 15 or 20 dB steps.

During testing most children will glance, at least occasionally, to the window of the two-room suite for some sign from the clinician. Most often the reward received for cooperation is a smile, a nod, clapping of hands, or words of encouragement. The manner of testing must be adjusted and readjusted as the procedure continues.

My own experience has shown that initially using a carrier phrase like "Say the word . . ." or "Show me . . ." gives the child the idea of what to do and further use of the phrase is often unnecessary. If a carrier phrase is used, turning the dial down quickly by 10 or 15 dB after the phrase and just before the stimulus word is awkward for me. When the carrier phrase is necessary, I use a two-channel speech audiometer presenting both channels to the same earphone or loudspeaker, the hearing level dial set 10 to 15 dB higher in one channel than the other. After the carrier phrase is spoken, depression of the tone-interrupter bar defeats the channel transmitting the phrase and allows only the test word to be heard at the lower level.

If pictures are to be used as stimulus items, it should be determined in advance that the words are in the child's vocabulary. Parents may provide this information. Pictures on a flannel board allow for rapid elimination of a test word or substitution of a new one. Some children will point to the picture, others will touch it with a finger or pointer, still others will hit at it. Anything short of violence will sometimes have to be tolerated in the interest of diagnosis.

When tangible reinforcement for cooperation is used, an item such as a token or small edible item is handed to the child by an assistant on a fixed-ratio basis, usually averaging one reward for three correct responses. It is possible to use an automatic token or candy pellet dispenser, which is enjoyable for some children. Stimulus items are placed on a table with the clinician and child facing each other. When the appropriate responses are made, they are conveyed to the clinician seated at the audiometer, who releases the reward by activating a relay by remote control. When the clown device (described earlier) is used, children may sit or stand and are shown how to depress a body part when they hear that part named. Since the microswitch behind the movable part is wired in series with the programmer, the reward is delivered instantly after the correct response, which results in faster conditioning and slower extinction than is seen with other methods.

If children are wearing hearing aids, it is often a good idea to condition them to respond to the speech items in the sound field with their aids on. After an SRT is determined, measurement again with the aid removed from the ear allows for an estimate of the gain provided for speech. After sound-field testing the child will often have learned, because of repeated visits to the audiology center, to be unafraid and will frequently tolerate the earphones.

Children who wear hearing aids and who do not accept earphones may be tested by using an insert-type receiver. The receiver cord may be attached to the auxiliary output of the audiometer and the receiver itself attached to the child's own earmold and placed in the child's ear. Naturally some recalibration is necessary, and a slight correction factor will need to be applied. This procedure is useful in obtaining both speech and pure-tone thresholds, often with very little objection even from small children. The size and weight of the headset is just too formidable for some children.

Speech reception threshold tests are sometimes complicated by conductive and unilateral hearing losses, which are not uncommon in children. Audiologists who test children regularly are familiar with the rules for when masking is needed (see ASHA, 1979) and the appropriate use of effective masking. How to mask is a matter of personal preference, and mine has been stated elsewhere (Martin, 1986, Chapter 4).

Often children have less difficulty in taking speech threshold tests with masking than in taking masked pure-tone tests. It is hard to convince a young mind to ignore the loud uninteresting signal (masking noise) in one ear and to pay attention to a very soft, also uninteresting signal (pure tone) in the other ear. If the noise is explained away as a part of the listening game and the child is interested by or sufficiently rewarded for responses to speech stimuli, the masked SRT should not be difficult to obtain.

## Using the SRT with Children

The speech reception threshold is often the only test that can be performed on very small children. When this is the case, it is important to pursue conditioning for pure-tone tests until results are obtained and an audiogram can be constructed, since the SRT does not provide the kind of information about hearing sensitivity at different frequencies that is required for fully appropriate habilitation. If pure-tone data are available, SRTs should be attempted until results can be obtained. When both tests have been completed, they serve to verify each other's accuracy. It must always be borne in mind, when testing children, that even though the responses appear to be at threshold, they must be considered to be minimum response levels, which are often 5 to 15 dB above threshold. The SRT is an indispensable piece of clinical information that should be obtained whenever possible on children suspected of having a hearing loss.

# Word Discrimination

A question that all audiologists wish answered of their hearing-impaired patients is how well they hear and understand speech. Some information on the ability to hear speech may be gleaned from the SRT, but other special tests are required to determine how well speech is processed and discriminated. Such information is useful not only in the diagnosis of the type and severity of the hearing disorder but in the approach to and prognosis for aural rehabilitation efforts.

In her review of speech audiometric procedures for children Jerger (1983) discusses the traditional and modern requirements for such tests. First is the obvious fact that test items must be in the vocabularies of the children tested. Second is the manner of response required of each child. Third is the necessity to deal with the child's receptive language (RL) abilities. Fourth is consideration of "extra-auditory" or cognitive difficulties that may affect results.

The development of speech discrimination tests, such as phonetically balanced (PB) word lists, has been well documented and is known by readers of this book. Many children, even as young as 4 years of age, can be tested using adult PB words, although it might be added here that these are the children who present the least difficulty in testing in general and who often show the least severity in auditory defects.

Since many of the words on PB word lists are not in the vocabularies of small children, several attempts have been made to develop tests that are appropriate to this group. One of the first such attempts was by Haskins (1949), who developed four 50-item PB word lists for children of kindergarten age, often called the PBK lists. As a rule this test is performed with monitored live voice.

The usual reward for cooperation on a speech discrimination test with children is of a social nature—that is, praise, a smile, or other gesture of approval, much like the reinforcement used for speech threshold tests. Smith (1969) used systematic reinforcement for correct responses to speech discrimination items using an operant conditioning method. Both normal-hearing and hearing-impaired children showed substantial improvements in their speech discrimination scores. This illustrates that without proper reinforcement children may perform at levels that do not indicate their maximum discrimination abilities.

Written responses on PB word tests are, of course, out of the question for most small children. Verbal responses may be limited by the child's language disorder, articulation defect, motivation, or a number of other factors. To bypass these problems and still test the word discrimination of small children, Myatt and Landes (1963) developed a multiple-choice picture identification test for use with 4- and 5-year-old children. The lists were standardized on normal and trainable mentally retarded children. Lerman, Ross, & McLaughlin (1965) performed the Myatt and Landes test on hearing-impaired children and found it less than completely effective. Subsequently Ross and Lerman (1970) developed the *Word Intelligibility by Picture Identification* (WIPI) test.

The WIPI test is easily administered but requires two clinicians, or a clinician and an alert helper. Like other speech discrimination tests, it may be administered under earphones if the child permits or in the sound field. The helper shows the child a card with a matrix of six colored pictures. Four of the pictures have words that rhyme, the other two are presented as foils to decrease the probability of a correct guess. The child is instructed, through the speech audiometer at a level above the speech threshold, to touch one of the pictures. If the response cannot be viewed by the examiner, it may be relayed by the assistant. For each correct identification of a picture the child is credited with four percentage points. A total of 25 words in each test yields a possible maximum score of 100%.

In some ways similar to the WIPI test is the *Northwestern University Children's Perception of Speech* (NU-CHIPS) test (Elliot & Katz, 1980). A list of 65 pictorially represented words is presented to the child, with 50 items actually scored in test results. The 50 test items are phonetically balanced, and one or more test words may appear in a four-picture set.

There are differences between the PB word and WIPI-type approaches to auditory discrimination testing besides the obvious fact that the latter is pictorially represented. PB words represent an open-response paradigm, in which the child is forced to select an answer from an unlimited set of possibilities. Like rhyme tests used on adults, the WIPI is a closed-response set, the child's response being a forced choice. Jones and Studebaker (1974) compared the two types of response systems using a group of hearing-impaired children. They found that the closed response was more productive with children evidencing very poor word discrimination abilities and that closed-response test scores were highly correlated with data that depended on hearing function. Jones and Studebaker concluded that data from closed-response sets tend to demonstrate auditory speech discrimination difficulties in a more satisfactory way than data from open-response sets.

In a study comparing the word discrimination scores of normal-hearing children, Sanderson and Rintelmann (1971) found that higher scores were shown on the WIPI than on the PBK lists. Both tests revealed higher scores than the PB words of NU-6. These score differences tended to disappear with age. The conclusion drawn from this research is that the WIPI serves best for young children and that a combination of the WIPI and PBK lists works well for older children. NU-6 should be reserved for older children when a more discriminating test is required, such as for hearing-aid evaluations. Hodgson's (1973) data agree with my own clinical observations that conventional WIPI scores are higher than those for PBK lists or the WIPI presented as an open-message set.

Siegenthaler and Haspiel (1966) developed the *Discrimination by Identification of Pictures* (DIP) test as a closed-message approach to testing children. Children were presented with 48 cards, one at a time, each consisting of two pictures representing words that differed on the basis of production and acoustic parameters such as plosion, nasality, etc. One obvious difficulty with this test is that the probability of a correct guess remains 50% for each item. Nevertheless, the authors found this a means of identifying specific discrimination difficulties in children.

Using protocols similar to the Spanish speech threshold test of Martin and Hart (1978), Comstock and Martin (1984) developed a pretaped Spanish version of the WIPI. The test is delivered to the child on one channel of a speech audiometer in Spanish as the clinician monitors responses on the second channel in English. Due to the nature of the Spanish language, bisyllabic words were used. As in the WIPI, each of the 25 plates contained six pictures: four rhyming test items and two foils. Because both Spanish vocabulary and pronunciation vary considerably from one region of the United States to another, it is very important that such tests be developed with special attention to these matters. It was found that this method does allow for testing word discrimination on children whose language is different from the audiologist's. Research is currently underway to refine this procedure.

The *Auditory Numbers Test* (ANT) was developed by Erber (1980) for use with children who have severe speech discrimination losses. A closed-message test, ANT utilizes colored picture cards showing one to five items per card, and the children tested must have the words representing the numbers one through five in their vocabularies. This test can be performed rapidly and is done with monitored live voice.

Children with sensorineural hearing losses usually show signs of dysacusis. Often this discrimination difficulty is so great that monosyllabic words cannot be discriminated at all or, at best, very poorly. Egan (1948) showed what is so obvious today—that the greater the acoustic redundancy in a speech signal, the easier it is discriminated. Such redundancy increases with increased numbers of phonemes and syllables.

To improve the measurement of word discrimination ability on hearing-impaired children, Cramer and Erber (1974) used pictures of 10 spondaic words recorded on Language Master cards and presented to a single insert-type earphone. It took several sessions before all the children could be tested, but results were quite interesting. Scores were bimodally distributed, clustering in the 0–65% and 66–100% ranges. Pure-tone averages less than 93 dB (ANSI 1969) showed the higher score group-ings while pure-tone averages greater than 103 dB showed the poorer scores. A close relationship did not exist between degree of hearing loss and spondee recognition scores for children with losses in the 93 to 103 dB range. Those recognition scores varied as a function of repeated test-ing in three ways: stable performance, steadily improving scores, and inconsistent performance. In another study Erber (1974) also found that scores clustered in the high range (70–100%) for children with losses milder than 85 dB (ANSI 1969) and in the low range (0–30%) for losses greater than 100 dB. Scores for spondee recognition in children showing hearing losses between 86 and 100 dB were difficult to predict. Data similar to these were reported much earlier by Hudgins (1954) and Erber and Alencewicz (1976).

Because word recognition so often appears very poor in children with sensorineural hearing impairments, the visual channel is sometimes added to improve overall discrimination. It has been known for some time that visual cues augment auditory cues in the discrimination of speech. Ross, Kessler, Phillips, and Lerman (1972) found that, using the WIPI test, com-bined auditory and visual scores are better than the sum of auditory and visual scores alone. The score sheet accompanying the commercial ver-sion of the WIPI provides space for testing hearing alone, vision alone, and hearing and vision combined.

Erber (1972) illustrated that visual cues allow normal-hearing and severely and profoundly hearing-impaired children to discern informa-tion regarding the place of articulation of consonant sounds; they were able to separate bilabials from alveolar and velar consonants. Auditory cues alone presented no problems for the normal group, the severely impaired group could recognize voiced and voiceless plosives and nasals, and the profoundly impaired group showed poor perception overall. In the combined mode the group with profound loss showed only slight improvement over the visual mode alone while the other two groups per-formed nearly perfectly. Monosyllabic, spondaic, and trochaic words were presented in the presence of a low-frequency noise. Several signal-to-noise ratios were used. Subjects were children who had normal hearing, were moderately hearing-impaired, or were profoundly hearing-impaired. Once again, the profoundly impaired group was helped least by the audiovisual channel.

The testing of speech discrimination of children with severe hearing disorders with consequent language limitations is often not attempted because the difficulties to be encountered are predictable and often the clinician feels that the efforts will not be justified. Erber and Alencewicz (1976) discussed their approach to a complete audiologic evaluation of severely hearing-impaired children, including a new speech perception test. They describe 123 picture cards illustrating four nouns in each of three stress categories: monosyllables, trochees, and spondees. Children are first shown all the cards and asked to name each one to ensure that the words are in their vocabularies. They then identify each picture as it is presented audiovisually. Any word not in the child's vocabulary is replaced. These words are used to determine the speech detection threshold as well as the most comfortable and most uncomfortable levels of loudness. For the discrimination portion of the test each word is presented twice at the most comfortable listening level with no visual cues. Scoring is accomplished in two ways—according to the percentage of correct words and the percentage categorized correctly by stress pattern. The procedure is appropriate for children over 5 years of age. Perhaps the greatest value of this test is that it assists in selecting the appropriate ear for a hearing aid and in deciding whether binaural hearing aids would be appropriate.

Relatively new in the battery of speech discrimination tests for children is the Pediatric Speech Intelligibility (PSI) test (Jerger, Lewis, Hawkins, & Jerger, 1980; Jerger, Jerger, & Lewis, 1981; Jerger & Jerger, 1982). The test contains both sentences and monosyllabic words and minimizes the effects of receptive language by dividing the test into two formats. Format I sentences are used with children who have relatively low receptive language abilities while Format II sentences are designed for children with relatively high receptive language. The PSI will be further discussed in the section on tests for central auditory disorders.

There are times when no standardized test is appropriate for the measurement of speech discrimination. In children this may be true because of the child's inadequate language or because the discrimination problem is very severe. If children can be taught the concepts of "same" and "different," they may be tested with some gross speech sounds like sustained vowels. In this way it can be determined whether they can make any auditory discriminations at all, assuming that the stimuli can be presented above threshold without reaching discomfort intensities. A more formalized approach to the same-different approach was postulated by Kelley and Pillow (1979) in a test they call *Nonsense Syllable Discrimination Test* (NSDT), in which 50 syllable pairs (e.g., *ma-la, la-la*) are presented to the child, who selects from the two alternatives of same or different.

Ling and Ling (1978) described a simple test for young children with limited hearing. The test involves three vowels, /a/, /u/, and /i/, and two consonants, /s/ and /ʃ/. Ling and Ling feel that the test taps the hearing for particular formants and is useful as a quick check of a child's potential speech discrimination. For example, if a hearing aid cuts the low-frequency sound excessively, /u/ and /i/ will be less audible than /a/. If hearing above 2000 Hz is poor or if a hearing aid does not amplify well in the upper-frequency range, the /i/ will be inaudible for a child for whom no low-frequency information is provided. Audibility of /ʃ/ indicates potential hearing of the second formant of the vowel /i/. This test can be performed under earphones or aided and unaided in the sound field. If necessary, the test can be performed as the sole test of speech discrimination, or it may be used in conjunction with other tests of children's discrimination, such as the WIPI.

Earlier in this chapter the subject of the bone-conducted speech reception threshold was discussed briefly. It is also possible to measure word discrimination by bone conduction as well (Goetzinger & Proud, 1955). Such measurements are of value in severe mixed-type losses to determine speech discrimination ability when the level for air conduction cannot be made high enough to determine the maximum score. A high speech discrimination score by bone conduction also helps to alleviate any anxiety over whether the pure-tone bone-conduction thresholds may have been the result of tactile stimulation rather than auditory perception (Nober, 1970).

Speech discrimination measurements are important in the diagnosis of the type and degree of hearing disorder in children as well as in the decisions necessary for appropriate remediation, ear choice for a hearing aid, and so forth. When such tests can be performed, they should be. If for any one of a variety of reasons no speech discrimination estimate is available, the audiologist may have to proceed with the data available based on SRT and pure-tone results. In such cases a general rule is that the greater the sensorineural component of the hearing loss, the greater the discrimination problem.

Certain basic assumptions may be incorrect in the minds of many audiologists regarding speech discrimination testing. For example, Giolas (1975, pp. 48–49) points out that data collected on a subject under specific conditions of recording will not be the same with a different speaker. Kreul, Bell, and Nixon (1969) have shown that test difficulty changes with different speakers and carrier phrases but does not change with words uttered by the same speaker. They point out that the auditory test is not the list of words but rather the recording of these words, or, in the case of children seen for audiological testing, the manner in which the words are uttered using monitored live voice. The use of a properly monitored carrier phrase before each test word has been shown to influence word discrimination scores (Gladstone & Siegenthaler, 1971; Schwartz & Goldman, 1974).

## Procedure for Word Discrimination Testing with Children

Tests of word discrimination in children are usually performed following SRT and pure-tone tests. Speech discrimination tests are sometimes not performed on children because the child's cooperation has expired, because there are no tests appropriate to the child's age or language skills, or because the clinician feels that estimates of speech discrimination ability may be inferred from other tests. While the first two reasons may be acceptable, the third one does not appear to be, since speech discrimination tests should be used whenever possible, despite their various limitations.

Children should be given the most difficult test they are capable of taking. If vocabulary permits, adult PB words may be used. Kindergarten PB lists may be substituted if necessary. If the child's language, articulation of speech, or reticence proscribe vocal responses, the WIPI or a similar test is the next choice. In performance of the test the child should remain comfortably seated, and, if a closed-message type of test is used, a small table containing the test materials should separate the child from the clinician. Care should be taken to conceal the face of the clinician at the audiometer to avoid any speech-reading cues. If the situation remains pleasant the child may actually enjoy taking the test. The clinician sitting with the child simply repeats the name of the picture pointed to so the other audiologist can score the item correct or incorrect. Reinforcement for cooperation should be ongoing. We have found it useful to run an extra receiver to the test room in parallel with the monitor receiver at the audiometer. In this way the clinician with the child can hear, at a comfortably set loudness, the words that are said to the child. There is an additional advantage to this second earphone in that children are often comforted by the fact that their adult partners are wearing devices similar to their own.

There are times, even with cooperative children, when they fail to point to the appropriate picture because the stimulus word has not been discriminated. There are also times when this happens because the word is simply not in the child's vocabulary. The authors of the WIPI, as well as many other tests, recognize this and recommend that children be queried over incorrect items, but this is probably not done as frequently as it should be. Tests like the WIPI are useful in checking the effectiveness of hearing aids by estimating the synergistic effect of combining visual with auditory cues in the sound field.

Some of the objections to the WIPI include the fact that many of the test items are too easy to tax the mildly impaired auditory system where speech discrimination problems exist. The WIPI was designed, however, for the more severely impaired child with unintelligible speech and limited or absent writing ability. Furthermore, since the WIPI is usually performed using monitored live voice, it lacks the standardization of prerecorded tests.

Because so many children have conductive or unilateral losses, the problem of crossover is even greater for speech discrimination tests than it is for the SRT or pure-tone tests. It is difficult to know for certain just when the nontest ear is augmenting the discrimination score of the test ear. It should be feared that this may be taking place whenever the hearing level of the test, minus 40 dB (for the loss of speech energy as it travels around, across, and through the skull), exceeds any of the bone-conduction thresholds of the nontest ear. In such cases, appropriate levels of masking should be used. Experienced clinicians have their own systems for masking, and mine has been set forth elsewhere (Martin, 1986). Masking cannot be ignored in word discrimination tests of children any more than it can for adults, although the approach for the two groups may have to be different.

Adults requiring masking for word discrimination tests are simply told to ignore the noise in one ear while they repeat, or otherwise indicate recognition of, the words they hear in the other ear. Children may be told the same thing, or they may be told that the noise comes from the airplane engine and that they should make believe that it isn't there. Actually, and fortunately, masking for word discrimination is less distracting than for threshold tests, since the loudness of the speech signal is not affected to any significant degree by the noise, and any drop in discrimination score below what might have been obtained in the unmasked condition can be attributed to elimination of the contribution of the nontest ear.

## Using Word Discrimination Tests with Children

Tests of speech discrimination are often difficult to obtain on small children. In each case the audiologist should attempt to complete the most sophisticated test of which the child is capable. Results of speech discrimination tests allow for increased accuracy in diagnosis, in improvement in the fitting of hearing aids, and in the verification of other audiometric data. While efforts at auditory habilitation should certainly begin before speech discrimination data are obtained if these tests will be delayed, such results should be pursued and added to the other audiometric information at the earliest possible time.

# Central Auditory Disorders

For some time it has been known that children may suffer from a variety of lesions in the auditory system that produce difficulty in processing speech. These lesions may occur in the presence or absence of peripheral disorders that are more easily recognizable because of their effects on hearing sensitivity. Because of the acoustic and syntactic redundancy found in the speech message as well as the neural redundancy found in the auditory system, attempts at diagnosis of these disorders have led to a number of tests that stress the speech signal in such ways as to make it more difficult, yet possible, for normal patients to discriminate, while showing decreased scores on some patients with central nervous system disorders.

A very wide range of tests is becoming available for the diagnosis of central auditory dysfunction in adults, some of which can be used with older and more cooperative children. The signal may be altered by filtering, dividing portions of words or messages into different frequency bands to be fused binaurally, time-compressed, masked, or presented as words or sentences with simultaneous competition, rapidly alternating the signal from one ear to the other, presenting words or sentences at a number of sensation levels to determine performance-intensity functions, and so on. Naturally, the younger and more deficient in language a given child is, the more difficult such assessments are to make.

Many children who have been diagnosed as learning-disabled appear to have disorders of the central auditory nervous system. One difficulty found in comparing different test results on such children is the paucity of neuropathologic data (Musiek, 1985). Some children whose problems appear superficially unrelated to audition (as, for example, dyslexia) are determined to have lesions in the central auditory pathways.

## Central Auditory Speech Tests for Children

Older or more cooperative children may allow for monosyllabic word tests at several sensation levels so that a performance-intensity function for phonetically balanced words (PI/PB) can be constructed. Although the data are frequently variable in such cases, especially when hearing sensitivity is normal (Musiek, 1985), at times the PB max is reduced or a rollover function may be seen in the ear contralateral to a cortical lesion.

Speech tests with ipsilateral masking noise have been used with some success in identifying children with auditory processing difficulties. Any monosyllabic test suitable for the child may be used (PBK word lists, WIPI, adult PB word lists, etc.). Unlike adults, more favorable signal-to-noise ratios are required for children in order to obtain usable scores (Rupp, 1983). Keith (1981) suggests a signal-to-noise ratio of +9 dB for children. While some normative data are available, more such information is necessary before speech-in-noise tests can be performed with confidence in search of a diagnosis of central auditory disorders in children.

Since central auditory lesions should theoretically cause a delay in neural transmission time, patients with such lesions should have difficulty with time-compressed speech. Such tests have been developed using both sentences and monosyllabic words. As time compression is increased, children have more difficulty in discrimination, although, as would be expected, scores increase with age (Beasley, Maki, & Orchik, 1976). Learning-disabled children perform more poorly than their normal counterparts when rapid rates of compression are used (McNutt & Li, 1980; Manning, Johnston, & Beasley, 1977). Similar results were found for children with reading problems (Freeman & Beasley, 1978) and artic-ulation disorders (Orchik & Oelschlaeger, 1977).

Binaural fusion of filtered speech has been studied using children with specific auditory processing disorders. Martin and Clark (1977) found greater diotic enhancement over dichotic scores for their experimental group than for their normal control group. High- and low-pass bands of the WIPI were used. A similar study by Roush and Tait (1984) showed some diotic enhancement but revealed generally poorer scores in both diotic and dichotic conditions for language-learning-disabled children.

The staggered spondaic word (SSW) test of Katz (1962, 1968) has been used with children. Patterns resulting from these tests suggest specific disorders in different anatomical loci. Patients with temporal lobe disor-ders have little difficulty with the noncompeting words but show lower scores during the competing condition. Those with lesions in the brainstem show rather unpredictable scores. Brunt (1978) points out the difficulty in interpreting SSW scores on children under 11 years of age.

The synthetic sentence identification (SSI) test (Jerger, Speaks, & Trammel, 1968) has been used successfully to determine lesions of the brainstem (with ipsilateral speech competition) and the cortex (with con-tralateral speech competition). Since being able to read the list of 10 possi-ble sentences presented is part of the test, its use is limited with younger children (Willeford, 1978).

The *Pediatric Speech Intelligibility Test* (PSI) (Jerger, 1983) allows for the use of sentence tests on children who cannot read. The PSI appears to be gaining in popularity as a test for central auditory disorders in children. The test takes considerable time to perform on young children. Children must first be administered the *Northwestern Syntax Screening Test* (NSST) (Lee, 1971) to determine whether they are eligible for the PSI procedure and whether Format I or Format II would be more appropriate.

In general, children are administered Format I in the sound field and Format II under earphones. Four different measures are obtained for each ear (when earphones are used): (1) performance-intensity functions for words with ipsilateral competition, (2) performance-intensity functions for sentences with ipsilateral competition, (3) sentence tests with ipsilateral competition (sentences) at message-to-competition ratios (MCR) of +10 and 0 dB, and (4) sentence tests with a contralateral competing message (sentences) using MCRs of 0 and −20 dB. Because of the importance of proper test and administration, the reader is referred to the manual for the PSI test provided by Auditec of St. Louis, the vendor of the commercial version of this test.

Low-pass filtered monosyllabic words have been used successfully to test for learning disorders in children (Willeford, 1978). As has been found previously, for the test to be reliable for children very careful attention must be paid to the filter characteristics (Farrer & Keith, 1981). These tests can be carried out using PBK words or the WIPI.

Some version of the dichotic digits test has been used for more than two decades in diagnosis of patients with brain damage (Kimura, 1961a, 1961b). In this test digits 1 through 10 (except 7) are presented, usually two or more numbers to each ear simultaneously, via binaural tape. Those subjects with normal hearing and no central auditory disorders can usually correctly repeat approximately 90% of a list of 40 or more numbers (Mueller, 1985; Musiek, 1983) with a slight right-ear advantage. This test has shown some success with children who have language disorders (Sommers & Taylor, 1972).

Dichotic tests using certain consonant-vowel (CV) nonsense syllables are used on adults in diagnosing central auditory nervous system disorders (Berlin & McNeil, 1976). The vowel /a/ is preceded by stop consonants that are either voiced (/b/, /d/, /g/) or unvoiced (/p/, /t/, /k/). Normal adults can usually identify 60% to 80% of the CVs in their right ears and 50% to 65% in their left ears. Adult subjects with temporal lobe lesions show alterations in the normal right-ear/left-ear relationships and poorer or better-than-normal scores, depending on the precise locus of lesion (Cullen, Berlin, Hughes, Thompson, & Samson, 1975). The value of dichotic CV tests in children continues to be debated with both encouraging (e.g., Dermody, Katsch, & Mackie, 1983; Harris, Keith, & Novak, 1983) and discouraging (Roeser, Millay, & Morrow, 1983) findings.

## Using Central Auditory Speech Tests with Children

Many tests are available for testing children who may have disorders of the central auditory nervous system. The use of a single test or a small number of tests is generally considered insufficient in testing children for central auditory disorders. Auditec of St. Louis has produced a commercial version of what has been called the "Willeford Test Battery," which is standardized on children 5 to 9 years of age and appears to be widely used. This battery consists of tests of binaural separation, filtered speech, binaural fusion, and rapidly alternating speech. It can be expected that while some form of each of these tests will doubtlessly survive, they will evolve and change as new research data become available.

# Summary

Because speech audiometry requires that at least some degree of language be present, it is limited to children who are older than those who can sometimes be tested with pure-tone audiometry. When speech audiometry is possible in any form, from the most rigidly controlled to the most "arty," it should be carried out since it serves a number of useful and often irreplaceable functions. Speech audiometry includes measurements of speech detection, speech reception, speech discrimination, and special discrimination tests for central auditory disorders.

The speech detection threshold, although it has limited utility with children in predicting hearing loss, can be used if no other test can be performed. If other tests are available and considered reliable, an SDT adds little in the way of useful diagnostic information. It should serve as a test of last resort, to be performed only when more definitive tests, such as pure tones or speech reception thresholds, cannot be established at the time. It should never stand by itself as a diagnostic entity.

The speech reception threshold provides useful information regarding the accuracy of the pure-tone audiogram or as a stopgap measurement while the child is being conditioned to take the pure-tone tests. The SRT is never a substitute for the pure-tone audiogram, and testing the former without the latter in no way indicates that testing has been completed, no matter what the results. The SRT can be used with children to indicate the gain of a hearing aid, to estimate—with a modicum of accuracy—the kinds of communication difficulties a child has, and to hazard a prognostic judgment for aural habilitative or rehabilitative measures. The SRT is also useful in determining the appropriate level for speech discrimination tests.

Speech discrimination measures allow comparison between the receptive aural communication of the child and that of normal children and between the child's right ear and the left. In this way the diagnosis of conductive versus sensorineural hearing loss may be substantiated, the selection of which ear to aid with amplification can be made (if, for some reason, binaural aids are contraindicated), and statements about probable present and future communicative problems may be ventured. No method of speech discrimination measurement is truly satisfactory for children, and future research is needed in this area.

The diagnosis of auditory processing disorders is difficult and often inaccurate. At the present time the average audiologist does little about this problem. Normal hearing on the audiogram and normal speech reception and discrimination tests do not necessarily eliminate the possibility of a deficit beyond the peripheral auditory mechanism. The emphasis in recent years on research in this area is most encouraging.

# References

American National Standards Institute (1970). *American National Standard specifications for audiometers, ANSI S3.6-1969.* New York: American National Standards Institute.

American Speech and Hearing Association (ASHA). (1979). Guidelines for determining the threshold level for speech. *Asha, 21,* 353–356.

Beasley, D., Maki, J., & Orchik, D. (1976). Children's perception of time-compressed speech on two measures of speech discrimination. *Journal of Speech and Hearing Disorders, 41,* 216–225.

Beattie, R. C., Svihovec, D. V., & Edgerton, B. J. (1975). Relative intelligibility of the CID spondees as presented via monitored live voice. *Journal of Speech and Hearing Disorders, 40,* 84–91.

Berlin, C. I., & McNeil, M. R. (1976). Dichotic listening. In N. J. Lass (Ed.), *Issues in experimental phonetics* (pp. 327–387). New York: Academic Press.

Brunt, M., (1978). The SSW test. In J. Katz (Ed.), *Handbook of clinical audiology* (pp. 262–275). Baltimore: Williams & Wilkins.

Bunch, C. (1934). Methods of testing the hearing in infants and young children. *Journal of Pediatrics, 5,* 535–544.

Clawson, J. (1966). Threshold for pure tone and speech in retardates. *American Journal of Mental Deficiency, 70,* 556–662.

Comstock, C. L., & Martin, F. N. (1984). A children's Spanish word discrimination test for non-Spanish-speaking clinicians. *Ear and Hearing, 5,* 166–170.

Conn, M., Dancer, J., & Ventry, I. M. (1975). A spondee list for determining speech reception threshold without prior familiarization. *Journal of Speech and Hearing Disorders, 40,* 380–396.

Cramer, K. D., & Erber, N. P. (1974). A spondee recognition test for young hearing-impaired children. *Journal of Speech and Hearing Disorders, 39,* 304–311.

Cullen, J. K., Berlin, C. I., Hughes, L., Thompson, C. L., & Samson, D. (1975). Speech information flow: A model. In M. D. Sullivan (Ed.), *Central auditory processing disorders* (pp. 108–127). Omaha: University of Nebraska Medical Center.

Davis, H. (1970). Audiometry: Pure tone and simple speech tests. In C. H. Davis and S. R. Silverman (Eds.), *Hearing and deafness* (3rd ed., pp. 179–220). New York: Holt, Rinehart and Winston.

Dermody, P., Katsch, R., & Mackie, K. (1983). Auditory processing limitations in low verbal children: Evidence from a two-response dichotic listening task. *Ear and Hearing, 4,* 272–277.

DeWachter-Schaerlaekins, A. M. (1969). The influence of intelligence on speech audiometry tests. *Acta Otolaryngologica, 23,* 497–503.

Eagles, E., & Wishik, S. (1961). A study of hearing in children. *Transactions of the American Academy of Ophthalmology and Otology, 65,* 261–282.

Egan, J. P. (1948). Articulation testing methods. *Laryngoscope, 58,* 955–991.

Elliot, L., & Katz, D. (1980). *Development of a new children's test of speech discrimination.* St. Louis: Auditec.

Erber, N. P. (1980). Use of the Auditory Numbers Test to evaluate speech perception abilities of hearing-impaired children. *Journal of Speech and Hearing Disorders, 45,* 527–532.

Erber, N. P. (1974). Pure-tone thresholds and word-recognition abilities of hearing-impaired children. *Journal of Speech and Hearing Research, 17,* 194–202.

Erber, N. P. (1972). Auditory, visual, and auditory-visual recognition of consonants by children with normal and impaired hearing. *Journal of Speech and Hearing Research, 15,* 413–422.

Erber, N. P., & Alencewicz, C. M. (1976). Audiologic evaluation of deaf children. *Journal of Speech and Hearing Disorders, 41,* 256–267.

Farrer, S. M., & Keith, R. W. (1981). Filtered word testing in the assessment of children's central auditory abilities. *Ear and Hearing, 2,* 267–269.

Frank, T. (1980). Clinical significance of the relative intelligibility of pictorially represented spondee words. *Ear and Hearing, 1,* 46–49.

Freeman, B., & Beasley, D. (1978). Discrimination of time-altered sentential approximations and monosyllables by children with reading problems. *Journal of Speech and Hearing Research, 21,* 497–506.

Frisina, R. (1973). Measurement of hearing in children. In J. Jerger (Ed.), *Modern developments in audiology* (2nd ed., pp. 155–174). New York: Academic Press.

Frisina, R. D. (1962). Audiometric evaluation and its relation to habilitation and rehabilitation of the deaf. *American Annals of the Deaf, 107,* 478–481.

Giolas, T. G. (1975). Speech audiometry. In R. T. Fulton & L. L. Lloyd (Eds.), *Auditory assessment of the difficult-to-test* (pp. 37–70). Baltimore: Williams and Wilkins.

Gladstone, V., & Siegenthaler, B. (1971). Carrier phrase and speech intelligibility test score. *Journal of Auditory Research, 4,* 101–103.

Goetzinger, C. P., & Proud, G. O. (1955). Speech audiometry by bone conduction. *Archives of Otolaryngology, 62,* 632–635.

Griffing, T., Simonton, K., & Hedgecock, L. (1967). Verbal auditory screening for preschool children. *Transactions of the American Academy of Ophthalmology and Otolaryngology, 71,* 105–110.

Hardy, W., & Bordley, J. (1951). Special techniques in testing the hearing of children. *Journal of Speech and Hearing Disorders, 16,* 122–131.

Harris, J. D. (1980). Obtaining speech and pure-tone thresholds with young children. *Audiology and Hearing Education, 8,* 17–43.

Harris, V. L., Keith, R. W., & Novak, K. K. (1983). Relationship between two dichotic listening tests and the token test for children. *Ear and Hearing, 4,* 278–282.

Hasegawa, S., Yoshida, T., Ohashi, I., Manage, T., & Itami, E. (1974). The Verbal Auditory Screening Test for Children. *Audiology Japan, 17,* 148–155.

Haskins, H. (1949). *A phonetically balanced test of speech discrimination for children.* Unpublished master's thesis, Northwestern University.

Hirsh, I. J. (1952). *The measurement of hearing.* Highstown, NJ: McGraw-Hill.

Hirsh, I. J. (1962). Speech audiometry—special remarks. *International Audiology, 1,* 183–185.

Hodgson, W. R. (1973). *A comparison of WIPI and PB-K discrimination test scores.* A paper presented at the annual convention of the American Speech and Hearing Association, Detroit.

Hodgson, W. R. (1978). Testing infants and young children. In J. Katz (Ed.), *Handbook of clinical audiology* (2nd ed., pp. 397–409). Baltimore: Williams and Wilkins.

Hudgins, C. V. (1954). Auditory training: Its possibilities and limitations. *Volta Review, 56,* 339–349.

Hudgins, C. V., Hawkins, J. E., Karlin, J. E., & Stevens, S. S. (1947). The development of recorded auditory tests for measuring hearing loss for speech. *Laryngoscope, 57,* 57–89.

Jerger, J., Speaks, C., & Trammell, L. (1968). A new approach to speech audiometry. *Journal of Speech and Hearing Research, 33,* 318–328.

Jerger, S. (1983). Speech audiometry. In J. Jerger (Ed.), *Pediatric audiology* (pp. 71–93). San Diego: College-Hill Press.

Jerger, S., & Jerger, J. (1982). Pediatric Speech Intelligibility Test: Performance-intensity characteristics. *Ear and Hearing, 3,* 325–334.

Jerger, S., Jerger, J., & Lewis, S. (1981). Pediatric Speech Intelligibility Test. II. Effect of receptive language age and chronological age. *International Journal of Pediatric Otorhinolaryngology, 3,* 101–118.

Jerger, S., Lewis, S., Hawkins, J., & Jerger, J. (1980). Pediatric Speech Intelligibility Test. I. Generation of Test Materials. *International Journal of Pediatric Otorhinolaryngology, 2,* 217–230.

Jones, K., & Studebaker, G. (1974). Performance of severely hearing-impaired children on a closed-response, auditory speech discrimination test. *Journal of Speech and Hearing Research, 17,* 531–540.

Katz, J. (1962). The use of staggered spondaic words for assessing the integrity of the CANS. *Journal of Auditory Research, 2,* 327–337.

Katz, J. (1968). The SSW Test: An interim report. *Journal of Speech and Hearing Disorders, 33,* 132–146.

Keaster, J. A. (1947). A quantitative method of testing the hearing of young children. *Journal of Speech and Hearing Disorders, 12,* 159–160.

Keith, R. W. (1981). Audiological and auditory-language tests of central auditory function. *Central auditory and language disorders in children* (pp. 61–76). Houston: College-Hill Press.

Kelley, B., & Pillow, G. (1979). Nonsense syllable discrimination by picture identification with young children. *Journal of the American Auditory Society, 4,* 170–172.

Kimura, D. (1961a). Some effects of temporal-lobe damage on auditory perception. *Canadian Journal of Psychology, 15,* 156–165.

Kimura, D. (1961b). Cerebral dominance and the perception of verbal stimuli. *Canadian Journal of Psychology, 15,* 166–171.

Kreul, E. J., Bell, D. W., & Nixon, J. C. (1969). Factors affecting speech discrimination test difficulty. *Journal of Speech and Hearing Research, 12,* 281–287.

Lee, L. (1971). *The Northwestern Syntax Screening Test.* Evanston, IL: Northwestern University Press.

Lerman, J. W., Ross, M., & McLaughlin, R. M. (1965). A picture-identification test for hearing-impaired children. *Journal of Auditory Research, 5,* 273–278.

Ling, D., & Ling, A. H. (1978). *Aural habilitation: The foundations of verbal learning in hearing-impaired children,* Washington, DC: Alexander Graham Bell Association for the Deaf.

Lloyd, L. L., & Reid, M. J. (1966). The reliability of speech audiometry with institutionalized retarded children. *Journal of Speech and Hearing Research, 9,* 450–455.

Lloyd, L. L., Reid, M. J., & McManis, D. L. (1967). The effects of response mode on the SRTs obtained from retarded children. *Journal of Auditory Research, 7,* 219–222.

MacFarlan, D. (1940). Speech hearing and speech interpretation testing. *Archives of Otolaryngology, 31,* 517–528.

McNutt, J., & Li, J. (1980). Repetition of time-altered sentences by normal and hearing-disabled children. *Journal of Learning Disabilities, 13,* 30–34.

Manning, W., Johnston, D., & Beasley, D. (1977). The performance of children with auditory perceptual disorders on a time-compressed speech discrimination measure. *Journal of Speech and Hearing Disorders, 42,* 77–84.

Martin, F. N. (1986). *Introduction to audiology* (3rd ed.). Englewood Cliffs, NJ: Prentice-Hall.

Martin, F. N., & Checkles, E. (1983). Syllabic stress (trochaic vs. spondaic) and speech thresholds in normal and hearing-impaired children. *Journal of Auditory Research, 23,* 127–130.

Martin, F. N., & Coombes, S. (1976). A tangibly reinforced speech reception threshold procedure for use with small children. *Journal of Speech and Hearing Disorders, 41,* 333–338.

Martin, F. N., & Clark, J. (1977). Audiologic detection of auditory processing in children. *Journal of the American Audiology Society, 3,* 140–146.

Martin, F. N., & Hart, D. B. (1978). Measurement of speech thresholds of Spanish-speaking children by non-Spanish-speaking clinicians. *Journal of Speech and Hearing Disorders, 43,* 255–262.

Martin, F. N., Durbon, A. S., & Maddock, M. (1984). Tangibly reinforced speech reception and pure-tone thresholds in mentally retarded adults. *Tejas, 10,* 18–21.

Martin, F. N., Maddock, M. L., & Durbon, A. S. (1984). Determining SRT in mentally handicapped adults: A comparison of two methods. *The Hearing Journal, 37,* 21–26.

Martin, F. N., & Mussell, S. A. (1981). The influence of syllabic stress on children's thresholds for speech. *Journal of Auditory Research, 21,* 105–108.

Martin, F. N., & Sides, D. G. (1985). Current audiometric practices. *Asha, 27,* 29–36.

Martin, F. N., & Stauffer, M. L. (1975). A modification of the Tillman-Olsen method for obtaining the speech reception threshold. *Journal of Speech and Hearing Disorders, 40,* 25–28.

Martin, F. N., & Weller, S. M. (1975). The influence of the carrier phrase on the speech reception threshold. *Journal of Communication Pathology, 7,* 39–44.

Mencher, G. T., & McCulloch, B. F. (1970). Auditory screening of kindergarten children using the VASC. *Journal of Speech and Hearing Disorders, 35,* 241–247.

Merrell, H. B., Wolfe, D. L., & McLemore, D. C. (1973). Air- and bone-conducted speech reception thresholds. *Laryngoscope, 83,* 1929–1939.

Meyerson, L. (1956). Hearing for speech in children: A verbal audiometric test. *Acta Otolaryngologica* (Suppl. 128).

Mueller, H. G. (1985). Monosyllabic procedures. In J. Katz (Ed.), *Handbook of clinical audiology* (3rd ed., pp. 355–382). Baltimore: Williams & Wilkins.

Musiek, F. E. (1983). Assessment of central auditory dysfunction: The dichotic digit test revisited. *Ear and Hearing, 4,* 79–83.

Musiek, F. E. (1985). Application of central auditory tests: An overview. In J. Katz (Ed.), *Handbook of clinical audiology* (3rd ed., pp. 321–336). Baltimore: Williams & Wilkins.

Myatt, B., & Landes, B. (1963). Assessing discrimination loss in children. *Archives of Otolaryngology, 77,* 359–362.

Nober, E. H. (1970). Cutile air and bone conduction thresholds of the deaf. *Exceptional Children, 36,* 571–579.

Northern, J. L., & Downs, M. P. (1984). *Hearing in children* (3rd ed.). Baltimore: Williams and Wilkins.

Orchik, D. J., & Oelschlaeger, M. L. (1977). Time-compressed speech discrimination in children and its relationship to articulation. *Journal of the American Audiology Society, 3,* 37–41.

Ritchie, B. C., & Merklein, R. A. (1972). An evaluation of the efficiency of the Verbal Auditory Screening Test for Children (VASC). *Journal of Speech and Hearing Research, 15,* 280–286.

Roeser, R. J., Millay, K. K., & Morrow, J. M. (1983). Dichotic consonant-vowel (CV) perception in normal and learning-impaired children. *Ear and Hearing, 4,* 293–299.

Ross, M., & Matkin, N. (1967). The rising audiometric configuration. *Journal of Speech and Hearing Disorders, 32,* 377–382.

Ross, M., Kessler, M., Phillips, M., & Lerman, J. (1972). Visual, auditory and combined mode of presentations of the WIPI Test to hearing-impaired children. *Volta Review, 74,* 90–96.

Ross, M., & Lerman, J. (1970). A picture identification test for hearing-impaired children. *Journal of Speech and Hearing Research, 13,* 44–53.

Roush, J., & Tait, C. A. (1984). Binaural fusion, masking level differences, and auditory brain stem responses in children with language-learning disabilities. *Ear and Hearing, 5,* 37–41.

Rupp, R. R. (1983). Establishing norms for speech-in-noise skills in children. *The Hearing Journal, 36,* 16–19.

Sanderson, M., & Rintelmann, W. (1971). *Performance of normal-hearing children on three speech discrimination tests.* Paper presented at the annual convention of the American Speech and Hearing Association, Chicago.

Schwartz, A., & Goldman, R. (1974). Variables influencing performance on speech-sound discrimination tests. *Journal of Speech and Hearing Research, 17,* 26–32.

Siegenthaler, B. M., & Haspiel, G. (1966). *Development of two standardized measures of hearing for speech by children.* Cooperative Research Program, Project No. 2372, Contract OE-5-10-003. Washington, DC: U.S. Department of Health, Education and Welfare, U.S. Office of Education.

Siegenthaler, B., Pearson, J., & Lezak, R. (1954). A speech reception threshold test for children. *Journal of Speech and Hearing Disorders, 19,* 360–366.

Silverman, S. R., & Hirsh, I. J. (1955). Problems related to the use of speech in clinical audiometry. *Annals of Otology, Rhinology, and Laryngology, 64,* 1234–1245.

Smith, K. (1969). *An experimental study of the effects of systematic reinforcement on the discrimination responses of normal and hearing-impaired children.* Unpublished doctoral dissertation, University of Kansas.

Sommers, R. K., & Taylor, M. L. (1972). Cerebral speech dominance in language-disordered and normal children. *Cortex, 8,* 224–232.

Sortini, A., & Flake, C. (1953). Speech audiometry testing for preschool children. *Laryngoscope, 65,* 991–997.

Tillman, T. W., & Jerger, J. F. (1959). Some factors affecting the spondee threshold in normal-hearing subjects. *Journal of Speech and Hearing Research, 2,* 141–146.

Tillman, T. W., & Olsen, W. O. (1973). Speech audiometry. In J. Jerger (Ed.), *Modern developments in audiology* (2nd ed., pp. 37–74). New York: Academic Press.

Weaver, N. J., Wardell, F. N., & Martin, F. N. (1979). A comparison of tangibly reinforced speech-reception and pure-tone thresholds in mentally retarded children. *American Journal of Mental Deficiency, 5,* 512–517.

Willeford, J. (1978). Sentence tests of central auditory dysfunction. In J. Katz (Ed.), *Handbook of clinical audiology* (2nd ed., pp. 252–261). Baltimore: Williams and Wilkins.

Wilson, R. H., Morgan, D. E., & Dirks, D. D. (1973). A proposed SRT procedure and its statistical precedent. *Journal of Speech and Hearing Disorders, 38,* 184–191.

# PART III
## Management

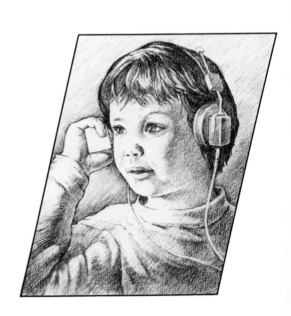

*K*nowledge of the etiologic factors and sequelae of hearing loss, as well as appropriate diagnostic procedures, are useless without correct amelioration when indicated. Too often correct history and diagnostic data are filed away on a child who never realizes the benefits to be derived from this information. The task of the habilitative and rehabilitative audiologist is usually to work around those auditory disorders that are irreversible. While these efforts involve the handicapped child directly, to a great extent they also include parents and significant others.

Too often the abilities of audiologists as counselors have been largely determined by their natural talents at communicating with people. In Chapter 9 David Luterman shows that audiologists can be good counselors if they become familiar with the deep emotions experienced by parents of handicapped children and become sensitive to the needs of these families.

Laurie Newton also deals with children through their families when she describes modern methods of auditory habilitation in Chapter 10. This clear, illustrative chapter is the result of the author's diverse experiences in dealing with habilitative methods. In Chapter 11 Antonia Maxon discusses the state of the art in amplification devices for hearing-impaired children, a critical aspect of auditory habilitation.

# 9

# *Counseling Parents of Hearing-Impaired Children*

## *DAVID M. LUTERMAN*

Counseling, as demonstrated for me in my training program, was something one did after testing the child and was invariably information-based. The usual clinical sequence was that the audiologist, or aspiring audiologist, would first take a case history, then try to separate the child from the parent so as to test the child without parental interference, and then "counsel" by informing the parents of the test results. Essentially this was a medical model. Implicit in this model was that the audiologist did not deal with parental feelings, that the affect area was the realm of the psychologist or social worker, and that the demonstration of feeling, more specifically crying, was to be avoided. I can remember discussing at length with my fellow students and supervisors "what to do when the parent cried." This was viewed almost in the same vein as a failure, the consensus being that one should have tissues available on the desk and quietly leave the room to let the parent compose herself (we never thought fathers cried). In practice, audiologists used content to distance the parents from the feelings area—by keeping the relationship in the cognitive realm, the audiologist could prevent or reduce the likelihood of a display of emotion that would embarrass both audiologist and parent. Implicit, and sometimes quite explicit, was the notion that people were so delicate that audiologists did not delve into the affect realm because they were not trained to do this (which is still quite true) and could cause some unspecified untold damage.

The medical model continues to be quite pervasive in our field, for it is comfortable and fits the experience of the instructors in our educational programs. The medical model often does work, and for certain families and situations it is very appropriate. For example, if an audiologist's tests suggest that a child has fluid in the middle ear space, the family should be referred immediately for appropriate medical treatment. A casual or laissez-faire attitude can result in prolonged infection, pain, rupture of the tympanic membrane, and consequent hearing loss. Diplomacy may be required when the audiologist believes that a child whose ear condition has possible dire consequences may be medically mismanaged. It is always a dilemma for the audiologist as to when to intervene directly in a child's best interest, and it is certainly appropriate at times to suggest a second medical opinion. The audiologist, however, needs to recognize the limitations of the medical model.

On the surface the medical model seems to be most efficient. At least one can block out a prescribed time so as to see the maximum number of cases in a given day, and audiologists can develop their set speech at the end of the testing sequence. One of my best set pieces, for example, used to be an explanation of the audiogram; I had another on how hearing aids worked; and one especially reserved for those parents with newly diagnosed deaf children was on the various approaches to education of the deaf and the schools in the area. I could fit each speech into a 10- to 15-minute time period and then send the parents off, feeling that I had fulfilled my clinical obligation and, perhaps as important, could see my next patient on time. There was no clinical fee for counseling—that was something tacked on at the end of the testing and was to be minimized. The set speech restricted the time spent and allowed the audiologist to get to the perceived area of his/her expertise: testing children.

This attitude still seems to be quite prevalent in our field. It is certainly implied in our educational programs when ASHA only recognizes time spent in direct client service toward the student's practicum hours. Time spent with the parents does not count and is minimized. This attitude also prevails in many employment situations in which work with parents is to be done on the therapist's own time and is not compensated.

Over the past 25 years of my clinical experience, I have come to see that the medical model is actually a very inefficient one—that the set speech I was delivering was not being "heard" by the parents. Upon their return for subsequent testing of their child, they would invariably ask me questions about almost everything I thought I had covered so well; when affect is very high, one cannot process information. Information is best processed when cognition and affect are in balance. When, for example, parents are stressed by having a child diagnosed as having a hearing loss, even when they "know" the child has the loss, affect overwhelms cognition—no matter how well prepared they seem to be for the diagnosis. Actually the very first reaction of most parents is one of relief that the child is only deaf and not retarded, which they have been most worried about; they are relieved that somebody finally believes them as they have generally had to convince relatives, well-meaning friends, and often the family pediatrician that there is something wrong with their child. The emotional response occurs when they learn that the hearing loss cannot be "fixed." Parents have reported to me that they couldn't remember what the audiologist said after she had emerged from the sound-proof room and told them that their child had a hearing loss and that the loss was not correctable.

In actuality, then, the medical/information-providing model is often inefficient—I have found that the time can frequently be best spent by listening to parents and allowing a release of the normal emotions surrounding the diagnosis of deafness in a child. We are dealing with people who are emotionally upset (normally so) rather than people who are emotionally disturbed, and the normal affect area is the proper realm of the audiologist. Strong feelings are a normal concomitant of any communication disorder, and the audiologist must be alert to the feelings of the client in order to be an effective clinician. The willingness to allow feelings to be part of the clinical interaction distinguishes for me the clinician from the technician.

## Parental Reactions

I have found over the years that one cannot go any faster with a child than the parent is willing or able to go. Audiologists limit truly effective case management when they become so overwhelmed by their anxiety to get a hearing aid on the child and to get the child into an educational program that they try to bypass the parental grief reaction by taking a very active management of the case. This invariably leads to passive and dependent parents and to ineffective long-term management of the child. I know a child psychiatrist who doesn't see any children—he finds that when he meets with the parents and helps them work through their own problems, the child's "problems" disappear. I feel very strongly that a similar attitude needs to pervade our field: if we pay careful attention to the parents and take time for them, especially in the early stages of diagnosis, then the children will do well in the long term. This may mean that the audiologist will allow some time to elapse between the diagnosis and the initiation of habilitation procedures, a hard thing for most audiologists to do. During this time the audiologists needs to be willing to allow the feelings of the parents to emerge. Effective counseling is a blend of supplying information and responding to the feelings as needed. Although parents in this situation seem to react on the surface in a variety of ways, certain basic emotions are almost universal in our culture.

Probably the most frequently used model to explain the parental process of coming to acceptance of their child's hearing impairment has been the mourning reaction articulated in the pioneering work of Kubler-Ross (1969) as a result of her observations of terminally ill patients. Her model of the grief process includes (1) denial, (2) anger, (3) bargaining, (4) depression, and (5) acceptance. Tanner (1980) has written a comprehensive article on the grief reaction and its relation to the speech pathologist and audiologist. I have used a similar model in my previous writings (Lutreman, 1979) and in lectures. I think it is a generally useful way of describing parental reactions, but I have grown wary of it—in that it presents a simplistic view of a very complex process and, as such, can be misleading. The stages of grief are not mutually exclusive, and there are no clear demarcation points as one moves from one stage to another. Acceptance itself is not a stage that is devoid of grief, as is implied in the model; it is characterized by a sadness that no longer immobilizes the parent. I find it useful to describe the various feelings that parents have and then to examine the implications of these feelings on parental behavior. In a later section I will deal with the clinical management of the grief reaction.

## Shock/Anxiety

The initial reaction to the diagnosis of deafness—or, more aptly, to the realization that the hearing loss is permanent—is shock. The shock reaction is a self-protective mechanism (much like denial) that is an emotional divorcement from the proceedings. One mother described it to me as seeing herself on a stage and going through the motions, almost commenting, "This is very interesting." At this point parents can still act and usually show a prodigious amount of movement (i.e., traveling to several doctors and having an infinite array of audiological examinations). However, the cognitive and affective aspects of their being are unhooked from each other. They cannot process much information; they are not psychologically owning the situation; they feel as if they are hollow shells or automatons going through the motions. They are attempting to keep at bay the very powerful feelings of being overwhelmed with anxiety and fear.

All parents, whether they have a handicapped child or not, feel inadequate at times in the face of the awesome task of raising a young child to responsible adulthood. When parents learn that they have a child with special needs, it means that they are going to be challenged to be a "special" parent, which provokes a great deal of fear. Parents never have to be reminded of their responsibility; they know it full well. The feelings of inadequacy lead the parent to seek a savior—someone to rescue them from their own felt inadequacies. As one father aptly put it, "I am looking to find a quarterback for my family." (He actually wanted a quarterback who would not make any mistakes!)

Audiologists all too often see themselves as the rescue agent and are all too willing to "call the plays." Doing so leads to convincing the parents that they really are inadequate—that they do indeed need someone to "call the plays." The only role I accepted for this family (and all families) was that of an enthusiastic fan—convinced of the parents' own competency to call a "good game," although not necessarily error free. Very early in the parent/audiologist interaction comes the plea for help to make the decisions for the family; this is a very delicate time. The audiologist must be helpful but in an indirect way that does not diminish parental self-esteem—not an easy thing to do in the face of so much pain and distress.

## Anger/Depression

Almost all parents of a hearing-impaired child are at some fundamental level quite angry. Anger comes about when there is a violation of expectations. Parents have many expectations about their unborn child, not the least of which is that he or she will be normal. When they find that the child is not normally hearing and cannot be cured, the parents feel cheated. They also wonder why they were singled out.

Invariably there is anger at the professional who does not cure the deafness and who does not rescue the parents from this awful dilemma. Anger also comes about when there is a loss of control—when we can no longer operate in our own best interests. Having a handicapped child means losing some measure of personal freedom. The father who could not accept a promotion in his company because to do so would mean moving to a community that had no programs for deaf children is angry. The family that does move in order for the child to go to a school for the deaf and consequently gives up much in their home community may also be very angry.

There is also an anger, almost rage, that comes about because of the frustration of not being able to cure their child. All parents I have met want at some level, one not always apparent to professionals, to do right by their child, want to make things better. I can remember so vividly going to the hospital to visit my daughter, who had broken her leg and was in pain, and realizing there was nothing I could do about it. I felt so angry and frustrated that I wanted to smash something. This is the anger in which one kicks the cat or puts a fist through a door. This type of anger is very often born of frustration and is frequently released toward others.

I have found that most people and families do not have good means for expressing anger. Anger is a very threatening emotion. When it is expressed, it is generally equated with loss of love. In actuality, there is a great deal of caring in anger; it implies that because this child means so much to me, I am deeply affected. Many families do not allow for an expression of anger and thus it is frequently repressed, which leads to depression. Audiologists, then, are very often dealing with depressed people who have a great deal of unexpressed anger. In depression, people often appear devoid of energy and feeling. Actually, the feelings are so intense that an immense battle is taking place within the person. The anger is seeking to emerge, and the person, not necessarily consciously, is trying to suppress the rage. This leaves little energy to do anything else. It is also true that when we choose to suppress any feelings, we tend to suppress all feelings, and the world becomes a rather gray place.

Most audiologists intuitively recognize that parents are potentially emotional volcanos that might erupt at any time. Very often the anger parents feel toward their situation is directed toward the audiologist. Most audiologists are more afraid of the anger emerging than they are of the grief. The use of content to distance the parent and the audiologist from the anger is very self-protective but not clinically helpful. Anger is a useful emotion. There is a great deal of energy in anger that needs to be released and directed toward working for the child's benefit. (It can also be directed toward working for programs that benefit all hearing-impaired children.)

The anger that is turned inward and becomes depression is not used in the best interests of the child. It festers and drains the parents of any useful energy. Audiologists who allow emotion to be part of their counseling experience need to be prepared for parents to be angry with them at some time in their relationship. This is very hard to do.

## Guilt/Resentment

Almost all mothers of deaf children feel at some level that they are responsible for the child's deafness. Guilt in general seems to be an epidemic among women in our society. They pick up guilt like a magnet attracting iron filings. I think this stems from child-rearing practices in which guilt is used as a means of controlling girls' behavior. One mother in a group said once, "I even feel guilty when it rains." When it comes to giving birth to a deaf or any disabled child, the opportunities for feeling guilty are manifold. Very often the cause of the deafness is not known (almost 50% of the time). Parental search for the cause frequently stems from their guilt feelings and represents a desire to fix blame somewhere else. This is a delicate time for audiologists when counseling the parents. Rather often audiologists inadvertently find themselves in the midst of a family fight seeking to fix the blame for the deafness on the other spouse. This is not to imply that the search is always a reflection of guilt. Parents are quite legitimately concerned about cause in determining whether to have more children. The audiologist needs to be sensitive to the family dynamics in choosing carefully the most appropriate response.

Almost all mothers of congenitally deaf children, in which there is no known etiology, have a guilty secret. It is almost impossible to have a nine-month pregnancy without something untoward happening that, in retrospect, cannot be blamed for the deafness. Thus, one mother felt she caused the deafness because she failed to take her vitamin pills; another, because she wore high heels and fell down; a third, because she went to a party and had several drinks. Although most of these guilty secrets are unfounded and cannot withstand rational examination, they lead to unwholesome behavior. Guilty parents are driven parents, almost always seeking the "cause" when it is no longer relevant and their energy can be better spent in child-management activities. Guilt-driven parents also tend to overprotect their child. They feel, "I let something bad happen to you once, and I'm not going to let it happen again." They do not let their child have the normal experiences necessary to develop the skills needed for responsible adulthood, which include taking risks and getting some "bloody noses" occasionally. The overprotection will extend to the therapy and audiological situations. These parents are not very trusting of professional competency, questioning the audiologist frequently and seeking other opinions when neither seem at all justified by the situation. It is very hard to maintain a long-term relationship with a guilt-driven parent.

The flip side of feeling guilty is feeling resentment. Guilt is such an uncomfortable feeling that we also resent the person or thing that is "making" us feel guilty. Guilt, when used as a controling device in relationships, as occurs in many families, usually leads to unhappy and poorly functioning families. The resentment simmers and generally leads to a sabotaging of relationships. Guilt-driven people usually "forget" to do important things, frequently miss appointments, and become unreliable. Resentments tend to lead to passive-aggressive behavior as opposed to anger, which can lead to action, where more energy is available.

The audiologist needs to be able to establish a caring, nonjudgmental relationship with parents so that sufficient trust can be established and the parents can feel free to share their guilty secrets. Very often these guilty secrets will not survive the light of rational examination, and information sensitively supplied can help the parents reduce the guilt. We can bestow no greater gift. Unfortunately there are parents who are reluctant to give up their guilt even when they have nothing rationally to feel guilty about. These parents must be helped to see that they can feel guilt and still behave in a manner that is helpful to the child.

## Vulnerability/Overprotection

For many parents, having a deaf child is the first bad thing that has happened to them. Very frequently this leaves them stunned and bewildered. If one lives long enough, something bad will happen; this is one of the facts of our existence. We tend to protect ourselves from the anxiety this fact engenders by thinking we are invulnerable. Since we are all at risk, our fantasy of being invulnerable is also at risk, and when the "bad thing" does happen, it increases anxiety, which can lead to overprotection. The parent begins to think, "Something bad has happened to my child once, and I'm not going to let any other bad thing happen again." For example, a mother whose normally hearing child was deafened because of meningitis would take a can of disinfectant with her every time she took her daughter grocery shopping and would spray the cart to get rid of any germs. Some sensitive listening on the audiologist's part can elicit some of these fears; by allowing the parent to talk them through, the audiologist can help the parent minimize nonfruitful behavior. The parent can now go to the supermarket without the disinfectant, but she is still panic-stricken whenever her daughter is ill. The topic of our vulnerability is always a very threatening one, especially among young audiologists who are about to become parents themselves.

## Confusion/Panic

Confusion is a normal stage early in the diagnostic process when parents attempt to acquire any new information. The vocabulary itself is so unfamiliar that they often become stuck trying to recall what a given word or term means and lose the meaning of the sentence itself. Terms such as "frequency," "decibel," and "audiogram" are not familiar to most persons. (Even the term "audiologist" is still pretty rare, and I have stopped telling people at cocktail parties that I am one as I am tired of trying to explain what audiologists do.) Yet audiologists use these terms quite freely with parents, defining them once and then assuming that the parents understand; they forget that it takes patience and time and that parents are approaching the learning process with a high degree of emotion, which limits their cognitive ability. In my experience, parental confusion and panic are not caused by too little information, but rather too much, too soon. Not only is information being supplied by the audiologist but they are also getting advice from well-meaning relatives, friends, and even strangers who notice their child's hearing aids and feel obligated to tell about their own experience. The parents feel very often as though they are drowning in a sea of information, much of it conflicting. This leads to a panic reaction that can be immobilizing: parents who cannot make a decision are frequently immobilized by their panic.

I have found it clinically useful to limit the information I give parents. As a rule of thumb, I do not give parents information unless they ask for it. I will generally ask them, "What do you need to know?" When I receive a response like "I don't even know enough to ask a question," which is not atypical in the early stages, I might respond, "It sounds like you are pretty confused and scared," then we can start talking about the feelings. Later, as emotions subside, content questions and answers will come. Content does need to be supplied by audiologists, but it has to be provided sensitively and slowly so as not to increase the parental confusion and panic.

## Denial

Probably there is no single reaction within the grief reaction that is so misunderstood and that confounds the parent-audiologist relationship more than denial. Denial must be seen as a very normal psychological reaction to a situation that is perceived as being overwhelming. It is self-protective and occurs spontaneously and unconsciously. For example, when I am driving my car and it begins to make strange noises, I respond by turning on the radio. On the surface this is very strange behavior. Even though I know that turning on the radio is not going to solve my car problem, it makes me *feel* better in the face of a potentially catastrophic situation because I can no longer hear the noises; that is, the noises no longer exist for me.

No matter how well prepared the parents may be for the diagnosis of deafness, there will be some elements of denial in their response and their behavior. When this denial is not understood by the audiologist, it looks as if the parents are being derelict in their duty and are hurting the child by not following through on the recommended clinical management. Denial extends to anything that will objectify the deafness (i.e., hearing aids, schooling, or any association with other parents who have deaf children). Parents who are reluctant to put a hearing aid on a child or to attend a signing class or a group session for parents of deaf children can be, and are almost invariably, seen by audiologists and educators as "bad" parents who are hurting the child. These are parents who are in denial. Invariably the audiologist's anger at the parents emerges as an admonitory lecture telling the parents how important it is to keep the hearing aids on the child and to attend classes. These lectures only serve to distance the parent from the audiologist and do nothing to help the parents give up the denial reaction. The parents will almost invariably agree verbally with the audiologist (they know the hearing aid is important), but "for some reason" they keep forgetting to put the hearing aid on the child. Thus begins an unwholesome cycle, with the parents looking more and more to the audiologist like "bad" parents and the parents trying to hide their behavior in the face of an angry and admonishing audiologist. This unhealthy relationship leads to both a frustrated audiologist and frustrated parents. Invariably in such situations there is a mutual "turn-off," and unfortunately it is not uncommon to see parents of adolescents who have never been allowed to work through the denial process and who have very impaired relationships with all professionals. Tragically they almost always have poor functioning children.

Denial must be seen as a function of feeling overwhelmed; it is a plea for help, a crisis of confidence. Thus, if I felt confident in my ability to fix engines, then I could psychologically afford to "hear" the engine noise. I would pull the car over to the side of the road and set about repairing it. In short, I would operate in a rational and approved manner; however, as long as I felt inadequate, I would need to protect myself by denying the problem. This is a normal reaction. Lectures telling me that I should not act this way are not helpful; in fact, they would just serve to increase my feelings of inadequacy. What I do need, and what all parents need, is someone to listen sensitively to my fear and to help me gain confidence in my own ability to solve my problems. When that happens, I can give up denial.

# The Audiologist's Reaction

All of the feelings experienced by the parents are also a part of the audiologist's reaction; under the skin we are all brothers and sisters. Audiologists often feel overwhelmed by the responsibility of determining a child's hearing loss and of counseling the family properly. This is especially true of the beginning audiologist who is still developing good test techniques and learning appropriate counseling strategies. Even veteran audiologists experience an anxiety almost akin to panic when presented with a child who promises to be difficult to test and a family that appears difficult to counsel.

Audiologists also experience anger. There is the anger they feel at the parents sometimes for not following through on a recommended course of action; there is the rage, frustration, and sometimes despair that audiologists feel when they can't make things better for the child or family or when they can't locate an appropriate placement. There is anger toward other professionals who insensitively and/or inappropriately treat the families. For example, pediatricians who fail to refer patients for testing or who inappropriately treat serous otitis media in children will arouse anger in audiologists. This anger is also a useful energy that can be used to educate other professionals. If repressed, it lends itself very often to depression and burnout.

Guilt is also a part of the audiologist's experience; I know of no responsible and competent audiologists who have no regrets about cases that they have handled. Mistakes are an inevitable part of the experience of all growing professionals. In one sense mistakes are "nuggets of gold." They are markers for what needs to be learned, indicating the next area of growth for the audiologist. I have learned far more from my mistakes than from my successes. My success I take for granted; my mistakes spur me on to new learning. Mistakes are seldom seen as valuable by practicing audiologists, perhaps a function of an educational system that penalizes mistakes so heavily. Consequently, many audiologists are burdened by the guilt of their errors. Fortunately for our field we are not brain surgeons and almost all of my patients have survived my mistakes quite well—some have even flourished, and so have I.

There are two common mistakes that audiologists make in counseling parents. One is the failure to listen and to credit parents with knowledge and ability. The other error that is made frequently is in regard to parents of mild to moderately impaired children. An audiologist who has been seeing profoundly deaf children is very often insensitive to the pain felt by parents of children with mild to moderate impairments. Any hearing loss is seen as a catastrophic event by the parents. Handicap is always in the eyes of the beholder. For some parents mild degrees of hearing impairments are seen as serious handicaps, and they need as much loving respect as parents of severely hearing-impaired children. The hearing loss and the parent's pain are not to be minimized.

Frequently when the feelings surrounding deafness in children are discussed, the painful and negative emotions are emphasized while the positive feelings and experiences are seldom described. To be sure, there is a great deal of pain and stress to be endured as part of the process of coming to grips with having a hearing-impaired child. Often overlooked are the marvelous opportunities for joy and growth that are also present. Very many parents come through the experience of having a hearing-impaired child with a clearer sense of themselves and a clearer sense of their priorities than they had before their child was diagnosed. Many parents find that their child's deafness has given their life meaning and direction. Their joy stems from actively participating in their child's growth—they take nothing for granted. When their child accomplishes a milestone, they rejoice with the knowledge that they helped put it there. I am always reminded of the Bertrand Russell quote, "To be without some of the things you want is an indispensible part of happiness."

In the same way, the audiologist experiences joy in workig with the parents of hearing-impaired children. In the very initial stages of diagnosis everything looks so bleak and hopeless to the parents that the audiologist very often becomes their lifeline. In well-managed families a marvelous reciprocal reaction begins to take place between the audiologist and parent and child. As the parent begins to "lighten up," in part because of the care and skill of the audiologist, the child begins to show progress, which further encourages the parents and leads to a more relaxed, open relationship between the parent and audiologist. My most meaningful clinical experiences have been in the intimate relationships that I have had with parents of newly diagnosed hearing-impaired children. It is very gratifying to witness and participate actively in a process by which people grow and fulfill their potential. I often tell parents that I will share some of their pain if they will share some of their joy with me.

# Clinical Management

Counseling begins at the moment of the initial contact with the parents and is continuous throughout the relationship. What needs to be established at the outset is what the major concern of the parents is and what their expectations for the audiologist are. Typically the parents will express some concern about the child's hearing (although one gets very surprising answers to the question "What concerns you most about your child?"). I don't try at this point to get a case history from the parents; I just let them tell me anything that they think is important—later on I may get the more specific details.

After the parents have shared their concern, I enlist them as coworkers in the task of determining their child's hearing status. As coworkers we all enter the testing booth. (I have also brought in other family members; if it gets too chaotic, I have the other members leave, but very often they are quite helpful.) Then I proceed to test the child. I describe how loud the test sound is in terms of decibels and in terms of environmental stimuli, and then I ask the parents whether they thought the child heard it or not. If we have some disagreement, I present the sound again until we are both satisfied that the child responded or did not respond. At the end of the testing I ask the parents what they think about their child's hearing, and we decide whether or not their child has a hearing loss. If we cannot agree, we resume testing.

Parents have recounted to me years later their feelings during this kind of testing process. They frequently report how painful it was for them to sit in the room and hear those loud sounds while their child showed no response. This procedure diminishes the denial mechanism (it does not eliminate it) because the parents see the hearing impairment objectified. Clinical procedures that separate the parents from the testing process will frequently increase the denial reaction by allowing the parents to fantasize about the testing (i.e., "Maybe they made a mistake—perhaps the tracings were switched," etc.). Thus any clinical procedure in which parents are separated from the testing—which tends to enhance parental denial—is poor from a counseling point of view. Although procedures that separate the parents might be more accurate in detecting and determining the hearing loss because there are no distractions to the audiologist, it is worthless if the parents cannot or will not accept the results. Parents have a need—much like that expressed in the folk custom of viewing the body at the funeral and then accompanying it to the cemetary—to see their child's deafness objectified before they can begin the grief process.

Another benefit of active parental participation in the diagnostic process is the strengthening of the bond between audiologist and parents. Parents have reported to me how glad they were that I was there helping them through the painful process. I was seen as an ally rather than an adversary. Audiologists who deliver the word to parents in the waiting room that their child is deaf, no matter how nicely done, are received with hostility. As in Shakespeare's plays, people very often beat the messenger when they don't like the message.

Another benefit of having parents help with the testing is that they are also being educated about the audiological process. Audiograms are much more meaningful to them when they are obtained in front of the parents' eyes. (I am not above having parents fill out their child's audiogram as we obtain it.) I prefer this procedure to trying to explain to parents what an audiogram is when they have not been part of the testing. They also obtain, from being part of the testing process, an idea of what their child can and cannot hear in the home environment, information that they can use in the habilitation of their child.

After completing the testing, if we have decided that the child is hearing-impaired, I make no effort to provide much information. As discussed earlier, it is usually not heard at this point. In response to "What do you need to know?" I usually get a few desultory questions that I answer minimally. I will also ask the parents how they feel; I often get a response such as "Numb." Occasionally parents will start to cry, and I will stay there with them. They have something to cry about, and they need someone to be there who is not trying to cheer them up or to focus their attention on content that they cannot absorb.

At this point I give them the name and phone number of parents of an older hearing-impaired child (they seldom call at first as they are still in denial) and set up an appointment to see them within a week. On subsequent appointments I supply more information as the parents ask for it and allow for more expression of their emotions by listening sensitively and nonjudgmentally to them.

# Listening

The essence of counseling lies in carefully listening to the parent, valuing the parent's competency, and sensitively supplying information as needed. I have described in detail elsewhere counseling theory and practice (Luterman, 1984), which is not within the scope of this chapter. In practice, very little more is needed beyond careful listening. (What is also needed is a warm, caring person, but I am not at all sure that this can be taught.) Listening is a skill that can be taught and that can also be learned. It needs to be seen by audiologists as a valuable skill; so often audiologists feel that they are effective, and therefore worthy of being paid, only if they are seen as actively doing. Listening is a matter of trying to hear the "faint knocking" that is underlying what the person is saying and that the person may not know is there. For example, parents frequently ask, "If this were your child, what would you do?" I often respond to this by saying, "It sounds like you are pretty frightened about making a decision right now. Why don't you sit down and let's talk about it."

Whenever I am asked a question, I try to take a moment to determine the feeling behind the question—or more appropriately, to determine how the world looks to this person at this time. Very often I will respond with content and answer the question directly. At times I may respond with a question if I suspect that the person is really seeking confirmation of a decision already made. This is especially true of anyone seeking advice; they usually have their minds made up and simply want my confirmation. It is much more efficient to elicit their decision than to blunder ahead trying to "advise" them. Parents who ask me whether oralism is better than total communication will usually get a response from me of "What have you been thinking about for your child?" I might also say, "It must be pretty frightening to be confronted with those choices." Which response they get would depend on my clinical judgment as to what that parent needed at the time. I could also respond with content by describing their options and some of the relevant research; seldom, however, do I burden the parents with my opinion. There is no one right response for a given situation; each response will move the relationship in a different direction, and clinicians must decide which way they want to go.

I have often found it helpful to try to change the person's perception of a situation by reframing it. For example, when parents complain about the lack of programs in their area, I might respond by pointing out what a marvelous opportunity they now have to establish needed programs. The ultimate goal of counseling is to help the parents make something positive happen as a result of having a hearing-impaired child, and reframing is often an important vehicle to helping them find a positive path to follow.

Very often it is quite appropriate to say nothing. I have a poster in my office which says, "It often shows a fine command of language to say nothing." As a matter of fact, some of the wisest things I have done have been to keep quiet. It is so presumptuous of us to think we have to have a response for every comment.

At workshops I am frequently asked in one form or another "Can counseling by an audiologist cause damage?" I think this question reflects the inadequacy and the lack of training that most audiologists feel when they step outside the narrowly prescribed technical aspects of our field. Webster (1966) has addressed the problem quite well:

> If counseling means the imposition of prescriptions without care for the person for whom they are prescribed one may indeed do damage. The non-accepting, non-compassionate clinician runs the risk of hurting parents; so does the one who focuses concern on the child to the exclusion of concern for the parents. The speech pathologist or audiologist who leaves to others the interpretation of the information his/her field has to offer may do parents great harm. The same can be said for the clinician with limited knowledge who gives faulty information.
>
> On the other hand, it is virtually impossible for one person to damage another by listening to him, by trying to understand what the world looks like to him, by permitting him to express what is in him and by honestly giving him the information he needs. In this view of counseling, the clinician serves as an accepting listener. He delays his judgment and tries to accept parents as they are and as they will become. (p. 33)

It is not enough for audiologists to learn just the technical aspects of testing—ours is a field that in order to be maximally effective requires the capacity to develop caring relationships with the people we are counseling and providing with services. We need as a profession to be humane. This means we need to select carefully the students we educate, and we need to provide students in our educational programs with interpersonal experiences that will promote personal growth and encourage a humanistic orientation toward the hearing-impaired and their families. We need to provide ongoing workshops for practicing audiologists to remind them of the human factor in the profession. It is so easy for us as a profession to bury ourselves underneath our equipment and our test techniques that we miss the heart and soul of our profession, which is providing a lifeline to people who desperately need the help of a caring fellow human being.

# Summary

Audiologists, by virtue of their training, have tended to view the counseling process as predominantly information-imparting without consideration of the emotional impact that the diagnosis of deafness has on parents. In order to be more effective clinicians, audiologists need to allow feelings to be part of the counseling process—when feelings are factored in and do not predominate, then information can be processed and utilized by the parents. The parental feelings of inadequacy, anger, guilt, vulnerability, confusion, and denial need to be considered by the audiologist. Diagnostic evaluations need to be conducted in such a way as to minimize parental denial by including the parents in all aspects of the testing. Effective clinical management requires that the audiologist sensitively listen to the parents and convey a sense of caring. Audiologists need to have confidence in the parents' ability to solve their own problems. As a profession we need to allow for personal growth both within our training programs and within our continuing education experiences so as to help create clinicians who are personally congruent and more effective in dealing with the emotional aspects of hearing loss.

# References

Kubler-Ross, E. (1969). *On death and dying.* New York: Macmillan.

Luterman, D. (1984). *Counseling the communicatively disordered and their families.* Boston: Little, Brown.

Luterman, D. (1979). *Counseling parents of hearing-impaired children.* Boston: Little, Brown.

Tanner, D. C. (1980). Loss and grief: Implications for the speech-language pathologists and audiologists. *Asha, 22,* 916–980.

Webster, E. (1966). Parent counseling by speech pathologists and audiologists. *Journal of Speech and Hearing Disorders, 31,* 331.

# The Educational Management of Hearing-Impaired Children

## LAURIE NEWTON

*T*he most important factor contributing to the linguistic competence of hearing-impaired children is their ability to use residual hearing. The better the hearing, the better the language. And the better the language, the better the prognosis for academic achievement. Educators have devised countless techniques to improve the language abilities of their hearing-impaired students. Not one can compete with improved hearing.

This situation places a hefty responsibility into the hands of professionals who influence the child's auditory capacity. Yet the majority of audiologists and educators serving hearing-impaired children do not understand the potential effects of comprehensive audiological management. In typical practice, each gives only token acknowledgement to auditory development. The audiologist typically tests, recommends a hearing aid, and sends the child off to school. The teacher may teach a 15- or 30-minute lesson from an auditory training curriculum. Neither tends to view hearing as a pervasive process, which is always interpreting and shaping and in a state of vulnerability to its environment. Therefore, neither may fully appreciate how attention to audition can make more difference than any other form of habilitation.

Not only are audiologists and educators estranged from the auditory process, they are frequently estranged from one another. Often they have never met. They may communicate occasionally by phone. Parents may have more contact with the audiologist since they usually take the child in for testing. Most teachers do not understand the test results that appear on the forms they receive from audiologists. Even fewer are able to evaluate the results in terms of their implications for speech perception. Many teachers do not consistently perform a daily hearing-aid check, nor are they attuned to more than the most obvious signs that the aid is not functioning properly.

Most audiologists know little about the home or school settings in which their pediatric clients function throughout the day, or how to adapt amplification in these various settings. They may not understand the implications of their test results for the acquisition of specific speech sounds. They do not know whether teachers and parents are monitoring the adequacy of children's amplification systems. They know little about auditory skill development or whether the teacher is facilitating this development. Most important, they underestimate the auditory and oral potential of many preschoolers with severe and profound hearing losses and consequently make educational recommendations that restrict the child's ability to develop these skills.

This chapter presents an interdisciplinary perspective for managing the hearing-impaired child. It focuses upon the audiologist's role as a member of the team of persons responsible for the child's development. It presents a new model for audiologists: to provide a portion of their service outside the clinical environment, closer to the real-life settings where hearing-impaired children actually use their hearing. Not every audiologist will need the complex skills required to serve hearing-impaired children appropriately. But those who do accept these children into their caseloads must acknowledge their potential for shaping the lives of children in profound ways. Recent attention to the development of a discipline in educational audiology offers hope for improved services to children. Audiologists trained during the 1980s may be better prepared to meet children's needs than were their predecessors.

This chapter begins with the critical first stage of habilitation: early intervention. Following is a discussion of educational considerations that affect the audiological evaluation. The audiologist's role in educational programming is then presented. Finally, services provided in the educational setting are discussed to familiarize audiologists with special areas of programming for hearing-impaired children.

# Early Intervention

The powerful results that can be accomplished through maximal use of residual (i.e., remaining, usable) hearing can be realized only if intervention begins at an early age. The auditory potential of a 6-year-old profoundly impaired child is very different from that of a child who is 18 months of age. It is probably true that an older child who has not yet learned to use residual hearing cannot become an auditory learner. However, most infants with severe to profound losses are able to achieve good use of residual hearing if managed appropriately.

Early intervention includes three components: early identification, early amplification, and early education. Early identification is essential, for without it no further intervention will occur. Hearing-impaired children should be identified as close to birth as possible, but at least by 1 year of age. Broad identification requires a hearing screening identification system at birth and in hospitals. Maternal questionnaire high-risk screening is the most commonly used screening system. An effective referral system must accompany the identification process (Clark & Watkins, 1985).

Early amplification interrupts the process of development without hearing. The auditory pathway provides stimuli that feed the growth of perceptual, cognitive, and psychosocial function. Before the child is aided, these processes continue to develop, but audition does not develop in parallel. Boothroyd (1982) describes the developmental asynchrony that can occur when skills in one area of growth develop out of parallel with skill development in other areas. There is also evidence that auditory neurons which are insufficiently stimulated lose their ability to perform their original function. This idea is related to the notion of critical ages— maturational periods during which the neurological system is most adaptable for growth. Once the critical age for development has passed, the potential to benefit from intervention is reduced. Failure to use sound may also influence the young child's psychosocial development. Parents may withdraw from a nonresponsive child. Deaf children may experience a reduced feeling of psychological safety in an environment that cannot be reliably monitored by audition.

Regardless of scientific verification, educators in daily contact with children see clear evidence of the effects of early auditory intervention in the receptive and expressive communication of their students. Many children who would have been functionally deaf prior to the advent of early amplification now function as hard of hearing. Many are able to receive an education in the regular classroom with supportive services.

Because we now recognize the importance of early amplification, we chastise pediatricians who delay the identification of hearing loss. Yet audiologists also contribute to postponed habilitation by delaying amplification. It is not uncommon for audiologists to schedule appointments for these children at the same time intervals as they schedule any other client. The protracted diagnostic process may then delay fitting a hearing aid for months. Such postponements should never occur. A child who needs amplification should be evaluated immediately and frequently. Some type of trial amplification should be fit as soon as an earmold can be obtained.

In addition to their responsibility for early amplification, audiologists are usually responsible for early referral for educational intervention. This situation happens because they are generally the first to know that the child has a hearing loss. It is important that the audiologist not wait until the nature of the hearing loss is completely defined, or the precise parameters of amplification determined, before referring the family to an educational facility. Postponing referral while the audiologist completes the diagnostic process can add months of additional delay. During this time the child and famly are losing the critical months so important to development. A more appropriate service model would include referral to the educational facility as soon as the hearing loss is confirmed. At that point the family can immediately begin to learn strategies for facilitating the acquisition of communication. The initiation of educational services helps many parents feel that they are taking an active role in helping their child, thereby facilitating their transition from feelings of helplessness to feelings of greater control and involvement. The audiologist will continue to see the child after educational intervention has begun. Coordinated efforts with the school program, including teacher reports on the child's differential response to various hearing aids, can contribute greatly to the audiologist's decisions regarding the child's auditory function.

In order to make appropriate educational referrals, audiologists and educators must learn to rely on more than children's auditory thresholds.

They must be attuned to the early characteristics that distinguish children with potential for speech discrimination from those with poor potential. Young children's performance should be observed over time, evidenced by changes in voice quality and prosody, ability to approximate speech imitations, and nonverbal responses to sound. Children who demonstrate no changes in these characteristics, even following 6 to 12 months of intensive auditory intervention, may lack sufficient residual hearing for use in language learning.

# Educational Considerations in Audiological Assessment

## Parent and Teacher Involvement

In traditional practice, the audiological test suite is the domain of the audiologist. Many audiologists prefer to evaluate children without the participation of parents or other service providers. When testing a young or difficult-to-test child, this procedure may be unwise. Isolated evaluation limits the benefits that parents and educators, as well as the audiologist, might gain from cooperative assessment. Most teachers or parents can learn with minimal explanation the types of behaviors that are appropriate and inappropriate to the evaluation environment. Only in rare circumstances is it best to exclude parents from the testing situation.

Including parents is beneficial from a psychological and educational perspective, as it establishes a team spirit, acknowledging their expertise regarding their child right from the start. Participation also decreases the anxiety that could develop as they sit in the waiting room with only minimal awareness of what is happening to their child. Since they then have little knowledge of what transpires, they must rely entirely on the audiologist's judgment, which may leave them feeling helpless, without power, and doubtful about the test results. Empowering parents with self-confidence as child-rearers may be the best gift a professional can offer parents. It is the parents who will make the most difference in the child's life.

Including parents during testing is the ideal way to begin parent education. When serving young hearing-impaired children, a large portion of the educational efforts are directed toward the parent rather than toward the child. If the parent is to be ultimately responsible for the child's development, we must allow them to become fully informed. They must view themselves as important contributors to the decision-making process affecting their child. Establishing these attitudes early will discourage later decisions to leave their child's development up to the schools or the professionals. Children of parents who leave their child's development to professionals rarely achieve as they might.

If parents are present during the evaluation, they will better understand the explanation and implications of results. They can hear the stimuli change in volume and pitch and observe their child's differential responses. Observing the electroacoustic analysis of their child's hearing aid, accompanied by simple explanations, provides an early introduction to concepts that may take years to learn well. Because of the many opportunities for repetition as the child returns for reevaluations, every parent who is taught can eventually obtain some degree of competence in understanding the audiological process.

Including parents and educators in the evaluation can be of benefit to the audiologist as well. They may be much more familiar with the child's typical behaviors and thus able to provide interpretations that would not occur to the audiologist. They can often better select activities that would engage the child during testing. They will be more familiar with the child's vocabulary, allowing the audiologist to obtain speech results when the child might otherwise appear untestable. Speech test results (comparing ears, hearing aids, hearing-aid settings, etc.) based upon even 10 to 15 familiar words provide more information than CNT (could not test)—the typical report on children who lack sufficient vocabulary to take a formal speech test. Finally, the presence of parents, educators, or caretakers during testing will provide the familiar, supportive environment which most young children need in order to perform optimally.

## Areas of Assessment and Their Relation to Auditory Development

A typical pediatric evaluation consists of immittance measures, pure-tone tests, and speech tests. When evaluating a hearing-impaired child, other types of assessment may also be relevant to linguistic development. Aided pure-tone and speech test results should be performed on a regular basis throughout the child's educational career. This information is of more value to planning than are unaided test results. It is always better to teach a speech sound through audition, rather than through alternate modalities, if the child can be helped to hear it. Aided thresholds help provide this information. For example, a child with aided thresholds of 30 dB HL, between 500 and 1000 Hz, will learn most characteristics of speech through audition. That is because a 30 dB aided threshold allows the child to hear most of the features of conversational speech (which occur at about 30 to 65 dB HL). If this same child's aided thresholds at 2000 Hz and above are only 70 dB, the child may have to learn high-frequency fricatives through visual and tactile channels. This is because the acoustic information of high-frequency sounds would not be heard even with amplification.

Audiologists can also use aided test results to evaluate whether the child's amplification is providing appropriate gain at all frequencies. For example, the teacher may tell the audiologist that a child with good aided thresholds in the middle frequencies is not acquiring mid-frequency consonant sounds as expected. Inspection of aided thresholds might suggest that too much gain in the low frequencies could be masking mid-frequency consonants. Another example would be aided thresholds falling just below levels that would permit the child to hear the high frequencies of normal conversational speech. The audiologist might explore earmold modifications that could provide greater gain in the high frequencies.

Aided speech tests help the audiologist and educator evaluate the child's ability to use residual hearing to hear and to discriminate speech. Usually a child with poor thresholds will have poor discrimination ability. However, two children may have identical audiograms, yet be very different in their ability to discriminate speech sounds. This difference may not be attributable to intelligence, linguistic competence, or education but rather to a difference in ability to process or interpret auditory information. Distinguishing between children with good and poor discrimination ability is very important to the prognosis of oral language acquisition and to decisions about the modality through which language can best be taught. Some form of speech threshold and discrimination testing should always be attempted, even if only informal assessment can be achieved. The audiologist might ask the parent or teacher to provide words the child knows and then use these in testing. If possible, these words should be selected to reflect different syllable lengths and/or speech sounds. Children can also be *taught* word-sound associations with pictures or toys that represent various sounds, such as *peep* (/i/), *moo* (/u/), *bah* (/a/), running water (/ʃ/), and a snake sound (/s/). Ling (1978) recommends performing the Five-Sound Test, which can be used to quickly check speech reception across the speech frequency range, during testing or at the beginning of a speech lesson. This test consists of having a child clap after (detection) or imitate or point to (discrimination) the sounds /i/, /a/, /u/, /ʃ/, and /s/ (or the pictures or toys representing these sounds, as described above) at a predetermined distance from the ear. Some audiologists use this test as a part of their test battery. Finally, speech test results should be interpreted in conjunction with reports of the child's ability to discriminate in the home and classroom since each contributes distinct and important information.

Audiologists may also be involved in evaluating the child's ability to perform other auditory behaviors related to habilitation. This could include the ability to approximate imitation of nonsense sounds, syllables, or prosodic patterns. If a child approximates an imitation, that is good evidence that he or she can discriminate it. If the imitation is not approximated, the failure may or may not be attributable to failure to hear the sound. The breakdown might occur in processing, integrating, or producing the sound.

Other areas of assessment needed for planning an auditory skill development program include localization and auditory comprehension. Localization skills are used for nonlinguistic tasks, yet are important to daily function. Comprehension is the highest level of auditory function, requiring perception, discrimination, and finally integration with the cognitive/linguistic system. A variety of tests are available for evaluating comprehension, such as the *Test of Auditory Comprehension* (Office of the Los Angeles County Superintendent of Schools, 1976), normed on hearing-impaired children, and the Glendonald Auditory Screening Procedure (GASP!) (Erber, 1982), a test which is not normed but was developed for hearing-impaired children. Both of these tests are used by teachers to place children into a curriculum of auditory skills.

A final area of assessment important to prognosis is observation of the child during spontaneous communication at home or in the classroom. This is the truest test of the child's ability to use hearing in the real world, where noise, distance, poor visibility, and other forms of interference impede ideal listening conditions. Ross (1982) presents a classroom observation instrument that guides the observer in evaluating the child's performance in a variety of communicative contexts. For infants who are not yet in school, the Ski*Hi program (Clark & Watkins, 1985) has formats to follow in making these assessments.

Many of these assessment procedures (comprehension, classroom behavior, imitation, etc.) are performed by the educator in planning an auditory skill development program. However, some teachers do not recognize the importance of assessing children in these areas, and others may not fully understand the auditory implications of children's performances on the tests. On the other hand, there are some teachers who are so skilled in auditory development that the audiologist could learn much from them. Here again, cooperation between the audiologist and educator will allow each to contribute his or her individual expertise, bringing the greatest combined resources to the child.

## Reporting Test Results

Audiological test results are usually first reported orally to parents. Audiologists who are able to adapt their language and explanations when presenting this information to less sophisticated audiences have achieved a very special and important skill. The audiologist should keep practicing and revising, with listeners of varying levels of sophistication, until a smooth, logical, simple format is developed. Practice will lead to a repertoire of language from which to draw, varying from simple to complex, in response to each unique audience. Diagrams and simple pictures may help. Learning to explain clearly and well is not typically taught in graduate school. Sometimes it can be learned by observing others. It is the audiologist who values the participation of parents and educators who cares enough to really communicate.

It is important to explain hearing capacity in relation to concepts that are relevant to the listener's world view. "Decibels," "hertz," or "frequencies" are important only as they relate to hearing speech or other sounds of importance. Audiograms are available that display the intensity and frequency of environmental and speech sounds (Northern & Downs, 1978). It can be very helpful to use these audiograms to show parents the location of normal speech sounds in relation to their own child's thresholds. A parent who does not understand this can be taken into the test room and allowed to listen to speech at different intensities, then helped to locate those levels on the audiogram. The parent can then be shown how a hearing aid with a certain amount of gain can make conversational speech louder, bringing it closer to levels where the child can hear. Some parents will understand how gain at different frequencies affects speech sounds differentially. For others, it may be best to begin by conceptualizing speech as occurring at a certain average level. These adaptations must often be made spontaneously during the conference as the audiologist obtains feedback on the listener's level of sophistication.

After the conference, the audiologist develops a written report of the test results. Clarity in test writing is another important skill. The report is typically the only record that preserves the results of the evaluation, thus making the testing worthwhile. A simple, well-written report can be used by the educator to improve programming for the child. Many are so complex and full of numbers that educators cannot benefit from the information. Some are so obtuse that they are unintelligible even to other audiologists. Reports should be written with the reader in mind. If school personnel or parents will be reading the report, it should be written for their understanding. Interpretations that relate findings to auditory, linguistic, and academic implications are essential. Although explanations may reduce the formality of the report, they should be included if necessary. Communication and improved service to children are paramount. The reader is referred to Ross (1982) for a good overview and examples describing report-writing for hearing-impaired children.

Throughout the evaluation and conference period, the audiologist should silently monitor the emotional status of the family. The initial diagnostic and amplification sessions can be a period of great anxiety, apprehension, or pain for parents. Each parent may be in a different state of acknowledgment and acceptance of their child's hearing loss. There may be tension and unresolved hostility between parents. Parents may experience lack of confidence in themselves, exhaustion, or feelings of intrusion into their family unit as they shuffle back and forth among doctors, audiologists, and educators, all of whom seem to know more about how to handle their child than they do. A great deal has been written about parents of hearing-impaired children as they proceed through the stages of acknowledgment and acceptance of their child's handicap. Every audiologist is encouraged to read a text such as Luterman's (1984) *Counseling the Communicatively Disordered and Their Families,* a sensitive account of parents' needs and the effects of those needs upon their children.

Sensitivity to the parents' status will help the audiologist judge the type and amount of information the parents are ready to hear. Emphasis on detailed academic matters during the early identification period may not be remembered by the brightest of parents. The audiologist who is not afraid of parents' feelings will communicate empathy and a willingness to listen to any type of communication the parent may be needing. Parents requiring more time than the audiologist can give may be helped by a counselor, a family service program, or the special educator. The parents' emotional readiness to accept their child's loss will underlie all their subsequent interaction with that child. For example, a child may refuse to wear the hearing aid long beyond the typical acceptance period. This is often interpreted as a problem with the amplification system. Another possible explanation could be that the parents are unconsciously avoiding use of the aid. The emotional status of parents must be of primary importance to the audiologist if effective child management is to proceed.

Deaf parents of hearing-impaired children may require special sensitivity. Their first need may be the services of an interpreter. Unless the audiologist has good sign language skills, it is best to solicit the services of an interpreter. Deaf parents deserve the same complete and adequate communication that hearing parents receive.

Although some deaf parents may wish for a hearing child, they are often more accepting and less estranged from their hearing-impaired children. Hearing-impaired parents vary greatly in their desire for their child to learn to use residual hearing and speech. They typically feel strongly about the issue, one way or the other. Parents who are opposed to deaf people learning speech will not support the audiologist's efforts toward this end. This can become a very difficult situation for the audiologist, especially if the child has good residual hearing. It is important to acknowledge the parents' reality in resisting the imposition of a goal that has been nothing but a psychological burden to them for the majority of their lives. They know how difficult it is to listen and speak, to try to "fit in with the hearing world." Explanations of how amplification and techniques for developing auditory potential have improved since they were young may or may not help. Once the child is enrolled in the school program, the parents may observe other children with similar losses who are using their hearing and learning to speak. Hearing grandparents or other relatives might help to provide an auditory environment for the child and encourage hearing-aid use. The teacher will have control over amplification used by the child during the school day, and this will allow many hours of listening. It is hoped that the child will come to appreciate the benefits provided by amplification and want to wear the aids. A child of hearing-impaired parents who sign should never be discouraged from using sign language, as this is unrealistic, unnecessary, and demeaning to the language of the family. Whether or not the child of deaf parents is educated in an oral or total communication program depends upon individual circumstances.

Whether parents are hearing or not, each child will become a product of his or her own individual family, with all its strengths and shortcomings. Professionals working with families can offer their expertise, but the family may choose to reject it. Except in extreme circumstances, the professional must acknowledge the parents' rights to choose for their family, and continue to work in support of the family and child.

# Transition into the Educational Setting

## The Audiologist's Role in Referral

Because audiologists are typically the first to identify children as hearing-impaired, they are generally responsible for initial referral to an educational facility. Referral should be made as soon as a child's hearing loss is identified. From that point on, management of the child's development becomes an interdisciplinary effort. Working in cooperation with other professionals requires unique interpersonal skills that may need to be learned.

Hearing-impaired children, especially those with additional handicaps, will be served by a wide variety of professionals. It is doubtful that all these professionals will always agree on all recommendations. Parents often feel torn by conflicting advice about which recommendations should take precedence or which are right. Professionals who serve these children must relinquish their view of themselves as primary or critical caretaker and devote the additional effort required to work together. Because this means additional time, patience, and compromise, professionals often prefer to work in isolation and send out reports. Then the parents and their children are left alone in the middle.

It is important that one member of the team become the central contact person for the parents. When this is not established, parents often feel confused about whom to contact for what. It is also important for parents to establish a bond with a primary service provider for their child, even though they will continue to contact and see all members of the team as appropriate. Because the educator is usually the person having the greatest regular contact with the child and family, this person can usually best assume this role. It is sometimes difficult for the audiologist to relinquish his or her role as the first and primary support system for the family. A close, mutual attachment may form during this early period of identification and hearing-aid fitting. It is important that the audiologist, as well as other professionals, show parents that they basically support the influence of the educator even if they disagree with certain recommendations. Dispassionate disagreement can be mentioned to parents, but major differences should be worked out between professionals, not through parents.

Audiologists are often in the position to recommend educational settings when referring children for habilitation. Their personal biases may influence objective data when choosing among educational options. They may feel that one program has better teachers or that one educational approach is superior to another. Audiologists must examine their consciences carefully to be certain that they are presenting fair recommendations to parents. Bias is acceptable if it is informed bias and takes individual differences into consideration. Unless the audiologist has considerable personal experience with a variety of options for educating hearing-impaired children, as well as knowledge about the individual programs available in the family's locality, extreme caution should be used in stating preferences. It is usually best to have the parents visit every educational facility where their child could be served. This acknowledges that the decision is not the audiologist's alone, and it can prevent later repercussions from dissatisfied parents. The parents must feel comfortable that they have considered every option and have made the decision.

Certain conditions may influence the audiologist to steer parents to one program as opposed to another. This should only be done when there are very obvious differences between programs that could seriously affect the child's development. The controversy between oral and total communication programs often biases referral agents in one direction or another. The relative benefits of these two approaches depend more upon the individual program's execution of these methods than upon the espoused methodologies themselves. It is essential that audiologists learn the difference between quality and mediocre applications of each of these two methodologies and evaluate the programs in their locality against these standards. Any child who has usable residual hearing (few young hearing-impaired children do not) should be placed in a program that puts strong emphasis on maintenance of amplification and on auditory and speech skill development throughout the day. This must be personally examined in both total communication and oral programs, as some total communication programs may have better auditory and speech programs than do some oral programs.

A young child with a hearing loss of 90 dB or better through 1000 Hz will often benefit greatly from an oral approach and not require the use of sign language. This prognosis could be severely impeded, however, by late identification and amplification; additional handicaps, perhaps even subtle in nature; a program and/or parents not skilled in oral language development; or very poor speech discrimination ability (the latter cannot be determined until after a period of educational instruction). The audiologist must weigh all of these variables when contemplating placement decisions. The advantage of a team approach is that the audiologist can be assisted by a group of people who together will work to reduce limitations and maximize oral potential (in both oral and total communication programs). But audiologists' contributions will work only if they can assure that teachers and parents have the skill to maintain attention to audition throughout the child's day.

## The Interdisciplinary Team Model

An interdisciplinary team approach is now advocated for serving most types of handicapped children. Federal education regulations require that evaluation of all handicapped children be made by a multidisciplinary team or group of persons, including at least one teacher or other specialist with knowledge in the area of suspected disability. Hearing-impaired children, especially those with additional handicaps, must be served by a variety of professionals in order to receive effective intervention. The depth of expertise required in each component of intervention is too broad to be provided well by only one or two individuals.

The primary team members serving every hearing-impaired child are the audiologist, the otologist, the educator, and the parents. Additional professionals should be used as needed. This may include the speech-language pathologist, the counselor or psychologist, the diagnostician, the geneticist, physicians addressing related disorders, the occupational or physical therapist, school administrators, and others. Different members may be of importance at different times during the child's development.

The degree of contact between professionals depends upon the questions needing responses by these experts. Older children with no additional handicaps who make good use of residual hearing, are progressing well in school, and have adequate family support may need no more than annual contact between teacher and audiologist. Young and recently identified children require regular contact between educators and audiologists. Children with special problems may benefit from a specifically planned multidisciplinary team evaluation, staffed by a variety of pertinent team members. The benefits that can be obtained when professionals come together to serve children are unmatchable. Team management is also a most invigorating, rewarding experience for the professionals, who can grow in their own knowledge from exchange with other professionals approaching the same handicap from a different perspective. The reader is referred to Matkin, Hook, and Hixson (1979) for a review of the multidisciplinary approach to the evaluation of hearing-impaired children. A team approach can be used during the treatment phase of service provision as well.

## Home- versus Center-Based Programs

A major component of habilitative programs for children 0–3 years of age is parent education. The degree to which the educator also works directly with the child varies across programs. Most programs emphasize parental training, where the educator models certain learning experiences with the child, then the parent attempts the interaction with the child. Supporters of this training model generally stress the importance of providing all training in the home rather than at a school or center-based program. The advantages of such a program are that the parents retain full responsibility for the child and remain the central figure in the child's life, the child associates early communication development with the immediate, personal environment, and the parents are able to continue the program throughout the child's waking day. The Ski*Hi model (Clark & Watkins, 1985) is an excellent example of an effective home intervention program that focuses upon parent training.

Children identified at age 3 and above are often handled very differently from infants. They are frequently placed into a half- or full-day preschool classroom for hearing-impaired children, with comparatively little instruction programmed outside this context. Parents may be included only minimally.

The choice of a home- or school-based, parent- or child-focused training is often a predetermined characteristic of an educational program rather than a program variable that can be modified to suit individual children's needs. An ideal program would have all these options available. The availability of a continuum of services, from home- to center-based, would allow child placement based upon need. Some 2½-year-olds are able to benefit considerably from a few mornings a week in school with other hearing-impaired children. Some may benefit most from placement in a small day-care program with normally hearing children, supported by staff training from the special education teacher. Other children may be less ready for school, but their options may be minimal. Some parents cannot assume responsibility for educating their child. Others may feel intimidated or diminished in power when an outsider comes into their most personal living space to tell them how to parent their child. Many parents work full time and cannot spend much time with their children. A child with a significant hearing loss may be much better off in a half-day classroom with a trained educator (the other half in a small day-care program) than in an 8-hour day-care program with 25 other children. Finally, a center-based program gives parents of hearing-impaired children regular opportunity to meet and learn together.

Training should always be provided to parents of recently identified hearing-impaired children, regardless of the setting in which the child is educated and regardless of the child's age. Furthermore, there is no reason for parents' participation in their child's education to cease at any time during the child's schooling. Continued active parent participation requires special planning and attention from professionals, but it is a key ingredient distinguishing successful from average students.

## The Audiologist's Role in Habilitation

The audiologist's role in the overall habilitative process is not universally defined and varies considerably from program to program. Audiological services to school children generally take one of the following forms:

1. *Separate clinical services.* In this service delivery model, audiologists may never visit the schools. They have clients who visit them in their offices, some of whom are hearing-impaired children. Their only contact with the schools may be through parent report, their own written reports that go to teachers, or an occasional telephone communication. They often know very little about auditory trainers or about how children they serve use amplification in their daily lives. They know very little about auditory training or the relationship between amplification and speech development. The graduate program from which they received their degree probably placed little or no emphasis on these factors. Unfortunately, most hearing-impaired children are served by these audiologists.

2. *Contracting with schools.* Some audiologists who have a special interest in hearing-impaired children may contract with a school to serve the children in that particular program. Other local audiologists may reasonably become disturbed by one audiologist's monopoly on services to hearing-impaired children. If the contracted audiologist is good, however, and becomes familiar with the needs of the children, this arrangement can be a very good one for the school program. An audiologist who works with many hearing-impaired students will be more familiar with their special needs and with the nature of their educational program. It is also easier for the school to work with one rather than many clinics.

   Although contracting can be a good service-delivery model, many audiologists and school programs do not carry the services far enough. In addition to testing and evaluating hearing and hearing aids, the audiologist should be hired to work on a regular basis (at least weekly) in the school. The audiologist can serve as a consultant in implementing a complete audiological management program. This would include establishing a hearing-aid monitoring and troubleshooting program, monitoring the use of auditory trainers, advising teachers on auditory capabilities and implications, establishing and monitoring a program in auditory training, adapting amplification systems to maximize speech perception, and monitoring classroom acoustics and communication. If these additional services are not available, the children are probably not receiving maximal benefit from amplification.

3. *The school-employed audiologist.* Whereas smaller school programs may find contracting for audiological services to be the only financially sound method for obtaining these services, larger programs may hire their own educational audiologist to work on a full- or part-time basis in their school. Holding other variables constant (e.g., the competence of the individual audiologist), this service-delivery model will provide the best audiological program by far. Audiologists who are always present are a working part of the staff and play an integral, daily role in planning and implementing children's education. They have the time to observe children in classrooms, to work with teachers, and to monitor the way teachers integrate audition into the total educational program. They come to know both the special and regular classroom teachers in the school in a personal way; therefore, their suggestions are met with greater acceptance. Because they are not also employed elsewhere, the school program is the central focus of their professional commitment. Consequently, they are more likely to develop expertise in the relationship between audiology and education.

The educational audiologist is a newcomer to the field of audiology and a long-needed missing link to successful speech and language acquisition in hearing-impaired children. Our profession is coming to realize that satisfactory service delivery to hearing-impaired children requires unique, specialized skills that many audiologists do not have. And these are skills that make a significant difference.

# Services Provided in the Educational Setting

### Instructional Components

The education of hearing-impaired children contains many of the same components as that of all children. This includes the facilitation of cognitive, academic, physical, social, and emotional growth. The major area of dysfunction for most severely to profoundly hearing-impaired children is the acquisition of language. Poor language skills and consequential experiential deprivation may interfere with most other areas of development as well.

Whether or not cognitive development is affected by poor language ability is a controversial issue. It would appear that children with minimal ability to process linguistic information would absorb considerably less data upon which to operate cognitively. It may also be more difficult to encourage the awareness of new or abstract relationships. Deaf children do appear to learn concepts in the same sequence and in the same manner as hearing children do but at later ages (Meadow, 1980).

The general level of academic achievement is low in children with significant hearing losses. This too is due to the influence of linguistic incompetence upon subsequent learning in all content areas. Hearing-impaired students at age 14 show median achievement levels of third grade in reading comprehension and sixth grade in math (Gallaudet Research Institute Newsletter, 1985).

Some hearing-impaired children exhibit disorders in physical development. Deaf children are more likely than hearing children to have problems with equilibrium and balance, caused by the same etiological factors that led to their hearing loss. Disturbances in lateral preference (handedness) are also more prevalent in hearing-impaired children (Meadow, 1980).

In reviewing the social and psychological development of deaf children, Meadow reports that many independent studies have found them to be less socially mature than hearing children. Residential school life can further contribute to social immaturity because the child grows up in a restricted setting. Meadow suggests that findings of greater immaturity in hearing-impaired children may be related to parents' reluctance to encourage independence and consequent maturity, coupled with strong pressures for achievement. Communication problems also contribute to reduced social interaction, leading to frustration for deaf children and their parents. Finally, deaf children appear to have more adjustment problems than hearing children. Normal deaf children have been found to exhibit characteristics of rigidity, egocentricity, reduced inner control, impulsiveness, and suggestibility. Reports of emotional or behavioral disturbance range from about 9% to more than 20%, depending upon the specific variables being investigated. All these characteristics are significantly less prevalent in hearing-impaired children of deaf parents.

These areas of development are described to remind readers of the breadth of programming required for total management of hearing-impaired children. The remainder of this section focuses upon the primary area of need for most hearing-impaired children: linguistic acquisition, which includes the habilitation of language, audition, and speech. These sections are described in depth because many audiology students will have little acquaintance with these subjects during their academic or professional careers. Although all of these topics may not fall within the domain of direct service provision by audiologists, they are important issues that all audiologists encounter at various points in their careers.

Furthermore, a multidisciplinary approach implies a good basic understanding of and involvement in a broad level of service provision.

## Language

The most profound consequence of deafness is not the inability to hear but the inability to process and learn language. Educators have labored for over a century to determine effective procedures for teaching language to hearing-impaired children, often with uninspiring success. Great discrepancies are seen in approaches to teaching language. Two of the more significant issues deal with (1) methods of instruction, in particular, whether language instruction emphasizes the formal, structured analysis of syntax or whether it deemphasizes grammar and stresses natural, spontaneous communication, and (2) the most effective modalities through which to facilitate language, in particular, whether any form of sign language should be used in concert with oral communication and, if so, how that is best done. Each of these issues is discussed below.

As is the case for most controversial issues, various approaches may at times be appropriate. The greatest determinant of success is probably less related to approach than to the effectiveness of instruction while using any method. Each of these procedures, in the hands of a mediocre teacher, will produce mediocre results. And this, rather than limitations caused by hearing loss, may be the real reason that so many children are not learning language well. Many teachers graduate from teacher training programs with few effective procedures for teaching hearing-impaired children. Much of their academic work has been theoretical in nature, and they have not received the systematic attention to applying those theories that most new teachers require. In addition, few have participated in an apprenticeship of sufficient quantity and quality, under the tutelage of a master teacher. After observing a great many teachers, both during and after their preprofessional training, I have the impression that most practicing teachers model more heavily on their student teaching experiences than upon their academic training. This is especially true when the practicum setting is insufficiently coordinated with academic instruction, so the students do not experience the application of what they have been taught.

Adult limitations must be acknowledged as a key determinant in why deaf children have difficulty learning language. Teacher preparation and skill is one of these limitations. Lack of skilled instructional supervision in universities and in school programs is another. Parent education and involvement is yet another. Hearing-impaired children have the potential to acquire better language than we have seen, on the average, across this country. We know this to be true because in our better school programs they are doing so. To date, direct intervention with children has received the focus of our efforts. It may be that indirect intervention, with greater time and money directed toward the adults who serve these children, would have a greater impact on their achievement.

***Language-Teaching Methodologies.*** Many methodological approaches have been developed for teaching language to hearing-impaired children. These can generally be grouped into two categories: (1) those focusing on instruction of vocabulary and syntax through formal, structured language lessons and (2) those placing primary emphasis on teaching language through conversations in more natural communicative settings. Although each of these approaches is used at various times in most classrooms, typical programs emphasize one over the other when planning for language learning. Each of these instructional methods is described below. Following that is a section on environmental engineering, which addresses improving children's access to the linguistic model outside of classroom lessons.

*Structured language teaching.* The structured approach to teaching language grows from a long tradition of analyzing linguistic patterns in order to teach them to deaf children. When this approach first emerged, research in normal language development was meager, and educators relied on intuitive analyses of adult linguistic patterns rather than on how children might normally acquire language. Educators using these methods break language down into what logically seems to be its component parts (e.g., parts of speech, grammatical morphemes) and then systematically teach the organization of these components to children during language lessons. Adult language is seen as the standard by which children's linguistic attempts are judged, and the teacher provides correctional feedback to the children on how closely their productions match that standard. The impact of the natural communicative environment on language acquisition is given minimal attention during language instruction. Both the Fitzgerald Key and methods based on transformational grammar (e.g., the *Apple Tree* and other curricula that present sentence pattern analyses) reflect this approach to language instruction.

Structured approaches to teaching language are still prevalent in classrooms. Programs using these approaches tend to work on language during the language period, but rarely plan for systematically incorporating language learning during other times of the day. Language is generally taught with children seated at their desks, a teacher's stimulus followed by a child's response, in various degrees of drill-like exercises.

The written mode is often used to present and practice language patterns, as opposed to practice through spontaneous oral and/or signed communication. Topics addressed during instruction are generally determined by the teacher and take a back seat to the grammar and vocabulary through which those topics are communicated. In general, language is considered to be a school subject that can be taught through traditional pedagogical procedures.

Structural analyses of language may be appropriate for older children who are refining and learning about language they already attempt to use. Such instruction is analogous to English language arts, which is taught as an academic school subject to young hearing children who come to school with basic linguistic competence already mastered. It is inappropriate, however, to teach English language arts to children who lack primary developmental language skills. Children cannot learn to analyze language that they do not know.

*Natural language teaching.* Those espousing more natural procedures for facilitating language would argue that language development is best viewed not as a school subject but more akin to psychosocial development: it is a psychological process of interaction between people, which can only be learned in those true communicative contexts. Moreover, it is better "facilitated" than "taught." Natural approaches attempt to capture features of spontaneous communication when providing language instruction to hearing-impaired students. This includes a focus on the meanings or intentions the child is trying to communicate rather than only on the structures (i.e., vocabulary, syntax) through which communication is accomplished. Only true communication reveals the proper interaction of linguistic components (pragmatic, semantic, and syntactic), showing the child how to say what to whom in various settings. Although emphasis may be placed upon different components of language at various times, efforts are made to preserve the communicative atmosphere in which language is practiced.

Other features of a natural approach include its reliance upon principles of normal child language acquisition rather than adult intuitions about acquisition. Young children are not expected to study and learn language through analytical practice. Rather, they learn it by trying to use it in natural situations, making many mistakes as they go. Just as hearing youngsters cannot provide analytical explanations of the language they are learning, young hearing-impaired children may lack the cognitive (metalinguistic) ability to do this. Furthermore, such analyses are not typically necessary for language learning. The greater the child's hearing loss, the more need there will be for special planned practice of specific language patterns. In a natural approach, the teacher will contrive procedures that permit this practice to occur through planned but natural conversations.

Another characteristic of natural approaches is avoiding correction of language attempts as right or wrong. Normally developing children produce many patterns that are not adultlike as they acquire mature linguistic competence. For example, it is not appropriate for children at the two- to three-word utterance level to include grammatical morphemes such as *is, the,* or *a.* Whereas structured approaches require the child to include every word of the sentence, natural approaches wait until the child is developmentally ready to produce complete sentences. Furthermore, they avoid correction as a response to a child's utterance but focus on strategies that have been determined to facilitate acquisition in normally developing children. These strategies could include (1) continuing the conversation by providing a meaningful, related response or (2) expanding upon the child's utterance in a way that models adult forms but does not demand that they be parroted back by a child who is not ready to use them. Parents and teachers may impede communication development by continually stopping an eager child to make him or her "say it right."

In a natural language lesson the teacher's task is to invent conversational situations that naturally elicit the use of target language and then repeatedly simulate these situations with students. Conversation would not include written language at this point. The children would learn to practice the language communicatively during natural interaction with others. Teachers would gradually lead children to more correct productions through strategies such as modeling (e.g., by role switching), cueing, or expanding the child's utterance, followed by renewed interaction.

A natural language-learning approach helps children develop a more integrated linguistic system, since they are exposed to new patterns in a context that demonstrates a complete communicative interaction. Consequently, when they learn new language (e.g., a prepositional phrase), they are also learning where, when, and why to use it. Furthermore, language learned in a broader communicative context is more likely to generalize to use in other contexts than is language learned while seated at a desk or through following teachers' instructions.

*Environmental engineering.* Natural and structured approaches to language acquisition each address methods for presenting particular language principles to hearing-impaired children. Hearing children, in contrast, are not taught language by certified teachers. They become proficient language users by merely experiencing communication during their daily interactions. Theoretically, then, if hearing-impaired children could simply be given access to this environmental linguistic model, which exists all around them at all times, no systematic language instruction would be required. Improving access to the linguistic model can be referred to as environmental engineering.

Hearing loss is not the only factor blocking the child's access to the linguistic environment. Adults impose considerable limitations for the child as well. Analyses of adults' language have shown that adults modify and/or reduce their language when communicating with deaf children in ways that they do not speak to normally hearing language learners. These changes alter the data available to the child for learning language. Researchers have recently suggested that differences in input may be the source of the linguistic deficiency so commonly observed in deaf children.

Mothers of deaf children have been described as more didactic, dominant, and intrusive, and less flexible, permissive, and approving than mothers of hearing children of comparable age (Schlesinger & Meadow, 1972). They use fewer questions, ask for fewer suggestions, and use less language showing solidarity and agreement (Goss, 1970). They also leave out words and grammatical morphemes when communicating in sign language. Hearing-impaired children must observe consistent and contrastive use of language structures in the linguistic environment in order to make correct hypotheses about the use of those structures (Crandall, 1978).

Teachers' language to deaf children has also been analyzed. They too exhibit controlling relationships and dominate interaction with deaf children (Craig & Collins, 1970). Descriptions of the grammatical characteristics of teachers' sign language have uncovered nonsystematic use of any linguistic system. Teachers using fingerspelling only (the Rochester Method) formed only 20% of the letters of the spoken text in accordance with the finger-spelling chart (Reich & Bick, 1977). Marmor and Petitto (1979) examined the sign language used by teachers and found it to be predominantly ungrammatical with respect to rules of either English or American Sign Language. Many of the errors that have been described as characterizing deaf children's language were found to exist in the language that teachers used when communicating with their students. Omissions and differences were found not only in the representation of grammatical aspects of the spoken message but also in the content. In all, less than 10% of all utterances were executed in accord with rules of English grammar.

Descriptions of language input to deaf children suggest that significant differences might be found in examining any linguistic domain of adults' communication. In the semantic domain teachers have been described as relying on basic vocabulary rather than enriching and expanding the lexicon through use of synonyms, which convey finer shades of meaning, or more abstract words. Nonliteral language, which occurs in approximately 25% of sentences spoken to young hearing children, is infrequently used by teachers communicating through total communication (Newton, 1985).

The pragmatic domain of language also reveals differences in the way people talk to deaf children. Pragmatics refers to the influence of the linguistic and environmental context upon language use. Deaf children seldom have access to language in context. Persons other than close acquaintances often avoid communication with them. This is especially true for children who rely on sign language to comprehend communication. Deaf children may observe mature language use primarily within the limited domain of the classroom, where language is modified or directed specifically to their needs. If a child cannot process spoken language, he or she will never experience language as it is used in the real world. This will block access to how language varies in different contexts and with different speaking partners.

Many of these children's language-learning problems may be improved by modifying the linguistic environment to enhance access to the language model rather than through direct instruction. Such modifications should take precedence over direct language instruction, since the degree to which they are effective will reduce the need for language lessons, economizing on both time and expense. Engineering the environment to provide greater access to language includes:

1. Considering spontaneous communication to be an important part of language learning rather than thinking of the classroom and the language lesson as the primary place where language will be learned. This implies increased time for ''focused chatting'' with children and less time in drill, seatwork, or other noncommunicative activities. In addition, children should be encouraged to participate actively in communication as opposed to allowing adults to monopolize the talk.

2. Finding avenues for other people (children, family, extracurricular personnel, etc.) to communicate with the child; placing children in situations where they can experience the communication of others, such as in small groups.

3. Focusing more on the content rather than the structure of language; using language for discussing, questioning, problem solving, and social interaction.

4. Finding ways to use language learned in the classroom in other activities, both in and out of the classroom.

5. Maintaining an excellent audiological management program (addressing both amplification and the development of auditory skills). The

more a child can hear, the greater the access to the natural communicative environment.

6. For children using total communication, ensuring that everyone interacting with the child on a regular basis (parents, school personnel, siblings, peers) learns to sign proficiently; that everyone tries to sign in the child's presence, regardless of whether the child is participating in the conversation; and that everyone uses the same sign language system and that this system marks every aspect of the English language.

*Communication Modalities.* Controversy over the best modality for teaching language to hearing-impaired children has existed since the time that educators first explored methods for teaching them. Educators differ in their judgment on whether children should learn language solely through audition and speech or whether some form of manual communication should be included in instruction.

Oral education was used almost exclusively in school programs prior to the 1970s. Although children achieved great success at the handful of special schools with a systematic devotion to that method, the majority of severely and profoundly impaired children educated in public school programs failed to make significant gains. Today those same special schools that promoted oral education are among the few remaining programs that do not use some form of sign language for instruction.

During the 1960s, the available alternatives to oral communication were (1) American Sign Language (ASL), a language that is very different from English and is used by the deaf adult community or (2) a pidgin sign system used by most hearing people when talking with deaf people. Pidgin sign is the use of ASL signs in English word order, omitting many grammatical components of both ASL and English. Educators were reluctant to teach language through sign language because of its failure to transmit essential features of English grammar. It would also be impossible to speak one language (English) while simultaneously signing another language (ASL). Therefore oral language could not be developed. In response to this dilemma, educators developed, in the late 1960s, a sign language system that would code each English word and word affix in English word order. Many different forms of manually coded English (MCE) were developed (e.g., Signing Exact English [Gustason, Pfetzing, & Zawolkow, 1972] and Seeing Essential English [Anthony, 1971]). These signed English systems are not true, natural languages, functioning as vehicles of communication within a social community, as are English and ASL. Rather, they have been "invented" in order to teach the English language to deaf children through a modality that is more accessible to them. Using an MCE system, a communicator can say and sign a message simultaneously. Using speech and signs together is referred to as combined or simultaneous communication.

Another force contributing to the shift away from an exclusively oral approach to education was the linguistic study of American Sign Language, which came into visibility during the same time period as did the MCE systems. As linguists discovered the legitimacy of ASL as a complete, true language that was not inferior to but merely different from English, the deaf community aligned its identity with this special, unique language. The ardor with which the deaf adult population espoused ASL for deaf people led many hearing educators to reevaluate their previous stance of isolation from manual communication. Hearing adults who were not affiliated with education grew to value ASL for its individuality and expressiveness as a language. The attractiveness of ASL as a language, its easy acquisition in deaf families, and its symbolism for the identity of the deaf community have become mixed with the issue of using signs to teach English to deaf students.

Consequently, no systematic procedure for using signed communication exists in school programs today. Deaf children still lack access to the English language, both because of their hearing loss and because adult models rarely use complete English sign systems when communicating with them. Children taught through various modes of combined (oral and manual) communication do not appear to be making the gains in language development that were predicted by introducing sign language into their educational program. Because of the inconsistent use of these systems, it is difficult to evelute whether lack of success is due to children's inability to learn English through combined modalities or to improper adult use of combined communication. Studies that have investigated children's use of signed English grammatical morphemes indicate that these forms are used by children if their adult models include them in their own communication with children. Confusion among educational leaders regarding whether to sign exact English grammar or whether to sign ASL has left the majority of teachers somewhere in the middle— signing a pidgin form that is neither English nor ASL—and uncommitted to the importance of consistency in the adult model. Similarly, most deaf children are learning neither English nor ASL.

Meanwhile, as combined communication has emerged as the dominant methodology in both public and residential school programs, oral education has not lain dormant. The major oral programs in this country have retained their allegiance to this methodology, and they continue to graduate deaf individuals with extraordinary communication skills. But oral education today is not what it was in the 1960s. New developments in amplification and in the use of residual hearing allow many children previously considered profoundly deaf to function and learn as hard-of-hearing children. The speech and listening skills of these children who were identified and trained early are amazing to observe. These successes have been observed in public as well as private schools, when there is parental and teacher commitment to maintaining consistent, effective amplification and to providing systematic listening practice throughout the day.

Auditory-oral education, with its emphasis on audition, is a new methodology—one that has not been tested as yet in the mainstream of public school education. Successful auditory-oral education would require a dramatic change in emphasis from present public school procedures. Great focus must be placed on early intervention, as success is doubtful once the critical learning period is past. Another area of primary emphasis would be in the area of audition. Audiologists with expertise in fitting and monitoring amplification for speech as well as in maintaining a dynamic auditory program would be key staff members of every program. Teachers' skills in auditory and speech development would be significantly upgraded. (At present few teachers feel competent in these areas or feel that such competencies are of major importance [Scott, 1983].) The portion of the school day allocated to developing these skills would be increased. And parent training would place greater emphasis on audition and meaningful communication rather than focusing on the learning of sign language (which should be easier for parents to learn than sign language).

Using auditory-oral communication, many more hearing-impaired children could use residual hearing to learn oral English. This would reduce the need for adding manual communication and reduce many of the barriers its use imposes: parents who can't communicate with their children, the dramatic unavailability of communicative partners outside the deaf community, and poor adult sign models from whom to learn language. No modality can compete with hearing as the best channel for learning the English language.

Even children who require support from sign language could receive many of these benefits if they learned to use hearing better. We know very little about whether children who use total communication can acquire the same listening skills that children in auditory-oral programs acquire. There are few total communication programs with the same commitment and expertise in auditory-oral development that is seen in oral programs. It is clear, however, that children in total communication programs that emphasize auditory-oral skills do use these channels far better than children in programs that pay only lip service to their development.

Exclusive auditory-oral communication will never be possible for all hearing-impaired children since some children do not have sufficient residual hearing. These are the children for whom combined methodologies are essential. However, combined communication is presently used with most children in programs for the hearing-impaired, not just those with untrainable residual hearing. It is not certain that signed English is easier for most hearing-impaired children to learn than is auditory-oral English, especially in light of recent developments in amplification and speech development. Until aural training receives the same emphasis in schools as has sign language, we will not know about the influence it might have in improving linguistic growth.

## Speech Perception

The more the child uses residual hearing, the less need there is for direct speech and language training because more of these skills will be acquired spontaneously. Attention to the development of speech perception skills includes (1) improving the child's potential for hearing speech by boosting the signal through amplification and reducing background noise and (2) training the child's ability to use residual hearing for understanding speech (auditory training).

Despite recent improvements in amplification and knowledge about the profound differences that appropriate, consistent amplification can make, the status of hearing-aid use in this country is poor. Studies of hearing-aid malfunction in classrooms have consistently revealed a failure rate of approximately 50% (Bess & Bratt, 1981). In addition, many children do not wear aids with regularity. Ross (1977) states that perhaps the greatest obstacle to maximum use of amplification for hearing-impaired children is "the widespread ignorance among professionals and lay people of what amplified sound is all about, and their apparent reluctance to correct the situation" (p. 7). When amplification is used, benefits are muted by failure to attend to interfering noise caused by poor room acoustics.

Auditory development depends upon this effective balance between signal and noise. Professionals may inaccurately view the development of speech perception as something that happens through lessons in auditory training. In fact, auditory training lessons are but a small component of auditory development—a time when the teacher can highlight particular aspects of the speech signal for special focus. The majority of what a child learns about hearing is acquired by listening to speech throughout the day. If the teacher fails to think of the child's full waking hours as the period for auditory learning, instruction will not contribute significantly to the acquisition of speech perception skills.

A variety of auditory training programs have been written to teach listening skills to hearing-impaired children. These are valuable for providing a model for auditory development and a systematic procedure for viewing the acquisition of skills. These curricula also provide examples of activities that focus upon specific listening skills. They are helpful so long as they are viewed as only one component of auditory learning.

Different models underlie auditory training programs and lead to differences in focus when training children in auditory skills. A program may consider the linguistic unit of analysis (e.g., connected speech, syllable length, vowel distinctions, consonant distinctions); the task level (e.g., detection, discrimination, identification, comprehension); psycholinguistic processes underlying auditory skills (e.g., memory, sequencing, figure-ground); and/or contextual features (e.g., open vs. closed set, amount and type of cueing or support provided, distance from speaker, noise vs. quiet). Each of these factors can be independently varied and affect listening abililty. In assessing speech perception skills, the evaluator tries to gain information on how each of these components influences the child's functioning. Formal tests of auditory ability are available, such as the *GASP!* (Erber, 1982) and the *Test of Auditory Comprehension* (Office of the Los Angeles County Superintendent of Schools, 1976), but no single test systematically evaluates all features. Informal assessment must be added to focus on the individual needs of children.

Programs also differ in their approach to training auditory skills. Some begin at the lowest task level (i.e., systematically proceeding from detection through comprehension), using the most elemental units (i.e., proceeding from syllable length to phoneme discrimination and then to meaningful connected speech). Others emphasize that the primary task is teaching the child that verbal passages have meaning and that meaning can be determined without perceiving all the acoustic/phonetic or linguistic components of the utterance. Such a program would focus on the comprehension of connected speech from the earliest stages of auditory training, highlighting phoneme recognition only as needed to clarify messages. It is probably best for a child to practice listening at both levels, minimal-pair syllables and words as well as connected speech, from early in the learning process.

It is also important that speech perception be coordinated with lessons in speech production. In addition to working on general auditory tasks, the teacher should formulate tasks that allow the child to listen to the specific speech targets he or she is working on. Finally, listening practice should be a planned component of various activities the child performs throughout the day.

## Speech Production

As is the case for language, deaf children's potential for developing intelligible speech remains untapped and unknown. Again, it appears to be our limitations as professionals and parents, rather than the hearing loss alone, that prevents most hearing-impaired children from acquiring better speech ability. Otherwise we would not observe success in children who do have the advantages of a good, consistent program combined with family support.

Recent developments in auditory and speech training have been overshadowed by attention to sign language in the hearing-impaired child's educational program. It is as if we can focus on only one thing at a time. Children often fail to acquire adequate speech skills because they are not educated under conditions that are conducive to the development of effective speech communication (Ling & Milne, 1981). Teachers admit that they receive minimal preparation in this area during preprofessional training. Their feelings of inadequacy lead them to avoid teaching speech to their hearing-impaired students. In many school programs, speech-language pathologists provide all of the speech training, so teachers feel no need to know about teaching speech. Speech is then not integrated into the child's daily communication. Thus speech acquisition remains a splinter skill with no real relationship to true communication. Hearing-impaired children logically see little use for such instruction.

The audiologist may contribute as much as any other professional to the child's ability to acquire speech. This is especially true for children with usable residual hearing, which includes many profoundly impaired children. If amplification is appropriately fit, the need for intensive speech instruction may be greatly reduced. The more profound the child's loss, the more he or she will require intensive speech lessons.

The most important service the audiologist can provide for hearing-impaired children is the appropriate fitting of amplification. In addition to knowing about selecting and modifying hearing aids, the audiologist must be familiar with speech acoustics in order to fit children appropriately. In particular, the audiologist should know the frequency and intensity information of individual speech sounds so that modifications can be made in amplification to assure maximum perception of any speech sounds within the child's range of residual hearing.

In order to estimate the speech sounds that an individual child may or may not hear, the child's unaided and aided thresholds can be plotted on an audiogram containing speech frequency information. The audiogram in Figure 10.1 depicts a child who would hear no conversational speech at normal distances (i.e., in quiet at a distance of 1 meter) without amplification (dotted line). With amplification (unbroken line), the child can hear many components of vowels and consonants. Some high-frequency consonants may remain imperceptible except at very close distances. Such information can help the audiologist make adaptations that will allow better perception of speech sounds. This child, for example, might be helped to hear more high-frequency information if provided with a hearing aid or earmold modifications that enhance high-frequency information. Other children may require increased gain at all frequencies if their present amplification fails to make speech sufficiently audible. Still other children may require reducing low-frequency gain when there is an imbalance between gain across the frequencies. As mentioned earlier, too much gain in the low frequencies could mask higher-frequency consonant information that the child is learning in speech.

Avenues for making speech sounds more audible through amplification should be explored before expending considerable time in speech lessons. There is no need to waste time teaching speech sounds if the child can learn many of them through aided audition alone. When the child is fit with appropriate amplification, speech lessons will be more effective. Speech, audition, and language should be consistently integrated throughout instruction so that the child experiences their relationship to one another during communication.

The greatest recent impact upon speech development for hearing-impaired children was made by Daniel Ling in his book *Speech and the Hearing-Impaired Child: Theory and Practice* (1976). This impressive work provides a framework for viewing speech development as well as systematic, specific procedures for evaluating and teaching speech sounds. Ling presents a progressive sequence of prerequisites for subsequent stages of development. The major stages of development are:

1. *Suprasegmentals.* Coordinated breath and voice control must be established before vowel sounds can be produced accurately and flexibly.

2. *Vowels.* Vowels form the central unit of the syllable. Consonants start and stop these vowel productions.

3. *Consonants.* Consonants shape the vowel and can rarely be produced in isolation without an adjacent vowel. The vowel in turn shapes the consonant.

4. *Consonant blends.* These blends usually combine and modify forms the child has learned as single consonants and therefore require more complex articulatory skills.

Each of these skill areas must be learned at two levels of development: phonetic and phonological. Phonetic instruction teaches the motoric production of speech sounds, independent of any words in which those productions may occur. Ling recommends developing these motoric skills

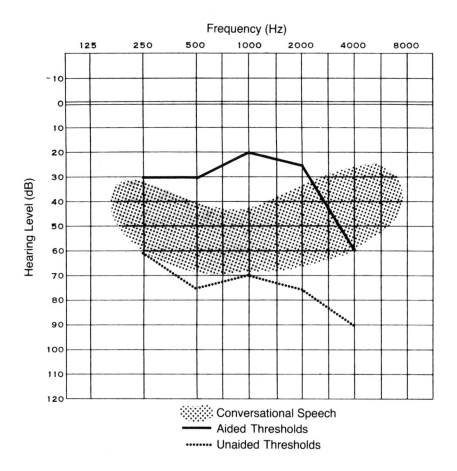

**Figure 10.1.**  Unaided and aided thresholds in relation to the intensity and frequency characteristics of conversational speech.

through the rapid imitation of nonsense syllables until the child can repeat and alternate those syllables so automatically that conscious attention is not required. At the second level of development, the phonological level, children learn to use the speech sounds they have acquired motorically in meaningful English words. This involves forming internal auditory representations of how sounds are patterned in words as well as learning to produce those words in isolation and in connected speech.

Because Ling's text focuses almost entirely on the development of phonetic, motoric skills, many educators and clinicians place insufficient emphasis on phonological development. Ling suggests that sounds which have been mastered at the phonetic level will spontaneously generalize to use in meaningful speech with minimal instruction. Such is not the case for many children, and they require systematic instruction at both levels. Furthermore, it is not clear that speech sounds always develop first in nonmeaningful speech. Several studies have shown that some children learn some sounds better at the phonological level and that generalization to meaningful speech is better fostered by phonological rather than phonetic practice (Abraham & Weiner, 1985; Dunn, Newton, Blackwood, & Marshall, 1984; Osberger, 1983). Although work on speech automaticity is important, automaticity can be acquired from word practice as well as through syllable drill. Hearing children develop automaticity while learning to produce meaningful words. Syllable drill is probably most important for profoundly impaired children, for whom simultaneous attention to speech and meaning is difficult.

Recent advances in teaching speech to phonologically disordered children (e.g., phonological process analysis) are beginning to find their way into speech instruction for hearing-impaired children (Hodson & Paden, 1983; Stoel-Gammon & Dunn, 1985). This body of knowledge can provide educators with good resources for teaching meaningful speech to hearing-impaired children.

# Instructional Settings

The majority of hearing-impaired children are educated in one of four primary settings: public school classrooms for the hearing-impaired, regular classrooms (mainstreaming), state residential schools for the deaf, and private schools for the deaf.

## Public School Classrooms for the Hearing-Impaired

Approximately 50% of school-age hearing-impaired students are educated in special classes for the hearing-impaired within the public schools. This setting allows the child to live at home and attend school with both hearing and hearing-impaired peers. The child is usually bused to a central program rather than enrolled in the local school program nearest the family home. The public school setting also permits flexible mainstreaming options for children, since they can easily move back and forth between the self-contained and the regular classroom at various periods of the day. Children who attend public schools have a greater opportunity to learn the social conventions of our society than those attending residential schools, since they can participate in regular family and school events.

Children with profound hearing losses who rely on total communication will usually benefit most from a large program for the hearing-impaired if they are to be adequately educated in the public school setting. Although hard-of-hearing children are almost always best educated in public schools, deaf children may become severely isolated and insufficiently served if left in a small program. They may find few peers or adults with whom to communicate. Special materials and teachers with expertise may be unavailable. These children will also be more isolated from support personnel (e.g., audiologists, speech-language pathologists, interpreters, counselors, etc.) who are skilled at serving hearing-impaired children. Special prevocational training will be less available in high school. In such cases, parents must seriously weigh the advantages of living at home and within the community against attendance at a residential school for the deaf. Another alternative is for the family to move into a large school district with good services for hearing-impaired children or locate a foster-home placement for their child in such a district.

## Regular Classrooms (Mainstreaming)

Most hearing-impaired children who are educated in the public school setting spend some portion of their school day in regular classrooms with hearing children. This mainstreaming may vary from participation in gym or art to full-day education in the regular classroom. Many hard-of-hearing children are taught exclusively in the regular classroom. Programs differ in the amount of support they provide these mainstreamed children. Many children have not been identified by special education programs and receive no support services. Julia Davis (1977) has described hard-of-hearing children as "the forgotten children" because regular educators may be quite unaware of their special needs. Children may sit through weeks of class with a broken hearing aid or may be unable to view the teacher's face. They may be reprimanded for inattentiveness or for day-dreaming.

Mainstreamed children who do receive special support services are typically removed from the classroom one or two periods a week for special work with an itinerant teacher of the hearing-impaired. They may also be removed for speech therapy. These services may or may not be coordinated with the remainder of the child's school program. There is controversy over whether the role of itinerant teachers should be to tutor children in classroom work or to provide training on communication skills. Somehow, both of these needs must be met. The itinerant teacher should also ensure that children's hearing aids are being checked and advise the regular classroom teacher on special considerations needed by hearing-impaired children in regular classrooms.

Traditionally, mainstreamed children have been those students who are bright and able to use residual hearing and/or speechreading well enough to benefit from regular instruction. Unfortunately, there has been little provision for bright, capable children who use total communication to participate in regular classroom instruction. This picture is beginning to change with the advent of a new professional group of educational interpreters. Public schools now employ interpreters to go with children to the regular classroom. In this way, children who use total communication can benefit from the same education as their hearing peers. It is important, however, that children selected for mainstreaming with an interpreter possess the prerequisite content and linguistic skills to keep up in the regular classroom even when the lesson is interpreted. Many hearing-impaired children are unable to meet this standard even when total communication is used, and they are lost in the regular classroom.

## State Residential Schools for the Deaf

Approximately 25% of school-age children are educated in state residential schools for the deaf. (There are also a small number of private residential schools, which are very different from state residential schools.) These children's auditory thresholds are often no poorer than those of children taught in self-contained public school classrooms. Children attending these residential schools generally represent one of the following subgroups: children of deaf parents; children whose families believe that they need the support of a specialized setting and of a deaf peer group with whom they can communicate through sign language more than they need to participate in mainstream society; children from small towns that cannot offer a comprehensive program; or older children who attended public school programs when they were younger, but now require the social and vocational opportunities offered at a school for the deaf.

State residential school programs are typically philosophically aligned with the views of the deaf adult community. They believe strongly in the importance of sign language for all severely and profoundly hearing-impaired children. Some members of their teaching staff may reject the use of manually coded English systems, believing that American Sign Language is the native language of the deaf and should not be subjugated to English. They believe that deaf children should learn English as well as ASL, often teaching English through the written form while using ASL and/or pidgin English for face-to-face communication. State residential schools for the deaf generally place less emphasis on the development of auditory and speech skills than do public school programs. The children generally have little or no opportunity to attend classes with hearing children, both because they are on a separate campus and because there is less value placed on integration as an educational option.

State residential school personnel generally feel that this is the only appropriate setting for deaf children's education. They believe that mainstreaming is often erroneously applauded and that, in fact, that setting may be the most, rather than the least, restrictive environment for a child who requires sign language for communication. Furthermore, they believe that deaf children should be raised in an educational setting where they can be full participants, not second-rate or handicapped. In the residential setting, the entire environment is oriented toward the needs of the deaf individual.

## Private Schools for the Deaf

A small number of hearing-impaired children are educated in private school programs. These programs are usually oral schools with a strong commitment to auditory-oral education. Although most of these schools have a sliding fee scale and admit disadvantaged children, they are also schools attended by the children of highly educated, dedicated parents who devote considerable energy and resources to their children's education. Graduates of these programs are generally quite successful compared to the average graduates of other programs.

# Summary

The most important factor contributing to the linguistic competence of hearing-impaired children is their ability to use residual hearing. Because audiologists play a critical role in the successful use of residual hearing, they have the potential for shaping the lives of these children in profound ways. Traditionally, audiologists have not been trained to provide the full range of services needed by hearing-impaired children. Recent developments in educational audiology have focused greater attention on the unique skills needed by audiologists who serve this special population.

Audiologists begin to participate in children's education on the day the child is identified as hearing-impaired. The proper approach to early amplification, communication with parents, and school referral can establish a sound basis for future development. Continued participation in interdisciplinary team management will help the child learn to use audition maximally when developing linguistic, academic, and psychosocial skills.

# References

Abraham, S., & Weiner, R. (1985). Efficacy of word training vs. syllable training on articulatory generalization by severely hearing-impaired children. *Volta Review, 87,* 95–105.

Anthony, D. (1971). *Signing Essential English.* Anaheim, CA: Anaheim Union School District.

Bess, F., & Bratt, G. (1981). Amplification in education: A perspective. In F. Bess, B. Freeman, & J. S. Sinclair (Eds.), *Amplification in education* (pp. 373–379). Washington, DC: Alexander Graham Bell Association for the Deaf.

Boothroyd, A. (1982). *Hearing impairments in young children.* Englewood Cliffs, NJ: Prentice-Hall.

Clark, T., & Watkins, S. (1985). *The Ski\*Hi model.* Logan, UT: Ski\*Hi Institute.

Craig, W., & Collins, J. (1970). Analysis of communicative interaction in classes for deaf children. *American Annals of the Deaf, 121,* 79–85.

Crandall, K. E. (1978). Inflectional morphemes in the manual English of young hearing-impaired children and their mothers. *Journal of Speech and Hearing Research, 21,* 372–386.

Davis, J. (1977). *Our forgotten children: Hard-of-hearing pupils in the schools.* Minneapolis: National Support Systems Project, Bureau of Education for the Handicapped, U.S. Office of Education.

Dunn, C., Newton, L., Blackwood, M., & Marshall, E. (1984, June). Phonetic and phonological assessment of speech: A comparison. Paper presented at the Alexander Graham Bell Association International Convention, Portland, OR.

Erber, N. P. (1982). *Auditory training.* Washington, DC: Alexander Graham Bell Association for the Deaf.

Gallaudet Research Institute Newsletter (Winter, 1985). *Today's hearing impaired children and youth: A demographic and academic profile.* Washington, DC: Gallaudet College.

Goss, R. (1970). Language used by mothers of deaf children and mothers of hearing children. *American Annals of the Deaf, 115,* 93–96.

Gustason, G., Pfetzing, D., & Zawolkow, E. (1972). *Signing Exact English.* Rossmoor, CA: Modern Signs Press.

Hodson, B. W., & Paden, E. P. (1983). *Targeting intelligible speech: A phonological approach to remediation.* San Diego: College-Hill Press.

Ling, D. (1976). *Speech and the hearing-impaired child: Theory and practice.* Washington, DC: Alexander Graham Bell Association for the Deaf.

Ling, D. (1978). Auditory coding and recoding: An analysis of auditory training procedures for hearing-impaired children. In M. Ross & T. Giolas (Eds.), *Auditory management of hearing-impaired children* (pp. 181–218). Austin, TX: PRO-ED.

Ling, D., & Milne, M. (1981). The development of speech in hearing-impaired children. In F. Bess, B. Freeman, & J. S. Sinclair (Eds.), *Amplification in education* (pp. 98–108). Washington, DC: Alexander Graham Bell Association for the Deaf.

Luterman, D. (1984). *Counseling the communicatively disordered and their families.* Silver Springs, MD: Fellendorf Associates.

Marmor, G., & Petitto, L. (1979). Simultaneous communication in the classroom: How well is English grammar represented? *Sign Language Studies, 23,* 99–136.

Matkin, N., Hook, P., & Hixson, P. (1979). A multidisciplinary approach to the evaluation of hearing-impaired children. *Audiology: An Audio Journal for Continuing Education, 4* (7). New York: Grune & Stratton.

Meadow, K. (1980). *Deafness and child development.* Berkeley: University of California Press.

Newton, L. (1985). Linguistic environment of the deaf child: A focus on teachers' use of nonliteral language. *Journal of Speech and Hearing Research, 28,* 336–344.

Northern, J. L., & Downs, M. P. (1978). *Hearing in children* (2nd ed.). Baltimore: Williams & Wilkins.

Office of the Los Angeles County Superintendent of Schools (1976). *Test of auditory comprehension.* North Hollywood, CA: Foreworks.

Osberger, M. J. (1983). Development and evaluation of some speech training procedures for hearing-impaired children. In I. Hochberg, H. Levitt, & M. J. Osberger (Eds.), *Speech of the hearing-impaired: Research, training, and personnel preparation* (pp. 333–348). Austin, TX: PRO-ED.

Reich, P. A., & Bick, M. (1977). How visible is visible English? *Sign Language Studies, 14,* 59–72.

Ross, M. (1977). A review of studies on the incidence of hearing aid malfunctions. *The condition of hearing aids worn by children in a public school program* (HEW Publication No. OE 77-05002). Washington, DC: Government Printing Office.

Ross, M. (1982). *Hard of hearing children in regular schools.* Englewood Cliffs, NJ: Prentice-Hall.

Schlesinger, H. S., & Meadow, K. (1972). *Sound and sign: Childhood deafness and mental health.* Berkeley: University of California Press.

Scott, P. (1983). Have competencies needed by teachers of the hearing-impaired changed in twenty-five years? *Exceptional Children, 50,* 48–53.

Stoel-Gammon, C., & Dunn, C. (1985). *Normal and disordered phonology in children.* Austin, TX: PRO-ED.

# Pediatric Amplification

## ANTONIA BRANCIA MAXON

*A*mplification is the first step in any good auditory management program regardless of the client's age and type or degree of hearing loss. Selecting appropriate amplification may be more difficult with children than with adults, but this problem should not deter audiologists from proceeding rapidly and aggressively.

The concept underlying the provision of amplification for children is the need to maximize use of residual hearing in order to foster the natural development of speech and language. Residual hearing is the difference between the child's thresholds of audibility and thresholds of discomfort across frequency. This is the dynamic range in which a child can receive and make use of amplified sound. Good early use of residual hearing is necessary whether the child is being trained in an aural-oral or total communication mode.

Ross and Calvert (1984) warn that we can make hard-of-hearing children into deaf children through inappropriate amplification and management programs. They report that all too many of the advances in pediatric amplification have not been put into clinical practice. They conclude that there continues to be a lack of professional commitment to exploiting a child's residual hearing for communication.

The rationale for the earliest possible amplification is found in the concept of a critical period for development. Children must experience certain kinds of stimulation at particular developmental stages in order to acquire specific skills normally. Once a particular developmental stage has been passed chronologically, the effective utilization of that stage decreases. Limited early auditory experience can cause long-term negative effects from auditory sensory deprivation and reduction of the auditory motor feedback loop (Fry, 1978). This is not to imply that providing amplification after 2 years of age will not allow a child to make good use of hearing. It does, however, lend credence to the belief that amplification provided prior to that age will give the child the opportunity to acquire auditory-based communication skills more naturally. Therefore, all hearing-impaired children should be considered candidates for amplification as soon as the hearing loss has been identified. With identification of hearing loss now commonly occurring in infancy, the goal of providing appropriate amplification prior to 2 years of age is quite feasible.

# Types of Hearing Loss

In order to provide a hearing-impaired child with appropriate amplification, consideration must first be given to the type of hearing loss: sensorineural, conductive, or mixed.

## Sensorineural Loss

A child with a moderate, severe, or profound sensorineural loss is usually a candidate for amplification. Some disagreement exists regarding the use of amplification for children with mild losses and the benefits for those with some profound losses. The latter concerns are generally related to the ability to use residual hearing as the primary mode for reception of speech.

## Conductive Loss

Traditionally, hearing aids have been recommended less often for a child with a conductive hearing loss because most often the loss, such as that caused by otitis media, could be treated medically or surgically. When there is external ear structural malformation, the inability to use an ear-mold because of absent or malformed pinnae and/or external auditory meatuses limits the audiologist to bone-conduction hearing aids with their inherent problems. However, middle ear malformations, which may be surgically correctable by the teenage years, are readily managed with air-conduction (traditional) body or ear-level hearing aids. For the child with recurrent otitis media the decision to amplify is typically based on the pattern of the disease recurrence and/or the degree of hearing loss associated with its presence. Downs (1981) discusses the many problems experienced by children with recurrent otitis media and associated con-ductive hearing loss. She points out that for young children learning language or for school-age children, even a mild hearing loss can interfere with the reception of speech, thus impacting upon language acquisition and academic performance. The fluctuating nature of the loss is a further complicating factor in that the child receives auditory information in an inconsistent fashion. Downs (1981) suggests that amplification would pro-vide consistent hearing levels to children with fluctuating losses and ameliorate the associated problems.

The type of amplification selected, bone conduction or air conduc-tion, is also determined by the status of the disease. For example, in cases where the middle ear fluid is draining fairly regularly, a bone-conduction aid may be necessary because the ear canal has to be kept open to allow for drainage and to decrease the likelihood of infection. Close consulta-tion with the child's physician is essential.

# Degree of Hearing Loss

A child's audiogram should not be the sole determinant of amplification candidacy. In a study by Davis (1981), 50% of hearing-impaired children who should have had hearing aids did not, with the degree of hearing loss being a significant determining factor. She indicated that more severely impaired children were more likely to have amplification, although many children with profound losses, especially those represented by "corner audiograms," were not hearing-aid users.

Children with moderate to severe hearing losses are generally readily provided with some form of amplification, but this may not be so for children with either mild or profound losses. The speed and conviction with which profoundly hearing-impaired children are provided with amplification varies with the philosophy of their audiologist and/or their educational program. It seems unfortunate that any such question should arise since there is strong clinical evidence to demonstrate that, regardless of the severity of the hearing loss, appropriate amplification can provide some useful acoustic information. Even children with profound losses can get important supplemental cues for speech perception through the use of appropriate amplification (Erber, 1981). For example, in the case of a corner audiogram, amplification can minimally provide the profoundly hearing-impaired child with low-frequency cues (fundamental frequency and first formant) that yield information about pitch, voicing, nasalization, and duration. Availability of these acoustic cues, combined with a good management program, can result in the ability to use residual hearing for speech reception and to improve speech production. Ling's (1976) well-known work describes how successful a profoundly hearing-impaired child can be in making use of the acoustic cues of speech.

Amplification is crucial for children with profound hearing losses and should also be considered important for children with mild degrees of hearing loss. The introduction of amplification is often delayed when there is a mild hearing loss because the loss may not readily evidence itself. Fry (1978) points out that hearing-impaired infants will babble and even have "conversations" with adults as long as they can hear speech. The proximity of the speaker is particularly critical with mildly impaired children. Concerns about hearing sensitivity may be postponed until an age when they are mobile and more often at a distance from the speaker. The type of "hearing tests" carried out at close range (e.g., clapping hands or jingling keys) will not reveal a problem. Once identified, these children respond quite well to amplification because they have so much residual hearing. Children with unilateral hearing loss may not receive the special attention necessary to determine their amplification needs. The problems that exist for these children have gained particular attention over the last few years (Bess, 1982). Bess's work demonstrated that traditional management of unilaterally hearing-impaired children may be creating problems for them. He found that approximately half of the children he studied needed remedial educational services and/or had failed at least 1 year of school. He further demonstrated that when compared to normal-hearing children, those with unilateral hearing loss had more difficulty with sound localization and syllable recognition.

Since special problems exist for these children, the audiologist must consider the various management options that are available: (1) use of a monaural aid on the poorer ear, (2) use of a CROS (contralateral routing of signals) hearing aid, and (3) use of preferential seating/positioning without amplification. The option recommended should be dependent on the child's hearing as well as the daily listening situations. In order to use a monaural hearing aid, a child must have usable residual hearing in the impaired ear. When the poor ear is aided and the child listens to speech through both ears, it is important that speech discrimination ability not be negatively affected. It may be necessary to develop an auditory training program to determine whether an aid can be used on the poorer ear.

Often the residual hearing in the poor ear is nonusable. In order to overcome this problem, a CROS hearing aid is used, whereby the sound is taken from the poor-ear side (with a microphone at that ear) and directed, via a wire or radio signal, to a transducer on the good ear. There is typically no amplification, and the sound is delivered to the good ear through an open earmold that also allows that ear to normally receive sound. The CROS aid, therefore, allows the person to receive sound from both sides of the head.

Although the advantages of binaural hearing are not restored with either type of amplification described, the disadvantages associated with unilateral hearing loss can be reduced.

When a child has a unilateral loss, the decision to provide amplification is often difficult, especially prior to the child's entry into school. The parents may have been unaware of the hearing loss until it is detected at a preschool or prekindergarten hearing screening. At that time they must cope with the acceptance of the loss and then must work closely with the audiologist to determine whether amplification is appropriate and, if so, which type will provide the most benefit. Often amplification is not recommended prior to the child's placement in an educational setting because it is then that the detrimental effects of this type of loss become obvious to parents and school personnel. When amplification is delayed until entrance into school, the parents must be aware of the necessity of monitoring the loss and future amplification needs.

Clinical experience has demonstrated that for the child with a unilateral hearing loss the use of amplification must be established with a carefully planned and monitored trial period that allows the audiologist to assess the benefits of the aid. The time period consists of monitoring 3 weeks of unaided behaviors, then 3 weeks of aided behaviors, and finally 3 weeks of unaided behaviors. During the monitoring the parent keeps a log of various situations in which the child has difficulty, such as instances of one-to-one or group interactions, of background noise, of being at a distance from the speaker, of listening to the TV and radio or musical toys and tapes, or of experiencing visual distractions. The logs are kept for all three monitoring periods so that direct comparisons can be made. Should any problems arise that are specific to handling the hearing aid (e.g., feedback or changing batteries), they are noted and reported to the home visitor or audiologist.

# Configuration of the Hearing Loss

The configuration of the audiogram has a definite effect on the ease with which amplification can be selected. Generally, the flatter the audiogram, the more readily the loss is managed with amplification. When hearing is poorer in the high frequencies, the audiologist is faced with the difficult task of improving high-frequency hearing without overamplifying the low frequencies. As the slope of the loss becomes sharper, the task becomes more difficult, being most pronounced when hearing is normal through 500 Hz but with a loss at 1000 Hz and above. Since most commercially available hearing aids do not amplify frequencies above 5000 Hz, providing aided sensation levels at these high frequencies is often not possible. High-frequency emphasis aids used in conjunction with modified earmolds can help reach this goal, but with children the uncertainty of earmold modifications can be a problem.

Less common sensorineural configurations include the low-frequency hearing loss and the "cookie bite" or mid-frequency loss. The audiologist must be somewhat creative in these situations in order to provide the child with improved hearing levels without negatively affecting the quality of sound and speech discrimination. Obtaining some less commonly prescribed hearing aids on a trial basis will enable the audiologist to select the best amplification and settings for these atypical losses.

# Types of Amplification

## Binaural Fitting

Every child with a bilateral hearing loss should be considered a candidate for binaural amplification. In general the use of binaural amplification with young children has been shown to result in better acceptance of amplification, increased vocalization (which is important for speech and language development), improved localization ability, and improved spatial perception (Levitt & Voroba, 1980).

Markides (1977) has demonstrated that many of the advantages of binaural hearing can be maintained with binaural amplification. In general he found that binaural hearing aids allow for the ability to ''squelch'' reverberation and background noise, provide improved speech discrimination ability in unfavorable signal-to-noise ratios, and provide a 7–8 dB head shadow effect (with ear-level hearing aids). He also demonstrated that one body aid with a Y-cord was similar in performance to a monaural ear-level hearing aid and significantly poorer than a true binaural fitting. Markides further reported that subjects in his study with bilateral symmetrical hearing impairment received the most benefit from a binaural fitting because any ear that receives or can accept speech through a hearing aid that is 20 dB above its speech detection threshold can contribute to binaurality (10 dB for localization).

The use of binaural amplification continues to meet with resistance from some clinicians and researchers, especially when it is for infants and young children. The resistance centers around five major concerns: (1) overamplification may result in permanent or temporary threshold shift, (2) binaural advantages demonstrated with hearing-impaired adults have not been demonstrated with children, who may lack the ability to make use of the acoustic cues provided, (3) difficulty in obtaining individual ear information may result in overamplifying the better ear if a difference between ears exists, (4) body aids may not provide binaural advantages because the microphones are not at ear level or separated by the head, and (5) parents often reject the use of two aids for cosmetic reasons (Maxon, 1981).

Since these concerns have persisted over the years, it is important to address and respond to them. The question of overamplification is certainly serious, but the problem may be overcome by following careful and well-documented procedures for the audiological evelation and hearing-aid fitting. Careful selection of the electroacoustic characteristics in combination with a properly conducted management program can ensure that the pediatric client is not overamplified. M. C. Pollack (1980b) indicates that when an audiologist has carefully provided a child with amplification, any changes in threshold or speech discrimination must be the result of factors other than overamplification. As for the issue of binaural advantages, there is a need for research that directly addresses the restoration of binaural advantages for hearing-impaired children; however, to postpone binaural fitting until such data are available seems unreasonable.

It is virtually impossible to expect that a congenitally hearing-impaired infant or child would be able to learn to use interaural cues after years of monaural hearing-aid use. If binaural amplification is postponed, the child may never be capable of using these cues to a maximum (Ross, 1977). Another concern is the problem in obtaining individual ear information with children 0–3 years of age, but early binaural amplification should not necessarily be dependent upon earphone testing. A significant between-ear sensitivity difference can be minimally determined for a child by at least 7 months of age by measuring localization ability. When there is no individual ear information available, at worst the poorer ear is being underamplified since sound-field audiograms represent the better-ear response. As for the possible difficulties with body aids, there are reports in the literature that binaural advantages can be obtained with body hearing aids. Harris (1980) described work indicating that early binaural amplification (with body aids) and good early management can assure good auditory skills, including localization, in children as young as 1 year of age. When body aids are used in noise, auditory skills may appear better because the body-baffle effect provides a certain degree of directionality to the aids. This is not to argue against ear-level hearing aids with children, but often fitting difficulties may leave no choice except body-worn amplification. For such children binaural amplification with body aids is superior to bilateral amplification provided by one body aid with a Y-cord. Finally, a parent's concern with cosmetics should not be a deterrent to binaural amplification. Parents who are convinced of the advantages of a recommendation for amplification, whether it concerns type of aid or binaurality, will have no problem with accepting it. The audiologist who feels comfortable and sure of the recommendation will be able to guide the parents in understanding the justification.

There may be times when a single body aid with a Y-cord, "pseudobinaural" arrangement is recommended for an infant or a very young child. Although Markides (1977) reported to the contrary, clinical experience has demonstrated that such an amplification arrangement is superior to a monaural one because bilateral stimulation is provided. However, true binaural advantages cannot be provided because the signal is being received by only one microphone and so cannot deliver interaural differences to the two transducers. It is also important to note that with a Y-cord there will be a decrease (3–6 dB) in the output of the hearing aid because the signal is being split between two transducers.

Binaural hearing aids should be recommended even for those children with asymmetrical hearing losses. As M. C. Pollack (1980b) points out, binaural amplification should be considered whenever a client's needs require it. The hearing-impaired child will have such a need when developing communication skills and when in an educational setting. Monaural hearing aids will put them at a disadvantage and make the possibility of maximizing residual hearing a more difficult, if not impossible, task. There is evidence that more clinical audiologists are opting for binaural amplification with children and have recommended or fit binaural hearing aids for approximately 66% of those children they manage (Curran, 1985).

## Body, Ear-Level, and In-the-Ear Hearing Aids

An individual child's needs must be considered when examining the advantages and disadvantages of the different types of hearing aids presently available. In-the-ear (ITE) aids have become very popular with adults who have an acquired hearing loss; however, there are difficulties associated with prescribing these aids for children. Most of the ITE aids presently on the market require recasing whenever they no longer properly fit into the ear. Children have a recurrent problem with conventional earmolds because of continued change in the size and shape of their ears. Since ITE aids require a tightly fitting mold (the case), children will have great difficulty maintaining a properly fitting aid over time. This would mean repeated recasing, which would result in many periods of time when the child would be without one or both hearing aids.

Curran's (1985) survey of audiologists' amplification recommendations indicated that approximately 75% of all hearing aids recommended for children 0–5 years of age were ear-level aids, regardless of degree of hearing loss. Less than 3% of them were ITE. As the age of the child increased (from 6 to 18 years), the percentage of ITE recommendations increased; however, the majority of those recommendations were for older children (13–18 years) with mild hearing losses. Until these aids are made more flexible with regard to recasing, electroacoustic characteristics, and the telecoil, they cannot be readily recommended for young children.

The advantages and disadvantages of body and ear-level hearing aids have been thoroughly explored in the literature (M. C. Pollack, 1980a). The pros and cons with regard to the pediatric population are presented in Table 11.1.

In light of the relative advantages of body aids, it is not surprising that these aids have traditionally been recommended for children, especially for infants and children with severe and profound losses. Until relatively recently, ear-level hearing aids could not provide these children with the needed gain. Even with the increased power now available, fitting a high-gain aid on a small head is difficult because of the increased

**TABLE 11.1**
**The Advantages and Disadvantages of Ear-Level and**
**Body Hearing Aids for the Pediatric Population**

| Type of Aid | Advantages | Disadvantages |
| --- | --- | --- |
| Ear Level | Allows for hearing at the ears | Increased chance of feedback |
| | More flexible electroacoustically | More susceptible to damage |
| | Provides headshadow | Difficulty fitting small ears |
| | Better binaural advantages | Shorter battery life |
| | Possible to modify earmolds | Wind noise |
| Body | More durable | Chest-level hearing |
| | Reduced chances of feedback | Top-mounted microphones can get food and liquid in them. |
| | Provides body baffle | Clothing noise |
| | Longer battery life | Poorer high-frequency amplification |
| | Ear size not an issue | Cords susceptible to damage |

likelihood of acoustic feedback. Regardless of feedback problems, the advantages of ear-level hearing aids are often extolled because they provide sound detection at ear level and allow for the possibility of using earmold modifications to alter the electroacoustic characteristics of a particular hearing aid. The advantage of hearing at ear level cannot be denied, especially with respect to binaural amplification. The head-shadow effect increases the interaural differences and so results in better localization ability and eventually improved speech discrimination in noise. These advantages notwithstanding, it is still important to consider each child's individual needs.

## Bone-Conduction Aids

Traditionally, bone-conduction amplification has been in the form of body-worn hearing aids coupled to a bone vibrator. The use of the bone vibrator as the transducer results in limiting the gain, output, and frequency response that can be provided with this type of amplification. Relatively recent advances have resulted in coupling bone-conduction transducers to ear-level hearing aids, making them considerably more flexible. The vast majority of recommended hearing aids are of the air-conduction variety, but, as discussed earlier, there are a few conditions that would make use of bone-conduction hearing aids necessary.

# Earmold Acoustics

A great deal of research has gone into developing modifiable plumbing for earmolds. Lybarger (1980) points out that changes in gain, frequency response, and output occur because the earmold is the last step of the hearing-aid system. The fact that this research and its clinical application have not been conducted with children should not deter the audiologist from trying various types of earmold plumbing to determine whether they are effective for a particular child. The type of modification used will be dependent on the desired change in electroacoustic characteristics. The following is a brief summary of the effects of earmold modifications that have been demonstrated with adults.

## Tubing and Canal Length

The length of the tubing used to couple the hearing aid to the earmold has been shown to have very little effect on the frequency response characteristics of the hearing aid (M. C. Pollack, 1980a). The earmold canal length does have an effect on the frequency response characteristics of hearing aids. Specifically, an earmold with a short canal (0.2 cm) will reduce the amount of low-frequency amplification while improving higher-frequency amplification when compared to an earmold with a long canal (1 cm) (M. C. Pollack, 1980a). These changes may significantly affect the hearing-aid response characteristics when the aid is used for a child. For the child with relatively good low-frequency hearing, these effects may work to an advantage; however, the exact nature and degree of the effects cannot be determined without assessing the child's functional performance using a specific earmold and hearing aid.

## Venting

The vent, an opening to the outside of the earmold, is purposely employed to create changes in the frequency response characteristics or to provide the client with some pressure release. The placement, size, and shape of the vent is dependent upon the desired type of modification. The simplest type of vent is that which is used to relieve discomfort from pressure in the ear caused by the closed earmold. A small pinhole, about 0.6 mm for the adult ear, should decrease the discomfort without affecting the hearing-aid response (Lybarger, 1980).

All other types of venting are used for the specific purpose of changing the hearing-aid response. In general, venting will result in reduction of low-frequency amplification. The amount of low-frequency reduction depends upon the size (diameter) and angle of the vent. Typically, increasing the size of the vent results in greater reduction of low-frequency amplification. However, consideration must be given to the interaction between the vent size and the canal length of the earmold described by Lybarger (1980). The audiologist can use a trial-and-error method to determine what vent size is most appropriate for a particular child by using a "select-a-vent" or positive-venting valve in the earmold. Such devices allow for changing the size of the vent (through the use of plugs or a valve) and determining the functional performance of the hearing-aid system. It would seem wise to opt for such a system when selecting amplification for a child for whom venting appears appropriate.

Aside from the diameter and length of the vent, the audiologist can also choose its placement, either angled or parallel. M. C. Pollack (1980a) recommends the use of parallel venting when possible because it does not have a great effect on the hearing aid's higher-frequency response. When there is not enough space within the earmold canal, as can be true with children, a diagonal vent is necessary. In such a case the vent should intersect the earmold bore as close to the end as possible so that changes in high-frequency response and output of the hearing aid can be kept to a minimum.

## Damping

Damping is used to modify the resonances set up in the tubing of the earmold. Those resonances result in an uneven frequency response that does not occur without coupling to an earmold. Libby (1980) describes a series of mesh dampers (BF series) designed by Knowles to reduce the unwanted amplification boost that typically occurs within the mid-frequency range. As the damper, which can be placed in the tubing, earhook, or hearing aid, is moved further away from the transducer toward the tip of the earmold, there is increased smoothing and a lowering effect on the primary peak at 1000 Hz. A predesigned set of dampers can be used to control the frequencies affected, allowing for the determination of the need for dampers and their appropriate placement for a particular child.

### Configuration of the Canal Bore

The most commonly used canal bore modification is the horn (also called step or megaphone) type. By progressively increasing tube diameter toward the bore opening to the ear canal, it is possible to create an acoustic horn. Such a configuration improves the higher-frequency output and smoothes the output curve because of the widened mouth of the bore. Libby (1980) reported that in order to use the horn type appropriately, the earmold tubing must be at least 30 mm in length. Tubing of that length may well be impossible with a child, making the use of a horn unlikely. Furthermore, the narrowness of a child's ear canal will put limitations on the degree to which the diameter of the bore can be increased to form the horn.

# Nontraditional Amplification Devices

### FM Auditory Training System

These systems have become well established as crucial classroom amplification because they reduce the difficult listening conditions caused by distance from the speaker, background noise, and excess room reverberation. Figure 11.1 displays the body-worn receiver of an FM auditory training system. The microphone or transmitter can be seen in Figure 11.2. The negative room acoustics that exist in classrooms can also occur in the home, especially when the child is at a distance from the sound source. In order to overcome these problems, some audiologists have been providing infants and young children with FM systems as personal amplification. Figure 11.3 shows the use of an FM system with young children in the home. The reasons for recommending the system over traditional

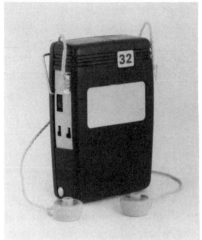 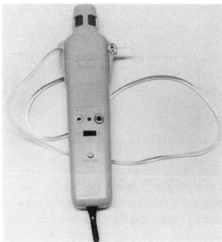

**Figure 11.1.** The body-worn receiver of a wireless FM auditory trainer. The unit is typically worn mounted on the chest. Courtesy of Instrument Distributors of America, Inc., White Plains, New York.

**Figure 11.2.** The microphone/transmitter of a wireless FM auditory trainer. Courtesy of Instrument Distributors of America, Inc., White Plains, New York.

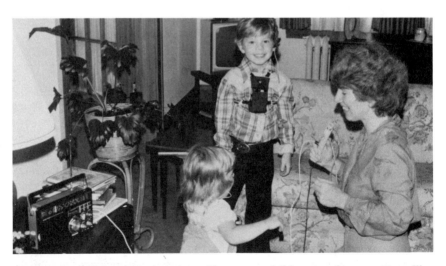

**Figure 11.3.** FM systems being used by young children in a home setting. The children are using the receivers, and the parent is using the transmitter. Courtesy of Instrument Distributors of America, Inc., White Plains, New York.

hearing aids are, of course, related to improving the signal-to-noise ratio for the child. Enhancing the listening conditions, the system allows parents more flexibility in providing good auditory input to the child. They do not always have to be close to ensure that their child hears what they are saying. Therefore, the system allows for a more natural interaction between parent and child, which is likely to result in more consistent, better-quality language stimulation. Outdoor activities can also be conducted more easily, enabling the child to be involved in natural play activities.

The major negative criticism of FM systems for use with infants and young children is that the transmitter (microphone) makes speech always sound as if it came from 8 to 10 inches away. Such a constant, nonchanging signal may cause the child difficulty in learning to localize the source of a sound as well as to make use of spatial cues. More research is needed to further explore the use of FM systems with this population.

## Vibrotactile Systems

There are some hearing-impaired children for whom conventional hearing aids cannot provide enough amplification. In such cases the audiologist is faced with difficult choices. For years there were no viable sensory aids that could readily be used, so these children often could not have any assistive devices. One of the sensory aids presently available and being used clinically is the wearable vibrotactile system. As early as the 1940s, devices that transformed an acoustic signal into a tactile display were available, but these early units were not practical because they did not allow for coding of continuous discourse. Their inherent problems included the fact that the skin was not capable of transmitting high frequencies and that speech was too fast to be processed. Recent advances, however, have resulted in wearable units that are designed specifically for the reception of speech, particularly connected discourse. One such unit, the TACTAID, is seen in Figure 11.4. The unit consists of a microphone, a processing unit, and one or more vibrators worn on the chest or abdomen. Typically, an intensive management program is provided with the unit in order to train the child to make use of the nonacoustic system for encoding speech and for developing language. Minimally such a unit will provide children with environmental information and alert them to the presence of sound. Some companies will provide a child with the unit on a trial basis and allow the audiologist to make a careful assessment of the appropriateness of the vibrotactile system.

## Cochlear Implants

This sensory aid has gained a great deal of attention since its relatively recent introduction. The apparatus has both internal and external components that consist of a receiver coil and electrodes (internal) and a microphone, transducer, and transmitter (external). Presently, devices have either single-channel or multichannel electrodes, which are used to stimulate the VIIIth-nerve fibers in their vicinity. In general the proponents of cochlear implants report that postlingually hearing-impaired adults demonstrate improved speechreading ability and closed-set speech recognition. There is, however, considerable controversy surrounding the

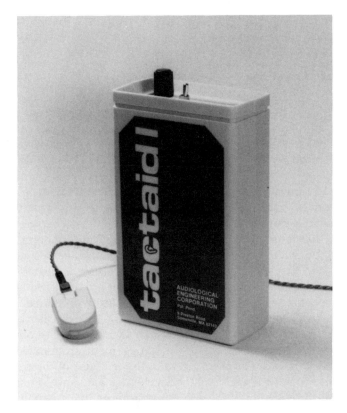

**Figure 11.4.** TACTAID, a wearable vibrotactile assistive device. The child wears the vibrator mounted on the chest. Courtesy of Audiological Engineering Corporation, Sommerville, Massachusetts.

use of implants with children, particularly with regard to judging candidacy. Since implants were designed to be used by adults who have profound hearing losses and who cannot use conventional amplification, there is considerable concern regarding the implant's ability to provide appropriate auditory cues for speech and language acquisition to children. Candidacy for adults has been well established; however, Simmons (1985) has presented reasons against considering hearing-impaired children candidates for cochlear implant. These reasons include (1) difficulty in determining that some children cannot benefit from conventional amplification, (2) necessity of surgical revisions, (3) difficulty in aligning external sections of the unit because prelingually hearing-impaired children cannot explain what they hear, (4) the possibility of significant improvement in the next decade regarding an improved signal, (5) possible damage to an ear that has some residual hearing, and (6) risk of cochlear infection resulting from the presence of otitis media. Simmons suggests that, as professionals working with hearing-impaired children, "what we can do is take as unemotional a view of implants as it is possible to do. We can try to intelligently influence parental decisions, making absolutely sure of motives and of residual hearing" (p. 63).

# Hearing-Aid Evaluation

Providing amplification for children is not as straightforward as it is with adults. Often the audiologist must make judgments about the type of hearing aids to recommend with relatively little audiological information. Clinical experience has demonstrated that the following should be available prior to recommending a specific hearing aid:

1. Unaided sound-field warble-tone response measurements

2. Unaided sound-field speech measurements

3. Acoustic immittance measurements

4. Medical clearance for amplification use

5. The child's own earmolds

Unlike the adult hearing-aid evaluation, the process with children is an ongoing one that begins with the audiological evaluation, at which time earmold impressions should be taken and an electroacoustically flexible hearing aid selected. In general, during the evaluation the unaided sound-field measures should be compared to aided sound-field measures (warble tones and speech) so that an estimate of functional gain of the hearing aids can be made. Since most of the procedures used with children are highly age-dependent, they will be discussed specifically for each age group.

## Infants (0–2 years)

An incredible change in behaviors and ability to respond to outside stimuli occurs during this age range. The change in response to sound, both in terms of the intensity at which an infant will respond and the type of responses that can be expected, will make it necessary to obtain minimal awareness levels (MAL) rather than threshold measurements. Table 11.2 demonstrates that the younger the infant, the louder a sound has to be to obtain a reliable response. It also demonstrates that there are differences in the intensities at which an infant will respond to tones and to speech. Thus MALs will allow the audiologist to determine whether the infant is responding at levels that are significantly higher (poorer) than those which would be expected for a particular age. The audiologist can use the information about the speech detection levels in comparison with the tone detection levels as an indication of the degree of hearing loss. For example, if a child is 4 months old and gives responses to tones and speech at 65 dB HL, then it can be assumed that the child has some hearing loss. By referring to expected MALs and a particular child's results, the audiologist can select the proper hearing-aid settings. The goal is not to increase the MALs to clinically normal limits for adults or older children but to provide amplification to afford the child as much speech information as possible.

## 0–6 Months

In order to obtain the unaided information, the audiologist must use a behavioral observation audiometry (BOA) technique using a test suite for that procedure (see Figure 6.4). The audiologist (and an observer) is able to observe the infant's reflexive responses (cessation of activity, frowning, cessation of vocalization, eyeblink, startle, etc.) and find the lowest intensity levels at which repeatable ones can be obtained (MALs). Frequency-specific information is obtained using warble tones. A speech awareness threshold (SAT) is also measured by finding the lowest intensity level at which the infant responds to speech (babbling, vocalization,

**TABLE 11.2**
**Auditory Behavior Index for Infants**

| Age | Warbled Tones | Speech |
|---|---|---|
| 0–6 weeks | 78 dB HL | 40–60 dB HL |
| 6 weeks–4 months | 70 dB HL | 47 dB HL |
| 4–7 months | 51 dB HL | 21 dB HL |
| 7–9 months | 45 dB HL | 15 dB HL |
| 9–13 months | 38 dB HL | 8 dB HL |
| 13–16 months | 32 dB HL | 5 dB HL |
| 16–21 months | 25 dB HL | 5 dB HL |
| 21–24 months | 26 db HL | 3 dB HL |

*Source:* Adapted from McConnell and Ward (1967).

etc.) through the use of behavioral observation audiometry. Since this basic information is readily obtained with even the youngest infants, it can be used as the basis for comparing responses with amplification.

Although it is important to obtain acoustic immittance measurement, the results should be judged carefully with infants in this age group. Cone and Gerber (1977) demonstrated that below 5 months of age adult norms cannot be used because the middle ear system is still very compliant. Since it is necessary to obtain medical clearance prior to providing amplification for all children under 18 years of age, any possible middle ear pathology can be diagnosed by a physician.

Clinical experience has demonstrated that the first hearing aids selected for this age should be body aids. The selected aids (and harness) are purchased, either through the dispensing audiologist or a hearing-aid dealer, and provided for a 30-day trial period. If a loaner hearing-aid program is available, then the following procedures can be conducted through it. At the scheduled hearing-aid evaluation the hearing aids, which have been set by the audiologist, are demonstrated for the parents, who are shown how to troubleshoot them, change the batteries, and put them on their child. It is important to have the parents carry out these tasks before leaving the office so that they know what to do at home. After the hearing aids are placed on the child, the family members are left essentially to themselves for approximately 1 hour. During this time the audiologist is observing to detect any immediate problems. Table 11.3 shows possible problems, manifested by specific behavioral reactions, that can occur during this initial introduction to amplification, along with solutions. No testing is conducted at this time because valid aided responses cannot be obtained until the infant has become accustomed to the aids and to listening to amplified sound. Testing will take place during the hearing-aid check. The parents are given a list of possible behaviors, much like those presented in Table 11.3, which they should be monitoring. They are

**TABLE 11.3**
**Behaviors, Problems, and Solutions Associated with**
**the Introduction of Amplification**

| Behavior | Problems | Solutions |
|---|---|---|
| Blinking, flinching to loud sounds | Output/gain too high; tolerance problem | Decrease output/gain |
| Pulling out earmolds | Child not used to earmolds | Use "Huggies" to facilitate use |
| | Poorly fitting earmold | Remake or trim earmold |
| | Sore ears due to allergies or poorly fitting molds | Have medical exam and/or remake with hypoallergenic material |
| Acoustic feedback | Cerumen plug in canal | Medical treatment |
| | Poorly fitting earmold | Remake mold with feedback-resistant material |
| | Middle ear fluid (flat tympanogram) | Medical evaluation |
| Pulling on or chewing cords | Cords are too obvious and attracting baby's attention | String cords through clothing or behind back; decrease cord length |

instructed to telephone the audiologist immediately if any concerns or problems should arise. Before the family leaves, an appointment is made for a hearing-aid check.

The hearing-aid check must be conducted within the 30-day trial period. It is important for the infant to become a good hearing-aid user—that is, using the aids all day—before the check is carried out. At that time, the infant's aided responses to warble tones (MALs) and speech (SATs) are obtained and compared with the unaided information. If an aided improvement in MALs and SATs is demonstrated, without over-amplification, then the aids are considered appropriate and the hearing-aid evaluation complete. If any problems exist, the audiologist must work at correcting them, and the hearing-aid evaluation continues until no significant problems are reported or observed. Possible problems discovered at this time are displayed in Table 11.4.

## 7–24 Months

Once a baby reaches 7 months of age, a conditioned orienting reflex (COR) procedure, one in which an appropriate response to an auditory stimulus is reinforced by a visual stimulus, can be used to obtained MALs. The setup displayed in Figure 11.1 remains the same, with the addition of a visual reinforcer (e.g., a lighted toy) placed on or near the loudspeakers. Reliable MALs can readily be obtained for warble tones, and an SAT is easily measured. Since it may still be difficult to obtain individual ear information, between-ear differences in sensitivity can be estimated through observation of localization ability. A significant between-ear difference can be ruled out by an infant's ability to localize at low sensation levels (SL). For example, after an SAT is obtained, speech is presented at 5–10 dB SL, alternating it between the loudspeakers. If the infant can readily turn in the correct direction, localization is assumed to be intact, indicating no significant ear difference. When no apparent ear differences are found, symmetrical binaural amplification can be recommended.

With this age group more complete audiometric and immittance information can be obtained prior to the hearing-aid evaluation. More reliable acoustic immittance measurements allow for a more complete description of middle ear functioning; however, medical evaluation is still necessary. Babies this age may not tolerate placement of headphones for prolonged periods of time. Although inability to maintain placement of the headphones will not interfere with obtaining a valid tympanogram, it is unlikely that stapedial reflex thresholds can be measured when the probe is hand-held.

**TABLE 11.4**
**Concerns That May Arise at the Hearing-Aid Check**

| Problem | Solution |
|---|---|
| Poor high-frequency amplification | Change the settings to allow for increased high-frequency gain. This may be the best setting until ear-level aids are used. |
| Overamplification in low frequencies | Reduce the low-frequency gain as much as possible. Select an aid with a different frequency response. |
| Startling to loud sounds | Reduce gain or output or low-frequency response. Select an aid with different electroacoustic characteristics. |
| Poor aided responses | Determine whether the baby has become a full-time hearing-aid user. If not, work on this problem with the parents. The baby may not have learned to make good use of hearing. Recheck in 2 weeks. Consider the possibility of changing amplification. |
| Dead batteries | Work on troubleshooting with the parents. |
| Baby using aid on low volume | Determine whether feedback is a problem; if so, remedy it. Determine whether the baby is reacting negatively to higher volume and remedy it. Determine whether parents are monitoring. |
| Food and liquid falling into microphone | Use a microphone cover. Body aids without them should not be recommended for infants. |

Usually the older babies in this age range will attend to the COR procedure long enough to obtain aided warble-tone and speech responses for an individual ear. If these measures cannot all be made in one test period, it is beneficial to schedule another appointment prior to the hearing-aid evaluation so that a complete assessment is made. The hearing-aid evaluation for these infants should be conducted in the same ways as that described above using the appropriate techniques.

There is the possibility that an older baby's response to speech at comfortable listening levels can be measured. Therefore, at the hearing-aid check, the audiologist can observe how well the child responds to being called by name, looking for Mommy or Daddy, waving bye-bye, etc. Minimally, the audiologist can look for alertness to sound at suprathreshold levels. The particular speech simuli used will be dependent upon what the baby is reportedly able to do as well as his or her age. The intensity level at which the speech is presented will be dependent upon the aided MALs and SAT.

For the younger infants in this age group, body-worn hearing aids are still the choice. For children closer to 24 months, ear-level hearing aids may be recommended, especially if the degree of hearing loss is, at maximum, moderate. The method for recommending, purchasing, and checking the hearing aids should be the same as that described for the younger infants (0–6 months).

## 2–3 Years

This is an age at which it is difficult to predict behavior. Depending upon the maturity of the child, either a COR procedure or a conditioned play audiometry (CPA) procedure should be used. The major difference in audiological information available for this age group as compared with that for younger ones is that it is more likely that individual-ear information has been obtained via headphones. With accurate measurements of each ear's sensitivity, setting the electroacoustic characteristics of the hearing aid can be determined without so much dependence upon trial and error. The child's acceptance of headphones will allow the audiologist to obtain complete acoustic immittance measures, including stapedial reflex thresholds, but again medical evaluation is necessary prior to a hearing-aid recommendation.

It is still not likely that the audiologist will be able to obtain a conventional measure of speech discrimination ability. Minimally, measures of response to speech can be made by using Ling's (1978) five-sound test in conjunction with either a COR or CPA procedure. These sounds (/a/, /i/, /u/, /s/, and /ʃ/) are presented at a comfortable listening level so that their audibility through the hearing aids can be determined. For children who are able to point to body parts or familiar objects, a gross estimate of their ability to receive various speech sounds through the hearing aids can be made by having them do so. Combining these kinds of procedures can give a fairly accurate estimate of the benefit the child receives from amplification.

Typically ear-level hearing aids would be recommended for this age group if a child has any degree of hearing loss but profound. The advantages of receiving sound at ear level, as well as the typically better high-frequency response of the aids, usually outweigh the disadvantages, such as acoustic feedback. Clinical experience has demonstrated that a child with a profound hearing loss, especially a corner audiogram, does better with body-worn hearing aids at least as initial amplification. The problem of trying to provide a profoundly impaired child with enough amplification without acoustic feedback occurring may be the deciding factor. Once again the recommendation, purchase, and check of the hearing aids would be the same as that described for the younger infants.

## 3–5 Years

Once a child reaches 3 years of age, a more traditional type of hearing-aid evaluation can be conducted. Prior to a hearing-aid recommendation, individual-ear thresholds can be obtained using a CPA procedure, and even if bone-conduction measurements are not carried out, complete acoustic immittance measurements should be available. Speech reception thresholds (SRT) can be measured through a talk-back or picture-pointing technique. For a child with a receptive vocabulary as limited as 5 words, an SRT can be obtained with a restricted number of familiar stimulus items that can easily be represented by pictures or toys.

Some measure of speech discrimination ability may be made by using either the measures described above or with a standardized technique such as the *Word Intelligibility by Picture Identification* (WIPI) (Ross & Lerman, 1971) or the *Northeastern University Children's Perception of Speech* (NU-CHIPS) (Elliot & Katz, 1980). For older children with more intelligible speech and larger vocabularies, talk-back procedures using appropriate lists such as the phonetically balanced kindergarten (PB-K) lists can be used. The greatest limitation in obtaining either unaided or aided speech audiometry measures is the linguistic ability of the child. If the child is severely hearing-impaired and is not identified until this late age, then language skills will ordinarily be very poor. Even if the child has been identified at an earlier age and this evaluation is for replacement hearing aids, the child's language may not be age-appropriate, so speech audiometry techniques designed for younger children may have to be used. There are also those children who do not depend solely on hearing for reception of speech. In such cases, an auditory-only measure of speech discrimination would not provide the audiologist with the pertinent information necessary during a hearing-aid evaluation. (It should be noted, however, that such measures can be very valuable during management when trying to determine how well a child uses aided residual hearing.)

For children in this age group, ear-level hearing aids are most likely the amplification of choice, but body aids should not immediately be ruled out for children with corner audiograms. It is hoped that most children will have been identified prior to 3 years of age and that this hearing-aid evaluation will be for replacement aids. However, children with mild or high-frequency hearing losses may be identified at this age, necessitating the use of the initial hearing-aid evaluation procedures described for younger children.

When the hearing aids are being recommended for a child who is an experienced user, the audiologist can select a few appropriate hearing aids and carry out aided warble-tone and speech measures to determine which of the hearing aids is best suited to the child. It may be necessary to carry out this procedure over a few test sessions because of a child's difficulty in attending to the task for the necessary length of time. It is better to schedule several sessions than to rely on measures that are made when the child is tired. Conducting a more traditional hearing-aid evaluation allows for comparisons of functional gain across frequency. These results can be used to recommend the electroacoustically flexible aid that is providing appropriate amplification. Consideration should also be given to any necessity for interfacing with amplification worn at school.

Once a recommendation is made, the hearing aids should be purchased with a 30-day trial period. When the aids are received, they should be placed on the child; however, a hearing-aid check by the audiologist should not be conducted until the child has used them for at least 2 weeks. This will provide the opportunity to evaluate any behavioral changes brought about by the hearing aids. Any problems should be reported to the audiologist, who can determine whether they are remediable or whether different hearing aids should be evaluated. Table 11.5 displays not only the problems likely to occur when providing amplification to children in this age group but also possible solutions.

There are a number of measures used in adult hearing-aid evaluations that cannot be reliably obtained with young children. Some of those are often considered to be the most useful for hearing-aid recommendations—such as uncomfortable loudness levels (UCL) and most comfortable loudness levels (MCL). Even normal-hearing children have difficulty understanding the directions necessary to complete the measures. For the hearing-impaired child, whose language level is most likely reduced, and certainly the preverbal child, it would be impossible to obtain any reliable UCLs or MCLs.

**TABLE 11.5**
**Problems and Solutions Associated with Providing Amplification**
**for Older (3–5 years) Children**

| Problem | Solution |
|---|---|
| Poor aided response in the high frequencies | Increase high-frequency response of the aid. Modify the earmold if possible. Consider changing the hearing aid. |
| Overamplification in the low frequencies | Reduce low-frequency response of the aid. Modify the earmold if possible. Use filtered tone hook if possible. Consider changing the hearing aid. |
| Feedback | Remake earmolds with feedback-resistant material. Remake earmold with tragus lock. Check for cerumen in canal and refer child to physician if it is a problem. Check for middle ear effusion with tympanometry and refer child to physician if there is a problem. Reduce output of the hearing aid. |
| Rejection of the hearing aid | If an experienced hearing-aid user, this may be a problem of becoming accustomed to a new hearing aid. If a new hearing-aid user, work with parents on ways to increase usage. |
| Using the aid on low volume | Gain is too high and needs to be reduced. There is too much low-frequency amplification, so frequency response needs to be changed. Parents are not monitoring the aid and should be instructed to do so. |

## Special Populations

When the hearing-impaired child is multiply handicapped or mentally retarded, the audiologist has a more difficult time in recommending appropriate amplification. These children may be difficult to test so that reliable results cannot be readily obtained. It may be that there are a number of professionals involved and the parents are overwhelmed by the prospect of yet another "expert" and "device" to handle. In these situations the audiologist may have to spend a good deal of time helping the parents understand the benefits to be gained and the relative ease with which amplification can be used on a regular basis. It is also important to make clear that hearing aids are not the answer to all of the child's problems. The parents have to understand that their child's speech, language, and cognitive problems may not necessarily be related to the hearing loss and so will not be solved by the hearing aids.

Even when realistic goals and understanding of the benefits of the hearing aids are established, the child may be difficult to test and assess for amplification. When behavioral audiological measures cannot be conducted, the child should be referred to an audiologist for auditory brainstem response (ABR) audiometry measures to obtain as much information about the status of the auditory system as possible. If the audiologist who conducts these ABR measures reports the presence of a significant hearing loss, then amplification can be recommended. ABR measures should not be relied upon for determining electroacoustic characteristics or for conducting any portion of the hearing-aid evaluation. It will be necessary to carefully monitor the child's aided reponses through a close involvement in the management program to determine what benefits are being obtained. Certainly the well-documented limitations of ABR for describing use of hearing and assessing aided responses should be taken into consideration (Weber, 1983).

The pediatric population, especially those difficult to test, may be considered a good group with which to use real ear measurements for conducting hearing-aid evaluations. Real ear measures of hearing-aid electroacoustic characteristics have gained a great deal of attention recently because they overcome the problem of using a 2 cc coupler to predict ear response. The concerns about validity of coupler response when working with adults is even greater with children because estimating gain and frequency response for a small ear canal is even more difficult. The placement of the earmold in the ear canal will have an effect on the ear canal resonances and therefore affect the sound that reaches the ear. Real ear measurements allow for actually measuring, via a probe, the sound delivered to the ear (Frye, 1986). Pursuing the use of these measurements with children could help overcome the problems associated with depending on manufacturer's specifications and the child's behavioral responses to recommend a hearing aid. Clinical application with children and infants has not been widespread and needs further study.

## Follow-up Management

As mentioned earlier, hearing-aid evaluations with children are an ongoing process that involves management planning. It is important for the audiologist to consider the following points whenever a child is provided with amplification:

1. The audiologist should remain accessible to the parents, child, and educators after the hearing aids have been provided.

2. Every effort should be made to provide the parents with accurate estimates of what to expect from the child in response to the hearing aids on both a short- and long-term basis. Such expectations should center around response to sound in different listening situations, localization ability, and difficulty in relation to noise and distance.

3. Parents should be encouraged to troubleshoot the hearing aids on a daily basis and to make minor repairs or call the audiologist when necessary.

4. The audiologist should address the concept of auditory training with the parents—that is, the need for the child to learn to use residual hearing. The need for consistent amplification use should be stressed.

5. The parents should be provided with information regarding the necessity of good linguistic input. They should be encouraged to become involved in the child's speech and language development regardless of the degree of hearing loss or mode of communication.

6. The audiologist should be comfortable in guiding the parents with respect to alternative educational placements. The parents should be provided with information regarding the alternatives for methods of communication and/or sensory aids when necessary.

# Case Histories

### C. J. (14 Months)

*Reported Problem.* At 3 months of age, C. J. had been diagnosed at another clinic as having a severe hearing loss. A loaner hearing aid was provided through that clinic at 6 months of age.

*Background.* Binaural power body aids were recommended by and purchased through an early intervention program at another clinic. C. J. had been using the aids for several months prior to initial evaluation at our clinic and was reportedly doing well with them. The child's mother reported that C. J. responded consistently to being called and understood "no." C. J. responded with an appropriate gesture when hearing "hi," "bye-bye," and "oh no." C. J. was using reduplicated babbling with a variety of consonants and vowels.

*Initial Evaluation.* Aided sound-field results using the binaural body aids were obtained using a COR procedure. They demonstrated aided responses to warble tones and a speech awareness threshold (15 dB HL) that were considerably better than would have been expected from the reports of the other clinic (previous results had indicated an unaided SAT of 80 dB HL). Unaided results obtained at this time showed considerably better warble-tone responses as well as a better SAT (50 dB HL).

*Recommendations.* It was recommended that the hearing aids be reset to reduce the output and gain and that ear-level amplification be considered in order to improve high-frequency gain. Continuation of a program of natural language stimulation through parental input was also recommended.

*Discussion.* Although C. J. was diagnosed as hearing-impaired at a very early age, the diagnosis with regard to the degree of loss was misleading. The early identification and amplification were good, but the original audiologist was not considering the normal development of auditory response patterns and was treating the hearing loss to be greater than it actually was. This case indicates the need for good follow-up procedures to regularly monitor the child's behavioral responses to the amplification as well as the regular audiological/amplification reevaluations. The flexibility of the particular body aids originally recommended allowed for some adjustment of output and gain; however, it was not possible to improve the high-frequency response characteristics. Ear-level hearing aids would allow for better high-frequency amplification. Since C. J.'s loss was not as severe as originally thought, the likelihood of acoustic feedback was greatly reduced.

At 3 years of age C. J. received binaural ear-level hearing aids (although improvement in high frequencies could not be obtained with the body aids, the parents were not in a financial position to purchase new hearing aids prior to that time). Aided performance demonstrated a relatively flat functional gain response. An aided speech discrimination score of 84% at 50 dB HL (auditory only) was obtained on the Word Intelligibility by Picture Identification (WIPI) test. C. J. is presently enrolled in a special language stimulation preschool program for five half-days per week and a regular nursery school for five half-days per week.

In both settings C. J. uses an FM system provided by the town. A recent speech and language assessment (conducted at age 5) demonstrated age-appropriate use of grammatical forms. Vocabulary is several months below chronological age expectations, and speech is judged to be intelligible. C. J. will be attending regular kindergarten and will continue to use the FM system. These most recent assessment results indicate how well C. J. uses residual hearing and how the benefits of early amplification and management have positively affected speech and language development as well as educational performance.

## L. L. (21 Months)

*Reported Problem.*   Bilateral auditory atresia with significant conductive hearing loss was reported. The family had recently moved to the area from another region of the country.

*Background.*   A normal pregnancy and delivery were reported. L. L. had no abnormalities except for the bilateral congential atresia. At 6 weeks of age the pediatrician referred the child for behavioral audiometry and auditory brainstem response (ABR) audiometry. Only behavioral measures were made at that time, and results indicated reduced hearing levels. Tomograms indicated severe malformation that would need extensive reconstructive and cosmetic surgery. As a result, the pediatrician recommended immediate amplification. The child was referred to an ear, nose, and throat specialist for medical clearance. That physician responded that a body aid with a bone-conduction transducer is not typically used with a child until 4 or 5 years of age, after which time surgery is considered, so the medical clearance was not given for L. L. The pediatrician chose to disregard this advice and referred L. L. for further audiological and amplification evaluations.

At 3 months of age L. L. was seen for ABR testing, and results indicated sufficient residual hearing to allow for significant benefit from bone-conduction amplification. At 7 months of age L. L. received a body aid with a bone-conduction transducer, which resulted in aided behavioral response levels in the 20–35 dB HL range. At 21 months of age the family moved to the area serviced by the University of Connecticut clinic. L. L. started in a preschool language stimulation program and early intervention program for the hearing-impaired.

*Initial Evaluation.*   Aided results obtained with COR procedures demonstrated responses to warble tones at 20–25 dB HL across frequencies. An aided SAT of 15 dB was obtained. A speech and language screening indicated that L. L. passed all items for both comprehension and expression.

*Discussion.* Follow-up evaluations have demonstrated that L. L. continues to receive considerable benefit from amplification. The possibility of an FM system is being considered for school. At the last evaluation L. L. was using ear-level aids with bone-conduction transducers on a trial basis and appeared to receive appropriate amplification from them. This arrangement was more appealing to the parents than the use of body aids. Evaluations conducted at 2 years and 5 months of age continued to show good aided responses to tones and a WIPI score of 80% at 45 dB HL. With the new arrangement L. L.'s general development and speech-language skills were evaluated as being at least age-appropriate.

The critical factor for this child was the virtually immediate diagnosis of the hearing loss and the pediatrician's understanding of the need for early amplification. Another factor in L. L.'s favor was the nature of the hearing loss—conductive—which responded so well to amplification. Finally, L. L.'s parents have continued to pursue every avenue in obtaining help for their child, and their work has certainly been rewarded.

## B. G. (3 Years, 5 Months)

*Reported Problem.* A speech-language evaluation through the school system resulted in a diagnosis of delayed speech and language development. B. G. was referred for an audiological evaluation to rule out any related hearing problem.

*Background.* B. G. was a low-birth-weight (2 kg), full-term infant who was jaundiced and spent 1 week in a neonatal intensive care unit. General physical development was age-appropriate and there was no history of middle ear problems. There was a family history of childhood hearing loss on the maternal side of the family.

*Parental Report.* The parents did not think that there was a hearing problem because B. G. responded to sound. They reported that B. G. was late in starting to talk and that language development was slow. Communication was primarily by gesture until 1 year prior to the evaluation. At the time of the evaluation articulation was very poor, and B. G. was often misunderstood. B. G. was in a preschool program and had been described as rowdy and disruptive.

*Initial Evaluation.*   Reliable individual-ear results were obtained with conditioned play audiometry (CPA), which demonstrated normal hearing at 250 Hz (20 dB) and 500 Hz (20 dB) and a moderate to severe sloping sensorineural hearing loss at 1000 Hz (60 dB) through 8000 Hz (90 dB). SRTs of 30 dB HL were obtained bilaterally as well as severely reduced speech discrimination scores on the WIPI. Normal acoustic immittance results were obtained. All results were duplicated at the reevaluation 1 week after the initial assessment.

*Recommendations.*   Immediate fitting of binaural high-frequency emphasis ear-level amplification with wide-bore, vented earmolds was recommended. Earmold impressions were taken and sent for fabrication. A hearing-aid evaluation to select the appropriate aids was to be scheduled within 1 week of receiving the earmolds. Furthermore, it was recommended that B. G. continue in the preschool program with emphasis directed toward auditory management by the speech-language pathologist. A home-based speech and language management program to assist the family in accepting the loss and working toward appropriate goals was suggested.

*Discussion.*   The family had a very difficult time accepting the hearing loss. They could not understand that good low-frequency hearing was what enabled B. G. to respond, particularly to environmental sounds. To them, the fact that B. G. could sometimes hear meant that there was no hearing loss and that therefore hearing aids were not needed. They did not keep the appointment for the hearing-aid evaluation, and a follow-up telephone call revealed that they were getting another opinion. They were encouraged to do so as soon as possible. With the help of the school system's speech-language pathologist the parents were able to begin to comprehend B. G.'s problem, but unfortunately this process took almost 4 months.

When the family did return, new earmold impressions had to be taken, and variable venting valve (VVV) molds were received within 2 weeks, at which time a hearing-aid evaluation was conducted. Bilateral high-frequency emphasis hearing aids were ordered and received within 2 weeks. B. G. has now been aided for 11 months, with the parents and the school system reporting positive results. There were no problems with acceptance of the aids on the child's part, and once the parents understood the hearing problem, they too accepted the aids.

At the latest amplification check, B. G. was demonstrating significant improvement in high-frequency aided hearing and no overamplification in the low frequencies. B. G.'s aided WIPI score was 68% at 50 dB

HL, but the errors tended to be related to the child's reduced vocabulary levels. B. G. should be entering kindergarten in the fall, but promotion was questionable because of delayed language and social skills. The school system has purchased a wireless FM auditory trainer for B. G. that is specially modified to provide appropriate amplification for this atypical hearing loss.

This case demonstrates the problems that arise when the family does not believe that a hearing loss exists. Such a problem is not unusual with this type of loss. The delays in diagnosis and management of the loss are directly reflected in the child's communication and social problems. It is important to note that if the high-risk characteristic for hearing loss (low birth weight) had brought about immediate follow-up, the loss would have been identified and amplification adopted earlier. Possibly the child's speech, language, and academic problems could have been avoided or at least reduced.

# Summary

Providing appropriate amplification for infants and young children is a complex process. The audiologist must make use of what is known about hearing aids, the effects of hearing loss on speech and language development, and pediatric assessment in order to make a good recommendation. Once the hearing aids are provided, the audiologist must remain closely involved with the family, not only monitoring the child's performance but providing information and counseling to the parents.

Early provision of amplification, preferably binaural, is crucial for a child to maximize use of residual hearing, especially for speech and language development. Although this process is involved and sometimes trying, its outcome is always rewarding.

# References

Bess, F. H. (1982). Children with unilateral hearing loss. *Journal of the Academy of Rehabilitative Audiology, 15,* 131–144.
Cone, B. K., & Gerber, S. E. (1977). Impedance measurements. In S. E. Gerber (Ed.), *Audiometry in infancy* (pp. 99–115). New York: Grune and Stratton.

Curran, J. R. (1985). ITE aids for children: Survey of attitudes and practices of audiologists. *Hearing Instruments, 36* (4), 20–25.

Davis, J. (1981). Utilization of audition in the education of hearing-impaired children. In F. H. Bess, B. A. Freeman, & J. S. Sinclair (Eds.), *Amplification in education* (pp. 109–120). Washington DC: Alexander Graham Bell Association for the Deaf.

Downs, M. P. (1981). Contribution of mild hearing loss to auditory language and learning problems. In R. J. Roeser & M. P. Downs (Eds.), *Auditory disorders in school children* (pp. 177–189). New York: Thieme-Stratton.

Elliott, L. L., & Katz, D. R. (1980). *Northwestern University Children's Perception of Speech*. St. Louis: Auditec of St. Louis.

Erber, N. P. (1981). Speech perception by hearing-impaired children. In F. H. Bess, B. A. Freeman, & J. S. Sinclair (Eds.), *Amplification in education*, (pp. 69–88). Washington, DC: Alexander Graham Bell Association for the Deaf.

Fry, D. B. (1978). The role and primacy of the auditory channel in speech and language development. In M. Ross & T. G. Giolas (Eds.), *Auditory management of hearing-impaired children*, (pp. 15–44). Baltimore, MD: University Park Press.

Frye, G. J. (1986). High-speed real time hearing aid analysis. *Hearing Aid Journal, 39* (6), 21.

Harris, J. D. (1980). My love affair with Ruth Bender: A history of binaural aids for babies. In E. R. Libby (Ed.), *Binaural hearing and amplification* (pp. 259–273). Chicago: Zenetron.

Levitt, H., & Voroba, B. (1980). Binaural hearing. In E. R. Libby (Ed.), *Binaural hearing and amplification* (pp. 59–80). Chicago: Zenetron.

Libby, E. R. (1980). Smooth wideband hearing aid responses: The new frontier. *Hearing Instruments, 31* (10), 18.

Ling, D. (1976). *Speech and the hearing-impaired child: Theory and practice.* Washington, DC: Alexander Graham Bell Association for the Deaf.

Ling, D. (1978). Auditory coding and recording: An analysis of auditory training procedures for hearing-impaired children. In M. Ross & T. G. Giolas (Eds.), *Auditory management of hearing-impaired children* (pp. 181–218). Baltimore, MD: University Park Press.

Lybarger, S. F. (1980). Earmold venting as an acoustic control factor. In G. A. Studebaker & I. Hochberg (Eds.), *Acoustical factors affecting hearing aid performance* (pp. 197–217). Baltimore, MD: University Park Press.

McConnell, F., & Ward, P. H. (1967). *Deafness in childhood.* Nashville, TN: Vanderbilt University Press.

Markides, A. (1977). *Binaural hearing aids.* New York: Academic Press.

Maxon, A. B. (1981). Binaural amplification of young children: A clinical application of Ross's theory. *Ear and Hearing, 2* (5), 215–219.

Pollack, D. (1980). Binaural hearing aids in an acoupedic program. In E. R. Libby (Ed.), *Binaural hearing and amplification* (pp. 249–258). Chicago: Zenetron.

Pollack, M. C. (1980a). Electroacoustic characteristics. In M. C. Pollack (Ed.), *Amplification for the hearing-impaired* (pp. 21–90). New York: Grune and Stratton.

Pollack, M. C. (1980b). Special applications of amplification. In M. C. Pollack (Ed.), *Amplification for the hearing-impaired* (pp. 255–308). New York: Grune and Stratton.

Ross, M. (1977). Binaural versus monaural hearing aids. In F. H. Bess (Ed.), *Childhood deafness: Causation, assessment, and management* (pp. 235–249). New York: Grune and Stratton.

Ross, M., & Calvert, D. R. (1984). Semantics of deafness revisited: Total communication and the use and misuse of residual hearing. *Audiology, 9* (9), 127–145.

Ross, M., & Lerman, J. W. (1971). *Word Intelligibility by Picture Identification,* Pittsburgh: Stanwix House.

Simmons, F. B. (1985). Cochlear implants in young children: Some dilemmas. *Ear and Hearing, 6* (1), 61–63.

Weber, B. A. (1983). Pitfalls in auditory brain stem response audiometry. *Ear and Hearing, 4* (4), 179–184.

# PART IV
## The Public Schools

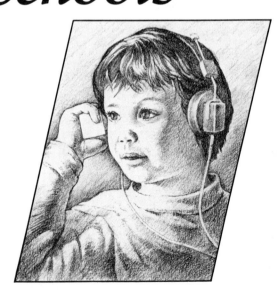

*T*he focus in the preceding chapters in this book has been on very young children. As the final two chapters reveal, the responsibilities of the pediatric audiologist continue well into the school years. These responsibilities involve the identification of hearing-impaired children as well as appropriate remediation.

In Chapter 12 Polly Patrick presents both historical and modern approaches to identification audiometry in the public schools, based on her broad clinical experience in this area. Procedures to find children with medically significant ear conditions or with hearing impairments that can interfere with normal progress in the classroom are explored. In Chapter 13 Victor Garwood details the audiologist's responsibilities to students with a hearing loss, and then illustrates a variety of ways to meet the challenge of public school audiology.

# Identification
# Audiometry

## POLLY E. PATRICK

$S$creening programs for the detection of educationally significant hearing loss have been established in the public schools for more than 50 years. The public schools have accepted, perhaps by default, the responsibility for health screening—that is, testing hearing and vision and maintaining health records with regard to immunizations and communicable diseases. The reasons for this role are obvious—that is where the children are! However, it has often taxed an already overtaxed system to expect adequate health management from programs designed to be basically educational in nature. Periodically, reports appear that are critical about the practice of school hearing screening. Are they efficient? Is screening really necessary? Are most programs operated according to established guidelines? Although hearing screening has a long history, it has not been without controversy. In addition to discussing some of these problems with hearing tests, this chapter examines the rationale for hearing screening and suggests a workable and efficient model for implementation.

# History

Group testing gained popularity for a time (Hollien & Thompson, 1967; Johnston, 1948; Reger & Newby, 1947) but proved to be expensive and impractical for widespread use. The requirement of a written response made group testing inappropriate for children below the third grade, thus eliminating its effectiveness with the majority of children needing testing.

Speech materials were recommended (Griffing, Simonton, & Hedgecock, 1967), with subsequent study indicating them to be insensitive to high-frequency hearing loss (Mencher & McCulloch, 1970). Despite these reports, the use of speech materials has persisted and is often the "last resort" when dealing with language-delayed children through the use of picture identification. One should be aware of inherent limitations of speech materials, however, when recording screening results.

In 1961 a national conference on the status of identification audiometry was convened. Out of that conference came the first recommendations for uniform implementaton of audiometric screening programs (Darley, 1961). With some modification, those guidelines are the basis for many school programs today.

A survey reported by Bess and McConnell (1981) indicated that screening is mandated by law in only 22 of the 50 states. However, every state has mechanisms in place to accomplish screening. The programs are generally administered through the state departments of health and/or education. In the unregulated states the decisions regarding procedures, testing criteria, and screening personnel are delegated to the local or regional educational authorities.

# Prevalence

Why screen hearing? In order to justify the use of a screening instrument, one must determine whether the disorder to be detected is common and/or detrimental to the health and educational experience of the population. Significant hearing loss has been estimated to be present at birth in 1 out of 1,000 infants (Northern & Downs, 1984). Several investigators have demonstrated middle ear disease to be prevalent in the birth-to-6-year categories, with estimates ranging from 4% to 8% of this age group exhibiting reduced hearing as a result (Eagles, Wishik, & Doerfler, 1967; Howie, 1975; Renvall, Liden, Jungert, & Nilsson, 1973; Savory &

Ferron, 1982). When these groups are combined, the frequency of hearing loss becomes approximately 1 in 25, at least for the younger children, making it a highly prevalent disorder. These findings indicate that screening should begin at an earlier age than the typical kindergarten class. Unfortunately, we find that a majority of screening programs begin at that level simply because that is the earliest time that most systems have ready access to the population (Wilson & Walton, 1978).

# Infant Screening

As technological advances have made mass screening of infants feasible, the practice has become increasingly more widespread. Armed with the recommendations of the Joint Committee on Infant Hearing regarding the establishment of screening programs following high-risk registers (American Speech-Language-Hearing Association, 1982), several state agencies have instituted such programs. Mahoney (1984) reported that six states currently have mandated programs involving birth certificate questions with follow-up recommending hearing tests for those identified. Eight other states have regional programs actively participating in infant screening. While a majority of the states are still without organized programs for infant screening, the increasing prevalence of journal articles and platform presentations concerned with this subject attest to the level of professional participation in the area.

As an advocate of early identification and remediation, I heartily recommend the use of infant screening programs for hearing loss. However, since these methods are discussed elsewhere in this text, the scope of this chapter will be limited to the traditional school programs.

# Choosing a Test Instrument

A screening test by definition is not diagnostic but simply a tool by which individuals at risk for a certain disorder can be identified and referred for diagnostic evaluation. An effective screening test must be reliable and valid (Paradise & Smith, 1978). Reliability is defined as the ability of a test instrument to yield consistent results over time with both large numbers of people and with test-retest results for a single individual.

Validity, on the other hand, describes a test's performance in accurately identifying those individuals who have the disorder under investigation. Validity is made up of the components of sensitivity and specificity. Sensitivity is commonly defined as the percentage of time the test identifies abnormals versus the number of abnormals it fails to find. Specificity is the accuracy with which normals are recognized as normal. A good screening test must have an acceptable interaction between sensitivity and specificity. A test having high sensitivity and low specificity will result in unnecessary referrals as a result of a high false positive rate, with many normals being labeled as abnormal. Conversely, a test with low sensitivity and high specificity will fail to identify a significant number of abnormals, thus yielding a high false negative ratio.

Throughout the last five decades, the following questions have been asked regarding hearing screening:

1. Can we effectively identify those children who have significant hearing loss?

2. Is it practical to screen for middle ear disorders?

3. What is the school's responsibility in implementing and maintaining these programs?

With these factors in mind, let us attempt to design an adequate screening program.

# Pure-Tone Screening Audiometry

## Goals

The goals of screening audiometry are threefold:

1. To identify those individuals who have sufficient hearing loss to compromise communication and/or learning in the typical classroom.

2. To find and send for medical management those students who have middle ear pathologies.

3. To perform these tasks in the most cost-effective and efficient manner.

Sounds simple enough, doesn't it? Unfortunately, the realities of mass screening, referral, and follow-up are anything but simple. While I concur with the notion of utilizing screening audiometry in tandem with immittance testing, these two components will be discussed separately.

The most recent guidelines for identification audiometry (American Speech-Language-Hearing Association, 1985) give very clear and concise suggestions for implementing a screening program. We will dissect these guidelines with some solicited criticisms and, admittedly, biased suggestions for compliance.

## Population

The American Speech-Language-Hearing Association guidelines are designed primarily for children from the age of 3 through the third grade. Several investigators have demonstrated that since a majority of children with significant hearing loss have been discovered by the third grade, the necessity as well as the cost-effectiveness of mass screening is significantly reduced after this point (Corliss & Watson, 1961, March; Downs, Doster, & Weaver, 1965). I agree with this principle in general, with the following provisos:

1. All children from the ages of 3 through third grade are tested every year.

2. All children who failed previous screening procedures (with follow-up) should be screened the next year, regardless of age.

3. All children new to the school system should be screened as part of their entry, regardless of age.

4. Children who are identified as having potential learning problems and speech and/or language problems should be screened, regardless of age.

5. Students involved in potentially noise-hazardous activities (i.e., industrial arts, wood shop, band, or orchestra) should be screened every year. This also affords an excellent opportunity to introduce the benefits of noise protectors.

We live in a transient society, particularly in urban areas. Many directors of health screening in metropolitan districts report that it is difficult if not nearly impossible to ensure proper rescreening unless it is mandated. For that reason many systems use a testing schedule based on kindergarten through grade 3 every year with alternate-year testing of grades 6, 8, and 10.

## Procedure

Despite claims to the contrary, an efficient and valid group screening test has not proved to be effective. Problems with these tests are well known: setup time, use of written responses, etc. Maintenance of equipment is a big factor since many groups appear to have difficulty keeping one audiometer and two earphones calibrated, let alone a dozen. The one-tester, one-listener situation still appears to be the most efficient manner of testing.

A manual testing mode is recommended. The flexibility of this method particularly lends itself to the testing of young children. I would discourage the investment in expensive "computerized" screeners, which call for the listener to press a button that in turn is read by the equipment and then delivers a printout to the examiner. While this idea certainly has merit for individual record keeping, the time spent in training the child and resetting when false positive/negative responses occur could become a real encumbrance with 50 restless 5-year-olds waiting to be tested. Although the majority of screening programs may be directed by audiologists, they are actually performed by nonaudiologists (i.e., school nurses, PTA volunteers, or teachers). The simpler the equipment, record keeping, testing procedures, and interpretive decisions, the more efficient the program will be.

## Signal

Pure-tone signals should be used. The question of speech versus pure-tone signals has long since been put to rest (Mencher & McCulloch, 1970), although responses from some states have indicated rare but persistent use of the *Verbal Auditory Screening for Preschool Children* (VASC) test (Griffing et al., 1967). The test signals of 1000, 2000, and 4000 Hz are adequate if the program includes immittance testing as well as pure-tone screening (Katt & Sprague, 1981). However, if audiometric screening is used solely, 500 Hz should be included.

The screening level should be set at 20 dB HL for all signals (ANSI 1969). A survey of various agencies involved in screening shows a disparity with regard to test frequencies and levels, with some utilizing differing levels for 4000 Hz and 500 Hz. Usually the reasons given are the problem of overreferral that occurs with "failing" an individual at 20 dB HL at 4000 Hz as well as the common problem of poor acoustic environments influencing the thresholds at 500 Hz. These are valid points but of questionable merit.

First, an elevated threshold at 4000 Hz can be a precursor of progressive sensorineural hearing loss or a warning sign of possible early damage due to noise exposure. I have seen several youngsters under the age of 12 who show signs of noise-induced hearing loss. The causes are generally traced to farm implements in this rural state. However, an increasing number give a history of exposure to motor bikes or habitual use of stereo or portable cassette headsets. Elevation at 4000 Hz should not be ignored even if it is not medically treatable or a real impediment to communication. This finding should be explored as a method to intervene for noise protection and to act as a baseline for future screening.

Second, the testing environment should be managed, if at all possible, to meet the requirements of the test and not the reverse.

## Testing Environment

Usually screening is assigned to large cavernous areas like gyms and auditoriums, where testing procedures will not interfere with regular school activities. This assignment is well intentioned but not always advantageous to the screening condition. The tester should always assess the situation with the aims of the best acoustic environment possible and avoid "making do" by raising the level of the screening signal. A visit to the test site prior to the screening day can often accomplish this goal. Most school administrators are amenable to suggestions for improving test situations if they are given a little warning. A backstage dressing room or even a large closet is preferable to the auditorium, the gym, or the cafeteria, where preparations are being made for lunch. The library is usually an excellent choice and can often be scheduled with some advance planning.

Table 12.1 shows the approximate allowable octave-band noise levels for hearing screening. In reality, few if any hearing screeners arrive at the test site with a sound level meter in hand. Therefore, they must depend on daily biologic calibration to determine the appropriateness of the acoustic environment. Testers should previously assess their own ability to detect the presence of the signal. This, of course, requires normal hearing and a quiet environment. The procedure should be performed at the beginning of every test session and at every different site. If the signal cannot be detected, the acoustic environment is suspect and should be modified. This practice also serves to ensure day-to-day performance of the equipment. While this step may sound elemental, personal experience has shown that it is often overlooked. In 1981 a colleague and I screened the hearing of approximately 400 athletes at the XIVth World

**TABLE 12.1**
**Approximate Allowable Octave-Band Ambient Noise Levels (SPL) in Micropascals for Threshold Measurements at 0 HL and for Screening at Recommended ASHA Levels***

| | Test Tone Frequency (Hz) | | | |
|---|---|---|---|---|
| | 500 | 1000 | 2000 | 4000 |
| Allowable ambient noise for threshold at 0 HL | 21.5 | 29.5 | 34.5 | 42.0 |
| Plus ASHA screening level | 20.0 | 20.0 | 20.0 | 20.0 |
| Resultant maximum ambient noise allowable for ASHA screening | 41.5 | 49.5 | 54.5 | 62.0 |

*Based on ANSI 53.1-1977 (see American National Standards Institute, 1977).
*Source:* Data from American Speech-Language-Hearing Association (1985).

Games for the Deaf. In reviewing the audiograms provided by the various countries prior to the games, we made the puzzling discovery that all of the members from a certain Eastern Bloc country showed no measurable hearing in their right ears. Subsequent screening indicated that this finding was probably due to a malfunctioning right earphone at the original test site rather than to a tendency for young socialist athletes to develop unilateral hearing loss.

## Audiometric Equipment and Calibration

The standard MX-41 earphone cushion is recommended and appears to be widely used. Some people still mistakenly believe that the "aural dome" ear cushion provides better attenuation of ambient noise than the standard ear cuff. Not only has this been shown to be in error (Benson, 1971) but the oversized headsets are difficult to manage and provide real opportunity for placement error in very young children. One may end up testing cheeks instead of ears, and a significant number of false-positive findings can occur from collapsing ear canals caused from undue pressure on the soft tissue of the pinnae.

Audiometers used for screening should meet the ANSI S3.6-1969 requirements (American National Standards Institute, 1970). Regular calibration is essential to the success of any screening program. Annual "factory calibration" is an absolute minimum, with calibration checks of the sound pressure level made at 3-month intervals (American Speech-Language-Hearing Association, Committee on Audiometric Evaluation, 1982). To reiterate, daily listening checks are mandatory. One can never assume that equipment is functional simply because it worked previously. Typically, screening audiometers receive harsh treatment in being transported to various sites and touched by many different hands. The potential for damage is high: headsets are dropped, wires are pulled, and electrical connections are stressed. Daily inspection and biologic checks can prevent many wasted hours or invalid test results.

Provision should be made for regular cleaning of the earphone cushions since there is often an opportunity for contamination during mass screening (Talbott, 1969). Care must be taken to avoid disinfectants that could damage the cushions. Most equipment manufacturers will recommend proper cleaning methods.

## Testing Procedures

In a public school screening program, the tester's best friends are the classroom teachers. They know their pupils and can provide an appropriate vehicle for instructing students about screening procedures. A little advanced preparation can save a great deal of time and effort. Students should be instructed regarding the task and expected response before arriving at the screening area. The teacher acts not only as a gatekeeper to funnel the children into the test but serves as an authority figure to control the noise and activity level of these lively souls. One method that has proved efficient for initial screening is to give each child a card bearing his or her name and the teacher's name. This card is given to the screener, who simply indicates a pass or fail for each child. These cards can be sorted at the end of the testing session for rescreening or notation on the child's health record.

Instruction should be kept as simple as possible. If the students have been prepared, a brief review of instructions is all that is necessary: "You will hear a little beeping sound. Every time you even barely hear it, raise your hand." More complicated instructions—such as raising the right hand for the right ear, the left hand for the left ear, or detailed description of frequency differences—tend to confuse the situation and can result in elevated responses. Generally, children 5 years old and above have very little difficulty with these instructions. The entire testing session, including earphone placement, testing, and marking of results, should require approximately 1 minute.


## Pass-Fail Criteria

The ASHA guidelines define failure as absence of response at any test frequency in either ear. Some agencies consider this definition too stringent and have developed a weighting system that gives certain frequencies more priority, much like earlier ASHA guidelines (American Speech and Hearing Association, 1975). Again, to simplify decision-making processes, all failures should be referred for rescreening.


## Rescreening

When ASHA's Committee on Audiometric Evaluation revised the guidelines on identification audiometry, it solicited opinions, suggestions, and program plans from a variety of state agencies including state departments of education, departments of health, and so forth. The topic of rescreening elicited more differences of opinion than any other. The ASHA guidelines suggest rescreening within the same session, if at all possible, with a maximum of a 2-week period allowable. Many respondents stated that rescreening within the session was impractical and time-consuming. One individual even offered the rather jaundiced opinion that same-session rescreening might increase the failure rate by encouraging students to remain out of the classroom for an extended time period. Others felt that the 2-week maximum was difficult to comply with because of heavy initial screening schedules. Some offered the view that if failure was due to misunderstanding of instructions, nothing was lost by deferring rescreening, and that if it was because of transient middle ear dysfunction, a longer time period allowed for resolution. Most considered a time lag of 1 month to be sufficient. While each screening agency must establish its own procedures, care should be taken with the rescreening component. The primary goal of the screening program is to identify individuals with hearing loss—not just for identification purposes but to enable targeted students to be referred for appropriate remediation. The longer the time period before rescreening, the greater the opportunity for them to "fall between the cracks" in the system. One month represents more than 10% of a child's total time in the classroom during the school year. In this period of time significant impact can be made on a child's educational experience because of impaired hearing (Northern & Downs, 1984).

The following guidelines represent an abbreviated schedule for pure-tone screening:

1. Test frequencies are 500, 1000, 2000, and 4000 Hz (500 Hz may be omitted if immittance testing is used in conjunction with pure-tone screening).

2. Screening levels are 20 dB HL (ANSI 1969) for all frequencies.

3. Equipment should be regularly calibrated, and daily listening checks are mandatory.

4. Failure is defined as no response at any frequency in either ear.

5. Failures are rescreened within 2 to 4 weeks of original failure.

6. Those failing rescreening should be immediately referred for complete audiologic or medical evaluation.

7. Accurate and timely follow-up records should be maintained.

## Pseudohypacusis

Occasionally every screener will encounter a child whose behavior and subsequent responses to the hearing tests are inconsistent. Usually in younger children the cause can be traced to a misunderstanding of the task or to a reluctance to respond. A brief explanation of the directions coupled with friendly encouragement will often resolve the difficulty. However, there are those children who simply choose to fake a hearing loss. The underlying reasons for this behavior can be as simple as a temporary desire for attention or as complicated as a significant psychological disorder. While the screening tester has neither the time nor, typically, the training to deal with severe functional hearing loss, one should be aware that the problem exists and that the following behaviors may serve as alerting mechanisms:

1. The child responds normally to instruction and/or informal conversation, then fails to respond to even elevated tones in either ear.

2. An exaggerated "listening posture" with facial grimacing and/or pressing the earphone against the ear can occur.

3. Poor eye contact is maintained with the examiner. Occasionally, a child will even break eye contact concurrent with tonal presentation.

4. Sometimes a child, usually very young, will give a negative nod rather than a positive response. In this case a "no" is as good as a "yes" if it is consistent.

It is important to resolve the suspected functional hearing loss at the time of the original screening episode, if at all possible. Often the original inconsistent responses are linked to a misunderstanding of the task. In our zeal to identify disorders, it is possible to convert a child who is merely confused into one with a nonorganic hearing problem. The student is labeled a potential hearing loss and receives certain rewards for this accomplishment in the forms of parental concern, teacher sympathy, preferential classroom treatment, and extra attention. The child may then feel that it is necessary to persist with the charade in order to maintain these benefits. This is a real burden over time and one that should be avoided.

Ross (1964) suggested a simple technique for identifying nonorganic hearing loss in children that is easily accomplished within a screening session. If inconsistencies occur, the examiner can quickly change the task from "listening" to "counting." A tone is randomly presented in short pulses at levels approximately 15 dB above the voluntary threshold and 15 dB below that level. The child is asked to count the number of tones. By diverting attention away from "hearing" and into another area, the functional component may surface. Obviously if the child correctly identifies the total number of tones presented, those below the voluntary threshold were heard.

If, after reinstruction, the suspected functional loss cannot be resolved, the child should be rescreened at a later date. It might be appropriate to identify these cases with some sort of code letter (known only to the examiners) so that special care could be taken at the time of rescreening. A failure upon rescreening should be handled like any other failure and referred for professional management. Discretion should be taken in reporting suspicions of pseudohypacusis to teachers or parents based on screening results. Many factors can account for this. A skillful audiologist can often resolve test inconsistencies without necessary alarm, or a trip to the family physician may be just the impetus to "shape up!" Again, the responsibility of the screening tester is to identify, not diagnose.

# Acoustic Immittance Screening

Although pure-tone screening audiometry has been a common procedure for many years in the school setting, acoustic immittance testing is a relative newcomer for screening purposes. While immittance is a standard test in virtually all clinical settings, Bess and McConnell (1981) found that it is mandated by law in only 11 states. This is probably a significant underestimate of its use, however, since many states leave the decision regarding testing modalities to the local districts. A poll of the three major school districts in the Oklahoma City area indicated that immittance testing is used in two out of three although its use is not mandated by law.

The questions surrounding the use of middle ear analysis primarily center on whether the screening is intended to find educationally significant hearing loss or to identify middle ear disease. After years of investigation, the answer would appear to be "Both."

Several investigators have demonstrated a causal relationship between middle ear disease and learning delays (Brooks, 1976; Gerber & Mencher, 1980; Northern & Downs, 1984). Since many school systems have accepted the responsibility of health management for this population, the use of this sensitive measuring device is both valuable and cost-effective. As in the early days of pure-tone screening, there are controversies surrounding the use of immittance screening. Primary concerns include a lack of standardization of equipment, differing opinions on referral criteria, and inadequate information among testing personnel regarding the natural course and management of middle ear disease. However, the reality is that middle ear dysfunction is a significant problem among school-age children. It has been estimated that more than 400,000 ventilation tubes were fitted as a result of middle ear effusion in 1984, with the overwhelming majority of those procedures performed on children under the age of 12.

## Incidence of Middle Ear Disease

Otitis media is one of the most common diseases of young childhood, with some studies showing that as many as 95% of all children have had at least one episode by the age of 6 (Howie, 1975). Depending on the locale and the time of year, an average kindergarten class of 30 youngsters could have between 5 and 11 with significant middle ear effusion. While it is true that some cases of otitis media will resolve without medical intervention, many will not. All of us who have ever worked in a busy otorhinolaryngology practice can attest to the numbers of children seen with significant conductive hearing loss secondary to adhesive otitis resulting from an untreated episode of otitis media.

Certain groups of children are considered at risk for middle ear dysfunction and should be screened with immittance tests on a priority basis. These include:

1. Children with documented sensorineural hearing losses. Since these students have previously "failed" pure-tone screening, they are sometimes ignored with regard to the ongoing screening process.

2. Children classified as developmentally delayed or learning-disabled.

3. Children having cleft lip or palate or other craniofacial anomalies.

4. Native American children. The incidence of middle ear disease among American Indian children is very high, estimated to be approximately 30 out of 100 for preschoolers and only slightly lower for school-age children (Roberts, 1976).

5. Children with Down syndrome.

## Effectiveness of Immittance Screening

By now it is accepted by most that pure-tone screening alone will fail to identify a considerable number of individuals with middle ear problems. Several studies have demonstrated this fact (Haggard, Wood, & Carroll, 1984; Harkes & Van Wagoner, 1974; Hopkinson & Schramm, 1979; Paradise & Smith, 1978; Renvall, 1980), with some estimating an 80–90% efficiency rate when both pure-tone screening and immittance testing were used, as opposed to a 60–70% rate when pure-tone testing was used alone. The following variables cause this discrepancy:

1. Many children have better than normal hearing levels (better thresholds than audiometric zero) (Haggard et al., 1984). A 30 dB HL hearing loss from middle ear effusion could possibly result in a pass when pure-tone screening is the sole test.

2. Middle ear effusion in its early stages may not result in sufficient elevation of pure-tone thresholds to fail screening levels, thus allowing the situation to go undetected and untreated.

3. The all too frequent practice of raising the screening levels or eliminating 500 Hz because of a poor acoustic environment may fail to identify mild hearing losses.

So if acoustic immittance screening is so efficient, one might ask, why not use it altogether instead of pure-tone testing? There is very little correlation between the tympanometric shapes obtained in immittance screening and hearing levels. When the acoustic reflex is used as a determiner, the relationship improves, but it is still not sufficiently sensitive to warrant its sole use as a screening instrument, particularly when a single 1000 Hz tone is used (Haggard et al., 1984; Renvall, 1980).

In 1979 ASHA adopted guidelines for acoustic immittance screening (American Speech-Language-Hearing Association, 1979). These guidelines generally appear to be followed by most groups, with the exception of the recommendations regarding referral.

## Population

Because immittance testing requires only minimal participation from the individual, it can be performed on most 2-year-olds without difficulty. It also gives valuable information on those groups considered difficult to test. The ASHA guidelines recommend that acoustic immittance testing be used for nursery school (preschool) through fifth grade, with any child previously failing a screening being retested regardless of grade. A survey of the states using immittance screening indicates that most utilize it in conjunction with or as a secondary test after failure of pure-tone screening, thus following the original guidelines regarding population for pure-tone screening of kindergarten through third grade. However, since the enactment of PL 94-142, many school systems have become involved with preschool-aged children, making the use of immittance testing even more attractive.

## Equipment

There are many immittance screening instruments on the market today. Program directors should be sure that the equipment meets their own requirements with regard to ease of operation, maintenance, and calibration. An automatic constant-rate pump and recording system are recommended for screening purposes. Caution should be taken when choosing automatic tympanometers, as some of these devices will continue to print out a tympanogram profile even though the acoustic seal has been broken. Although a flashing or changing light may warn that the seal is compromised, this signal is often missed by an operator who is busy keeping a child still while monitoring a strip chart. This can result in unnecessary referral as well as a lot of wasted paper.

## Air Pressure

The recommended air-pressure range is from $+200$ to $-300$ mm $H_2O$. The greater negative range is to differentiate the significant number of children who display negative middle ear pressure with a peak from those having flat or rounded tympanograms.

## Acoustic Reflex Eliciting Signal

In compliance with the ASHA guidelines, most screening units utilize a 1000 Hz pure tone as the reflex-eliciting tone. A 100 dB HL signal is commonly used with a few units having a 95 dB HL signal. As previously noted, these levels are probably sufficient if used in tandem with pure-tone testing but may miss mild losses or high-frequency losses if used alone. The reflex is defined as a response (needle or meter deflection) that is concurrent with the presentation of a signal. In some automatic units the reflex may be demonstrated with a flashing light or a vertical mark on the strip chart recording.

## Ear Tips

Immittance screening units generally come equipped with the flange-type ear tips that fold back against the canal opening to create a hermetic seal. The tip is usually held snugly against the ear by the tester to maintain that seal. This type of tip is recommended for screening purposes over the rounded, individually sized tips that are inserted into the canal opening. The reasons for this preference are rather obvious. First, a variety of external canal opening diameters can be sealed with a single flange type, thus increasing speed and efficiency. Furthermore, the dangers of deep insertion into the canal with possible abrasion of canal wall and/or accidental retention of tip in the canal are minimized. Finally, comfort to the child is greater with a flange-type tip, thus improving cooperation.

Most manufacturers recommend procedures for the proper care of equipment and ear tips, and it is important that proper hygiene be observed. Tips should be scrubbed after every use with an antiseptic solution. Immittance testing should not be performed on an ear that shows signs of obvious drainage; instead, this child should be referred immediately for medical evaluation. The limited information obtained by immittance screening in such cases is insignificant compared to the potential for contamination and disruption of the screening process as a result of an equipment breakdown.

## Acoustic Reflectometry

In response to criticism concerning immittance equipment and testing, Teele and Teele (1984) introduced and developed an instrument called the acoustic reflectometer. This device resembles a large otoscope and is hand-held to the patient's ear. It consists of a signal generator, microphone, and signal processing circuitry. A tonal stimulus is swept from 1800 Hz to 7000 Hz. The instrument works on the principle of the quarter-wave theory—that is, the energy of the incident and reflective wave from the tympanic membrane is summated and cancelled with the lowest amount of energy (nadir) occurring at the point at which a quarter of the wave length of a reflected frequency is 180 degrees out of phase with the incident wave. The cancellation point is projected as a number, with 1 to 4 considered to be normal reflective values and greater than 4 indicative of middle ear effusion.

The reported advantages of this device are that it does not require a hermetic seal; it is unaffected by cerumen, except for complete impaction; and it can be effectively utilized with crying children. Teele and Teele reported a very high correlation with otoscopic findings of middle ear effusion. However, they reported a specificity rate of 79%, suggesting a possible problem with false positive referrals.

This instrument has achieved some popularity, particularly among pediatricians and family practitioners, because of its ease of operation. However, a later study reported by Buhrer, Hall, and Schuster (1985) indicated that the reflectometer was not adequate as a general screening tool and was the least sensitive testing method when compared with pure-tone screening, immittance testing, and otoscopic examination.

Obviously reflectometry is an interesting idea. As its use becomes more common, additional research will perhaps answer some of the questions still surrounding it. Utilized in conjunction with other screening methods, it may serve to fill a needed gap in the current equipment inventory.

## Pass-Fail Criteria

The pass-fail criteria for pure-tone screening are fairly straightforward. However, the standards for what constitutes failure for immittance testing fall within a gray area.

Table 12.2 summarizes the ASHA classification for pass-fail criteria (American Speech-Language-Hearing Association, 1979). Categories I and III are generally accepted by most organizations involved in mass screening. However, Category II, the at-risk classification, has been criticized by some as being too stringent, resulting in overreferral and/or unnecessary rescreening, or too complicated for untrained volunteers to handle, requiring excessive review by the screening director. There is also concern that labeling these children "at risk" rather than "failure" does not ensure timely rescreening and/or referral.

**TABLE 12.2**
**ASHA Pass-Fail Criteria for Immittance Screening**

| Classification | Results of Initial Screening | Disposition |
| --- | --- | --- |
| I Pass | Middle-ear pressure normal* or mildly positive/negative** and acoustic reflex present*** | Cleared |
| II At Risk | Middle ear pressure abnormal**** (and acoustic reflex present) Acoustic reflex absent (and middle ear pressure normal or mildly positive/negative) | Retest in 3 to 5 weeks. If tympanogram and acoustic reflex fall into Class I, pass. If tympanogram or acoustic reflex remain in Class II, fail and refer. |
| III Fail | Middle ear pressure abnormal and acoustic reflex absent | Refer |

 * Normal: Pressure peak in range ± 50 mm $H_2O$

 ** Mildly positive/negative: +50 to +100 mm $H_2O$/−50 to −200 mm $H_2O$

 *** Present: Pen or meter needle deflection judged to be coincident with the reflex-eliciting stimulus at levels of 100 dB HL for contralateral stimulation, 105 dB HL for ipsilateral stimulation at 1000 Hz

 **** Abnormal peak outside the range described for Classification I

*Source:* American Speech-Language-Hearing Association (1979, p. 286).

A survey of agencies performing screening shows a significant number who have simplified their pass-fail criteria for immittance screening to be consistent with the pure-tone guidelines. Table 12.3 shows an example of these simplified criteria. The ±100 mm $H_2O$ middle ear pressure peak is the point at which most otolaryngologists feel that treatment intervention is warranted (Howie, 1975). Therefore, it appears to be a good place for differentiation between normal and abnormal. However, some care should be taken when using this criterion as some children who pass the screening may be in the beginning stages of middle ear infections. If this simplified paradigm is used, it is very important that the acoustic reflex information be utilized and documented.

**TABLE 12.3**
**Simplified Pass/Fail Criteria**

| Classification | Test Findings | Disposition |
|---|---|---|
| Pass | Normal middle ear pressure* Acoustic reflex present** | Cleared |
| Fail | Abnormal middle ear pressure*** (reflex present or absent) Normal middle ear pressure (reflex absent) | Rescreen within 2 to 4 weeks. If results fall into Fail category after rescreening, refer for audiologic or medical evaluation. |

* Pressure peak occurring at ± 100 mm $H_2O$

** Meter response coincident with stimulation of 1000 Hz tone at 100 dB HL delivered either contralaterally or ipsilaterally

*** Pressure peak greater than ± 100 mm $H_2O$ or rounded or "flat" tympanogram

## Rescreening

Whatever pass-fail criteria are used, rescreening is a mandatory part of any immittance screening program. The transient nature and fluctuation of hearing loss in childhood middle ear disease is well documented. A fine line must be drawn between overreferral, with the attendant drain on professional and financial resources, and the necessity to ensure timely treatment and management for those children who require it. Although ASHA guidelines recommend rescreening within 3 to 5 weeks for the at-risk group and immediate referral for the failures, several studies have demonstrated a significant reduction in overreferral if all in Categories II and III are rescreened prior to referral (Roeser & Northern, 1981; Roush & Tait, 1985). Ideally, rescreening should be accomplished within 1 month of the original failure with appropriate referral made thereafter.

# Referral

Although identification is the primary responsibility of the screening program, the relative value and success of the program depends upon timely referral and accurate follow-up. Figure 12.1 represents a flowchart for screening, rescreening, referral, and follow-up.

In a majority of those agencies surveyed, referral is recommended to the parents for medical evaluation through the private physician. "Local realities" are often cited as the reason for this practice. While many speech and hearing personnel would prefer direct referral to an audiologist or an otolaryngologist, this is neither practical nor even possible in many situations. Moreover, the child's private physician is familiar with his or her overall medical history and is a known figure in the parent's lives. This often facilitates compliance with medical recommendations.

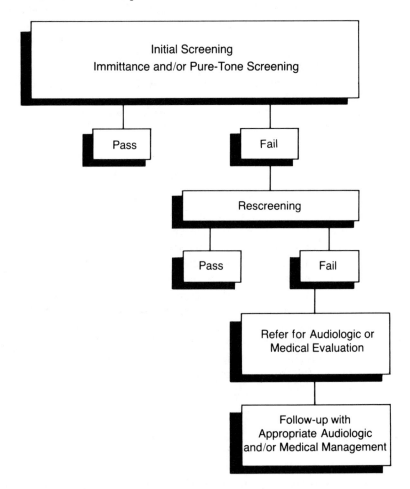

**Figure 12.1.** Screening flowchart

Notification to parents should impart the necessity for prompt attention without causing undue alarm. An example of such a notification form is seen in Figure 12.2. The information is transmitted with recommendation for follow-up. The form includes space for a brief notation by the examiner, who then returns the form to the screening director. One of the best forms that I have seen is made of sturdy paper perforated across the lower portion with the address of the referral source imprinted on the opposite side. After evaluation, the examiner simply notes the findings and recommendations and mails the post-card-size form back to the screening agency. While this type would be more costly than regular paper forms, the time saved in checking for lost forms would appear to be worth it. Since the screening director is responsible not only for the screening activities but for rescreening, referral, and follow-up, efficiency is important during every step.

# Training Personnel

Armed with guidelines, forms, and suggestions for implementation, the audiologist's next step in designing a screening program is to train those individuals who will do the actual screening. The following outline shows a suggested curriculum guide for screeners.

Hearing

    Basic anatomy

    Disorders of hearing

    Impact of hearing loss on speech/language/educational development

The Screening Program

    Program goals

    Test procedures

    Calibration and maintenance of equipment

    Administration, record keeping, and follow-up

School _____

Dear Parent,

Results of your child's hearing tests at school indicate a need for further evaluation. Medical examination by an ear specialist and/or family physician is recommended.

After your child's examination is completed, please return the physician's report of findings and recommendations to the school.

Please feel free to call me if you have any questions or need assistance in obtaining services.

Sincerely,

_____        _____

Date                       School Nurse

-----------------------------------------------------------------------------------

_____        _____    _____

Name of Student                            Grade      Teacher

SCHOOL TEST RESULTS:

|  | Right Ear |  |  |  |  |  |  | Left Ear |  |  |  |  |
|---|---|---|---|---|---|---|---|---|---|---|---|---|
| 250 | 500 | 1000 | 2000 | 4000 | 6000 | | 250 | 500 | 1000 | 2000 | 4000 | 6000 |

_____ Impedance (tympanometer) test results indicate potential medical problem.

PHYSICIAN'S REPORT TO SCHOOL:
Findings and Recommendations _____

_____

_____        _____

Date of Examination        Signature of Examiner

**Figure 12.2.** Notification to parents. From *Handbook for School Health Nursing*, 1983, Oklahoma City: Putnam City Schools Health Services. Reprinted by permission.

Special Areas of Responsibilities

Conditioning technique for very young or difficult-to-test children

Counseling parents

Interaction with professional and medical personnel

This training could be accomplished in 8 to 15 hours, with allowances made for a hands-on practicum. Screeners should be provided with manuals that can be used as reference. Usually, these seminars are best done at the beginning of the school year. In large systems with moderate personnel turnover, it may be prudent to offer the training courses every year. In other situations, less frequent offerings with shortened refresher programs may suffice.

# Testing Preschoolers

Although screening audiometry is generally used for school-age children, many screening programs are also involved with the younger ages, such as with Head Start programs and developmental preschool classrooms. The case has been made previously for the advantages of immittance testing with younger children. The reader is referred to Bess and McConnell (1981) for a lengthy list of suggestions to help keep little ones amused and sufficiently quiet so that immittance testing can be accomplished.

The following simple conditioning techniques can be utilized to ensure valid pure-tone screening:

1. Squeaky toys can be made to "talk" every time the tone is heard.

2. Blocks can be tossed in a bucket.

3. The child can be instructed to clap the hands as a response.

4. Mechanical toys can be used as a "reward stimulus" for response.

I would discourage the use of sweetened cereals or candy for conditioning since it is impossible in a mass screening to determine possible food allergies. Although examiners may feel that one would encounter a fairly large number of younger children who are uncooperative, this has not been my experience nor that of others. Hopkinson and Schramm (1979) reported that less than 1% of the 2,125 preschoolers in their screening study refused to be tested. A friendly smile and positive attitude will often modify noncompliant behavior.

## Cost-Effectiveness

When one calculates the cost of a hearing screening program, the following factors must be considered:

1. The salary of the examiners is the single largest cost, which is the reason many school systems give for using volunteers. However, someone must direct and supervise the program, making part of that salary accountable to the screening budget.

2. The cost of equipment and proper maintenance must be considered.

3. Supplies, particularly forms, are a continuing expense.

4. Less tangible costs, such as examiner's time, training time, and time spent in administrative tasks, must be calculated.

Cooper, Gates, Owen, and Dickson (1975) proposed the following formula for calculating cost per child of screening:

$$\text{Cost/child} = \frac{S}{R} + \frac{C + (M \times L)}{N \times L}$$

C = Cost of Equipment

S = Salary of screening personnel per hour

L = Life of equipment (years)

M = Annual maintenance cost

R = Screening rate per hour

N = Number screened per year

Depending on the sizes of the groups screened, the costs per child for pure-tone audiometric screening are usually about 30¢–40¢; immittance testing costs an additional 20¢–45¢. Naturally, bigger screening populations wil reduce the cost per child. Compared to hours of wasted teaching time, not to mention the loss of classroom participation that can occur from untreated middle ear disease, 75¢–85¢ per child seems to be a bargain.

## Summary

It is clear that the identification of hearing loss in preschool- and school-age children is an important aspect of general health care and educational management for these groups. Although the history of screening reveals difficulties and less than ideal results at times, the overall impact of these programs has been positive (Bess & McConnell, 1981; Brooks, 1976; Hopkinson & Schramm, 1979; Roeser & Northern, 1981; Vargo, 1980). The most critical features of a good hearing screening program are an adequate acoustic environment for testing, appropriately calibrated and maintained equipment, and competently trained and skilled testing personnel. Additionally, if timely referral and aggressive follow-up are provided, the potential for a successful program is very good indeed.

# References

American National Standards Institute. (1970). *American National Standard specifications for audiometers, ANSI S3.6-1969.* New York: American National Standards Institute.

American National Standards Institute. (1977). *American National Standard criteria for background noise in audiometer rooms, ANSI S3.1-1977.* New York: American National Standards Institute.

American Speech and Hearing Association. (1975). Guidelines for identification audiometry. *Asha, 17,* 94–99.

American Speech-Language-Hearing Association. (1982). Joint Committee on Infant Hearing: Position statement. *Asha, 24,* 1017–1018.

American Speech-Language-Hearing Association. Committee on Audiometric Evaluation. (1982). *Calibration of pure-tone air-conduction signals delivered via earphones.* Rockville, MD: American Speech-Language-Hearing Association.

American Speech-Language-Hearing Association. (1979). Guidelines for acoustic immittance screening of middle ear function. *Asha, 21,* 283–288.

American Speech-Language-Hearing Association. (1985). Guidelines for identification audiometry. *Asha, 27,* 40, 49–52.

Benson, R. C. (1971). Auraldomes for audiometric testing. *National Hearing Aid Journal, 24,* 14, 42.

Bess, F., & McConnell, F. (1981). The challenge of hearing impairment in children. In *Audiology, education and the hearing-impaired child* (pp. 82–107). St. Louis: C. V. Mosby.

Brooks, D. (1976). School screening for middle ear effusions. *Annals of Otology, Rhinology, and Laryngology, 85,* 223–228.

Buhrer, K., Hall, L. G., & Schuster, L. (1985). The acoustic reflectometer as a screening device: A comparison. *Ear and Hearing, 6,* 307–314.

Cooper, J., Gates, G., Owen, J., & Dickson, H. (1975). An abbreviated impedance bridge technique for school screening. *Journal of Speech and Hearing Disorders, 40,* 260–269.

Corliss, L, & Watson, J. (1961, March). A school system studies the effectiveness of routine audiometry. *Journal of Health Physical Education Record of NEA, 27.*

Darley, F. L. (Ed.). (1961). Identification audiometry for school age children: Basic procedures. *Journal of Speech and Hearing Disorders* (Monograph suppl. 9).

Downs, M. P., Doster, M. E., & Weaver, M. (1965). Dilemmas in identification audiometry. *Journal of Speech and Hearing Disorders, 30,* 360–364.

Eagles, E., Wishik, S., & Doerfler, L. (1967). Hearing sensitivity and ear disease in children: A prospective study. *Laryngoscope* (Suppl. 274).

Gerber, S. E., & Mencher, G. T. (1980). *Auditory dysfunction.* Houston: College-Hill Press.

Griffing, T. S., Simonton, K. M., & Hedgecock, L. D. (1967). Verbal auditory screening for pre-school children. *Transactions of the American Academy of Opthalmology and Otolaryngology, 71,* 105–111.

Haggard, M. P., Wood, E. J., & Carroll, S. (1984). Speech, admittance and tone tests in school screening. *British Journal of Audiology, 18,* 133–153.

Harkes, L., & Van Wagoner, R. (1974). Application of impedance audiometry as a screening instrument. *Acta Otolaryngologica, 77,* 198–201.

Hollien, H., & Thompson, C. L. (1967). A group screening test of hearing. *Journal of Auditory Research, 7,* 85–92.

Hopkinson, N. T., & Schramm, V. L. (1979). Preschool otologic and audiologic screening. *Otolaryngology, Head and Neck Surgery, 87,* 246–257.

Howie, V. W. (1975). Natural history of otitis media. *Annals of Otology, Rhinology, and Laryngology* (Suppl. 19), 67–72.

Johnston, P. (1948). The Massachusetts hearing test. *Journal of the Acoustical Society of America, 20,* 697–703.

Katt, D., & Sprague, H. (1981). Determining the pure-tone frequencies to be used in identification audiometry. *Journal of Speech and Hearing Disorders, 46,* 433–36.

Mahoney, T. (1984). High-risk screening for large general newborn populations. *Seminars in Hearing, 5,* 25–36.

Mencher, G. T., & McCulloch, B. F. (1970). Auditory screening of kindergarten children using the VASC. *Journal of Speech and Hearing Disorders, 35,* 241–247.

Northern, J. L., & Downs, M. P. (1984). *Hearing in children* (3rd ed.). Baltimore: Williams and Wilkins.

Paradise, J. L., & Smith, C. G. (1978). Impedance screening for preschool children—State of the art. In E. R. Harford, F. H. Bess, C. D. Bluestone, & J. O. Klein (Eds.), *Impedance screening for middle ear diseases in children.* New York: Grune and Stratton.

Reger, S., & Newby, H. A. (1947). A group pure-tone hearing test. *Journal of Speech and Hearing Disorders, 12,* 61–66.

Renvall, U. (1980). Screening procedure for detection of middle ear and cochlear disease. *Annals of Otorhinolaryngology* (Suppl. 68), 214–216.

Renvall, U., Liden, G., Jungert, S., & Nilsson, E. (1973). Impedance audiometry as screening method in school children. *Scandinavian Audiology, 2,* 133–137.

Roberts, M. (1976). Comparative study of pure-tone, impedance and otoscopic hearing screening methods. *Archives of Otolaryngology, 102,* 690–694.

Roeser, R., & Northern, J. L. (1981). Screening for hearing loss and middle ear disorders. In R. Roeser & M. Downs (Eds.), *Auditory disorders in school children* (pp. 120–150). New York: Thieme-Stratton.

Ross, M. (1964). The variable intensity pulse count method (VICPM) for the detection and measurement of the pure-tone thresholds of children with functional hearing loss. *Journal of Speech and Hearing Disorders, 29,* 477–482.

Roush, J., & Tait, C. (1985). Pure-tone and acoustic immittance screening of preschool aged children: An examination of referral criteria. *Ear and Hearing, 6,* 245–250.

Savory, P., & Ferron, P. (1982). Screening of hearing disorders in school children. *American Journal of Otolaryngology, 3,* 388–391.

Talbott, R. E. (1969). Bacteriology of earphone contamination. *Journal of Speech and Hearing Research, 12,* 326–329.

Teele, D. H., & Teele, J. (1984). Detection of middle ear effusion by acoustic reflectometry. *Pediatrics, 104,* 832–838.

Vargo, S. W. (1980). Auditory screening in the schools. *Journal of School Health, 50,* 32–34.

Wilson, W. L., & Walton, W. K. (1978). Public school audiometry. In F. N. Martin (Ed.), *Pediatric Audiology* (pp. 390–445). Englewood Cliffs, NJ: Prentice-Hall.

# 13

# Audiology in the Public School Setting

## VICTOR P. GARWOOD

$T$he practice of audiology in our public schools has burgeoned despite cyclic flurries in the federal political arena. Although statistics vary according to their sources, the number of public school audiologists seems to have increased over the past decade from around 700 to 1,000, or about 15% of a total of some 6,000 audiologists currently registered as members of the American Speech-Language-Hearing Association. The number of full-time school audiologists is not known. In a recent study Wilson-Vlotman and Blair (1986) found that 245 out of 415 individuals in the study sample were functioning as full-time audiologists in the schools. This study investigated demographic characteristics, practices, attitudes, and educational settings of this population. Berg and his colleagues (Berg, Blair, & Wilson-Vlotman, 1984) have compiled a directory that should be of interest to students and public school personnel. He lists 571 specialists, most of whom are school audiologists. The directory cites figures based on a survey of 86 accredited university training programs in audiology. Replies were received from 64 program administrators from 26 states that indicated training programs were preparing students for the case management role in educational audiology and providing a public school experience in educational audiology. At least 150 to 200 students received public school experience during 1982–83. The directory also cites state certification in 22 states and a total of 306 school districts with programs in educational audiology.

The impetus for these increases, of course, is intimately related to the passage of PL 94-142 in 1975 and, more recently, PL 98-199 in 1983. By these acts, the public schools became the primary providers of services for handicapped children of school age. Training programs for future professionals whose interest lay chiefly with school-age children should have therefore changed the foci of their curricula. Unfortunately, the politics of higher education have made such changes difficult to execute.

Local school administrators may still be confused about the role of the school audiologist. School administrators tend to assume that teachers of the hearing-impaired have sufficient time to deal with audiologic issues, not realizing that a standard teaching load is a full-time responsibility. Training institutions with audiologic curricula have made similar assumptions, stating that their training programs will adequately prepare students for entry into the public schools. As a former full-time audiologist in a large public school system, I have observed the absolute need for continuous observation and monitoring procedures by audiologic personnel within the school system. Generally speaking, schools are reluctant to exchange information with outside agencies, a consequence of legislation relating to the privacy of school records. Parents are reluctant to take their children out of school for clinical treatment while school is in session.

One of the first impressions of the new school audiologist is the enormous range of hearing impairments, ranging from mild unilateral to severely handicapping bilateral losses accompanied by a multiplicity of other problems. The audiologist will also find other problems: children whose hearing aids will not work; children wearing hearing aids who do not need them; children who reject body aids for ear-level aids; children with minimal impairment who are fitted with high-power aids; and children whose only exposure to amplification is with school-purchased auditory training units that are used only when school is in session. The audiologist will be shocked, and understandably so, by the high incidence of middle ear infections, along with severe sensorineural impairment, parental neglect, and generally poor hygiene. With regard to proper program placement, the audiologist will be startled by the lack of prior otoaudiologic evaluative data, which should, of course, be of paramount importance.

When knowledge of the availability of audiologic services filters down to the teachers, the audiologist is bombarded with requests to see their pupils, generally because of an amplification problem. One of the most disruptive problems and chronic concerns for the audiologist is the development of a priority system that will satisfy not only the teachers but also the counselors, nurses, and principals as well.

The rewards for conscientious clinicians become apparent when, because of their intervention, the child begins to succeed as an active participant in the educational process. The audiologist's services are always needed, despite the current wave of financial conservatism sweeping over our school systems. It may well be, however, that as they do their jobs, the relatively small force of audiologists presently employed by public schools will prove to be in an area where the requirements may far surpass all present clinical opportunities for employment.

Because the majority of school audiologists will be employed by large school districts, the thrust of this chapter will be aimed accordingly. Smaller districts will undoubtedly join forces to hire audiologists on a shared-time basis. Certainly all school districts share one area of concern— all have hearing-impaired children and few audiologists to serve them. By using the Los Angeles Unified School District as an example, I will describe some of the responsibilities, problems, and satisfactions of school audiologists at a moment in history that is characterized by significant changes in the management of handicapped children.

# A Decade of Progress, 1975–1985

This section assumes knowledge of the purpose of PL 94-142 and its impact upon the public schools. Essentially the law assures all handicapped children between the ages of 3 and 21 of a free and appropriate education in the least restrictive environment. What follows is a brief summary of events of relative importance to school audiologists since the advent of that legislation in 1975.

## PL 98-199 (1983)

The purpose of PL 98-199 was to amend PL 94-142. The amendments contained the following provisions:

1. To revise and extend ten discretionary program authorities.

2. To provide authorization levels for fiscal years 1984, 1985, and 1986.

3. To establish one new discretionary program in the area of secondary and transition services.

4. To establish the authority for the Secretary of Education to bypass the state education agency to provide services to private-school handicapped children in states where such services are prohibited by law.

Of particular interest to audiologists and speech pathologists is Section 623, titled "Early Education for Handicapped Children." This section provides additional financial incentives for states to develop model early childhood projects to aid handicapped children and extend services from birth to 3 years of age. This new initiative expands the current program and has been formalized in the Education Act Amendments of 1986 (PL 99-457) (99th Congress produces "landmark" legislation, 1987). Funding for grants is determined by a state's needs rather than the size of its population or demographic characteristics. The state plan must meet the needs of all preschool handicapped children.

Counseling achieves even more importance with the implementation of this law. The importance of counseling parents whose children are in the infancy stage is not to be restricted to the teacher of the deaf and hard-of-hearing child but also is to include the school audiologist, who can interpret test results and evaluate amplification requirements. The audiologist ranks with the pediatrician, otolaryngologist, and teacher as a member of this counseling team.

Of equal importance, Section 602 adds "speech- and language-impaired" in the definition of handicapped children. This section also adds a new focus on technical assistance in addition to direct services previously provided for deaf-blind children and youth.

Audiologists have been frustrated by the limits previously imposed by the minimum 3-year age level. Their concern must be translated into action at the district level. As a conservative estimate, I would say that several years may elapse before the states modify their own regulations to accommodate the provisions of this significant law.

## School Employees Versus Contractual Services

I hesitate to approach this sensitive issue because of my bias toward the use of full-time school audiologists rather than outside contractors. At the same time, I recognize the public and administrative pressures being put on all public services. The argument by our present administration seems to be that private contractual services are cheaper and therefore advantageous to taxpayers. "Civil service" is apparently anathema to a number of influential lawmakers, and they may be right. I prefer to defer this issue, cowardly, by considering this movement a sign of the times. Types and levels of services between the public and the private sector lack definition. We may also be forced to develop more precise definitions of medical versus educational approaches to communicatively handicapped children (and adults).

## Computers and Audiology

Now that we have been ushered into the age of the computer, any journal one picks up will have at least one article on the use of a computer for making our task easier, quicker, and more accurate. I find no fault with this argument. Software seems to be the crucial issue. School districts are being offered attractive bargains for hardware, but consultation in its use is apparently sparse, so computers may be gathering dust not only in the workplace but also in the home. Schools need computers to eliminate onerous statistical tasks, as well as special-purpose computers as augmentative communication devices for seriously handicapped children with orthopedic problems, but I balk at their use as instruments designed expressly to function as diagnosticians.

Special-purpose computerized devices in the area of auditory testing are beginning to show us hitherto unknown functions of the lower auditory pathways leading to the brainstem. As a matter of fact, there may even be a plethora of such devices in the present marketplace. This physiological test instrument shows much promise in exploring the neurological maturity of the auditory system. In California, for example, all children at risk in neonatal intensive care units who are eligible for and enrolled in the California Children's Program are mandated by law to be screened by this method or by "Cribometry," a computerized system of registering significant body movements in response to an auditory stimulus.

Computerized hearing-aid fitting is still in its experimental stage—a highly personal matter between the dispenser and the patient. We shall see whether the fitting process is an art or a "computer-friendly" science.

## Our Émigré Children

Our entire country is confronted with the tremendous task of educating immigrant children, some of whom have come to the United States with exotic diseases. Some of the diseases are irreversible, some chronic. A common problem, upper respiratory disease, has in general been poorly treated and is now a significant problem for public health agencies. In Los Angeles County, for example, 84 different languages and dialects are spoken in the home and on the streets. The city of Los Angeles is now divided by areas (and ghettos) where only a native language is spoken. These ethnic groups now account for the majority of children enrolled in the Los Angeles public schools. Bilingual and even trilingual teachers are at a premium. The impact of this situation is obvious to personnel in special education, where a close relationship must be maintained between the school, the child, and the family. The issue is particularly sensitive in the area of preschool education. Arguments are presented either to promote early instruction in the child's native language or to reject such a practice as being contrary to laws regarding language instruction in the public schools. Audiologists would be well advised to learn some basic foreign language skills through language tapes and develop auditory test materials in foreign languages relevant to their geographical area. A few East Asian word tapes, for example, have been developed in the Los Angeles area as speech intelligibility materials.

## Oral-Aural, Manual, and Total Communication

Manual communication has apparently become more prevalent as a communication instrument in our special schools. True, it is presented as a combined method (total communication) but remains chiefly manual. Increasingly, audiologists are learning and utilizing sign language and fingerspelling. It is an "exotic" language that has been well dramatized on the stage and television and has gained acceptance by the public. The University of Southern California, for example, has set up a two-semester undergraduate course sequence in manual communication. Surprisingly, the course has been offered each semester and is composed of students from a number of departments in the university. My former colleagues in the audiology unit of the Los Angeles school district are now becoming proficient in this art. It has its place in the schools, provided all steps have been taken at the early childhood level to investigate the oral-aural approach to communication. The basic problem with manual communication is whether its sole use will lead to social restriction and isolation.

## Amplification

The past 10 years have brought significant improvements in acoustic amplification and ear-mold design. Unfortunately, most of the advances have concentrated largely on miniaturization—not always an accurate criterion for excellence. This is not to say that technological advances such as input compression should be slighted as a distinct advance in electronic circuitry. But more significant are the advances being made toward the use of digital rather than analog circuits of hearing aids. We can hope that advances in the amplifier and the receiver will one day match the excellence of the electret microphone.

Vibrotactile aids are still on the market, despite the relative insensitivity of the skin and its pathways to the cerebral cortex as compared with the high sensitivity of the auditory system, an adjunctive system that has been only superficially explored. We may be surprised when we learn more of the basics of neurotransmitter physiology. In the meanwhile, clinicians report that the vibrotacticle devices are helpful for selected and seriously impaired children.

## Noisy Classrooms

The landmark studies of Cohen (e.g., Cohen, Evans, Krantz, & Stokols, 1980), although not nearing culmination, have delineated variables important in attenuating noise in our schools. Noise may have a greater negative effect on children wearing hearing aids than normal-hearing children. Their findings suggest that as the length of noise exposure increases, children are more, rather than less, disturbed by auditory distractions. Their studies related to schools under aircraft patterns are being extended to traffic noise and longitudinal data on children attending schools near airports. Audiologists should therefore notify administrators of the results of these studies when new classroom additions are in the planning stage.

## Implants

Although cochlear implant procedures and accompanying hardware were utilized in the early 1960s, it was well into the 1970s before the technique began to appear in the popular literature. The present status of some eight techniques of implant procedures has been reviewed by Miller and Pfingst (1984). In 1984 the House single-electrode procedure was approved by the Federal Drug Administration. Undoubtedly other approaches will soon be approved. Now that the technique has been performed on young children of school age, schools are now concerned with a number of questions. How are schools to deal with these children? How does the central nervous system translate these electrical signals into a linguistic code that can be perceived as communicative processing to a prelinguistic hearing-impaired child? After the surgeon has successfully implanted the electrode and after the hardware is connected, who is responsible for monitoring the device? Obviously a long unknown road of habilitation must follow. Auxiliary hearing aids? Sophisticated auditory processing devices? Yes and no. The nitty-gritty must be performed by the school. Day-to-day data must come from the school personnel: audiologists, teachers, psychologists, and linguists. Parents must also be trained to relay formalized observations to the schools. The procedure is still experimental and will remain so until we know much more about the parameters of speech recognition, perception, and production. Perhaps it is too much for the schools to handle at this time. The children, however, are there to be served and must be served. A solid link must be forged between the surgeon, the engineer, the audiologist, the linguist, and the teacher.

### Parents and Babies

The role of the parent or parent surrogate deserves a special section in any text on child behavior, but it is most pertinent when describing children with special needs. In the area of pediatric audiology I feel that no one has written better on the subject of counseling parents than Luterman (1979). This small book is one of those timeless jewels of inspired writing that are meant to be read and contemplated.

Counseling plays an important role in the Home-Based Infant Program designed for hearing-impaired children between birth and 3 years of age. This program, an integral part of the program for the deaf and hard of hearing in the Los Angeles city schools, was developed with federal and state discretionary funds. According to the coordinator for the program, "The primary intent of the Home-Based Infant Program is to stimulate the development of the child's language skills, and to provide parent education. [And] parents are the primary teachers of their very young child. To facilitate parents' success, the teachers provide appropriate techniques to stimulate language development, and serve as models for the parents" (Lieberman, personal communication, 1984). The program includes both the oral-aural as well as the total communication approach to speech and language.

# School Procedures

A new audiology program in the schools can produce considerable confusion at all levels of the school hierarchy. Personnel should be informed at an early stage that there are differences as well as similarities between audiologists and audiometrists.

The sole function of audiometrists in the Los Angeles Unified School District, for example, is to identify the hearing-impaired child by conventional pure-tone test methods and report such findings to the school administration. The audiometrist's academic preparation is specified by California law and consists of the successful completion of a few units of undergraduate preparation in audiometry and hearing conservation, with the additional specification of valid credentials, which may be earned in an area of health and development (e.g., teaching exceptional children). This program is highly restrictive and involves no clinical management.

In theory, audiologists pick up where audiometrists leave off. Their concern is the management of those children whose pure-tone screening results are above a normative threshold criterion specified by law. Children with unilateral losses, however, should be rated with a relatively low priority when compared with children possessing equal or greater bilateral losses. The actual priority differential may be directly related to regulation by third-party payees, such as the California Children's Program and Medicaid, which may not supply hearing aids to children with unilateral losses. At this stage, the school audiologist may have to assume the role of a clinical or diagnostic audiologist, performing additional diagnostic tests on individuals. Because the audiometer furnished the audiometrist is generally the portable pure-tone type, speech tests in sound-treated quarters are required.

In a sense, then, school audiologists are diagnosticians, although they may be generally restricted to those speech tests designated as conventional—that is, speech awareness threshold, word identification score, speech reception threshold under earphones and in a sound field. Immittance testing (tympanometry and acoustic reflex) is also a valuable assessment tool so long as access is provided to a physician who is skilled in the examination of the ear canal and tympanic membrane. The current training programs have now caught up with technology to the extent that audiologists know how and when to perform immittance testing. Special tests such as auditory brainstem response audiometry must be performed in quarters where medical support is immediately available. Practically speaking, the testing program, although necessary, should be secondary to the audiologist's other responsibilities, which will shortly be explained. If the pupil has a personal hearing aid, the schools may request a reassessment, both aided and unaided, even though the child has been tested in an outside clinic. It is at this point that a conflict may be generated between the school and the clinic regarding this retest procedure.

In my experience, clinics are usually very cooperative, particularly if the parents are unable to bring the child in for a reevaluation. The basic responsibilities of the school audiologist—in contrast with those of the clinical audiologist—are as follows:

1. Day-to-day or week-to-week monitoring of hearing-aid usage

2. Conducting hearing-aid performance checks

3. Conducting auditory training as a part of the school curriculum

4. Scheduling frequent and consistent conferences with classroom teachers

5. Monitoring the acoustic characteristics of the classroom and the school in general

6. Developing an auditory skills program.

It may well be that in the future clinical pediatric audiologists will restrict their function to diagnostic procedures, leaving the entire hearing-aid evaluation and follow-up procedures to the school audiologist (Garwood, 1979). Furthermore, the entire evaluation procedure, which consists of testing earmold impressions and subsequent hearing-aid fitting, may be performed in the schools. Such procedures for ocular problems are presently being implemented in the city schools of Los Angeles. Precedents have already been established in eyeglass fitting in one of the PTA clinics in the district. The same should hold true for the fitting and dispensing of hearing aids for the hearing-impaired. California's Children's Services Program has shown a supportive attitude toward this concept. In California, as with other states, the audiologist would be required to satisfy the current licensing law related to dispensing.

## Tests and Equipment

The requisites for adequate testing are expensive, whether the testing is done in permanent environments or in mobile units. In districts where agencies and hospitals are plentiful, it is unnecessary to purchase the sophisticated equipment available at such clinics. Purchases should be restricted to the level required for conventional pure-tone and speech testing. Such equipment should contain booster amplifiers and loud-speakers for hearing-aid checks and evaluations. Also required is an immittance measuring device with an X-Y plotter. A simple circuit with suitable toy stimuli for conditioned orienting response (COR) audiometry has proved most helpful. The test room should conform to ANSI specifications and be large enough to hold at least two people—the child and a second audiologist or aide for working with difficult-to-test children. An inexpensive and useful device to aid the test room assistant is a simple circuit containing a battery-charged amplifier-microphone for use by the control-room audiologist. Fed through the wall to a monaural headset, this device enables the tester to instruct the assistant without going through the master control panel of the audiometer. This device more than pays for itself in just one test session with a difficult child.

## Earphone Calibration—Sound Level Meter

In the long run, it will pay a school district to invest in a combined sound-level meter and artificial ear kit to calibrate earphones as well as evaluate noise levels in the classroom. An octave or one-third octave band filter accessory is desirable, as the audiologist may be called on to take measurements at locations where complaints are common: classrooms, cafeterias, hallways, playgrounds, auditoriums, and the neighborhood in general.

## Hearing Aid Analyzer

Devices for measuring the electroacoustic characteristics of amplification systems have undergone many changes over the years. Instead of an instrument rack composed of four or five expensive laboratory components at a fixed location, an array of portable units is now available. Such equipment may yield the type of information required for an overall estimate of hearing-aid performance. These units have also proved to be an essential adjunct to the understanding of amplification at the school level by personnel other than the audiologist who can gain some insight into the role played by the hearing aid. The anechoic chamber should be large enough to test both personal aids and auditory training units.

Although the school personnel involved in purchasing the equipment cited above may be appalled by the expense, none of the foregoing equipment is superfluous, and the cost is actually small when compared with equipment required for other programs for physically handicapped children. The justification for these expenses should be confirmed by the passage of federal and state laws mentioned previously.

## Amplification

*Hearing Aids.*   Within the varying legal definitions specifying hearing loss levels, the crucial task of the audiologist in the public schools is to be assured that the hearing-impaired child wears suitable amplification. If audiologic services are new to the district, a position paper on amplification should be presented to the schools explaining concisely the role of the audiologist as a member of the team skilled in the use of auditory amplification.

School audiologists may have little to say about the prior otoaudiologic evaluation and the hearing-aid fitting, but they are in the position to comment about the fitting as a positive factor in the educational process. There is nothing more discouraging than to find that children with beatific expressions on their face have no batteries in their cases or that the units have not been turned on. There is also the child who enters the classroom with the hearing aid in its box, not having used it since school was over the day before. Even more pathetic is the child who comes to school without the hearing aid because the parent "forgot." These examples, common experiences of school audiologists, are a reflection on prior care. The assumption is made that the child is "responsible," but hearing-impaired children, like all children, have to learn responsibility. The occasional trips to the otologist and the audiologist must be reinforced in the school. It is imperative that the school audiologist be trained for such a task.

Accomplishing this objective is not at all simple. The audiologist must work closely with each school principal to inform parents of their role in this situation. Parents should be not only notified of their responsibility to see that the hearing aid is working before the child goes off to school in the morning, but also encouraged, if not coerced, into attending both individual and group information and guidance sessions at the schools (Ross, 1976). Home visits may be required, but should be made only with the advice and approval of the principal. Often parents feel that once their child has completed a specialized preschool program, their responsibility is over and the school will take charge. Other parents have had their child in a residential school where presumably such needs were met.

When the child walks into the classroom, however, the legal responsibility for that child is vested in the classroom teacher, whether it is a special school, integrated class, or regular classroom. It then becomes the responsibility of the audiologist as a resource specialist to render such services as will augment the teacher's role, services that are mutually decided on by both parties. Oftentimes the role of resource personnel in the schools is not clearly defined. The classroom teacher working with handicapped children is confronted by such a formidable array of consultants that continuity in the educational process is almost impossible. It is essential that the audiologist assure the principal and the classroom teachers collectively that individual service is integral to the learning process and must occur at times of mutual convenience. The old criticism of "speech teachers yanking children out of the classroom" may well be leveled at the audiologist unless an intervention program is carefully planned in advance. By knowing a teacher's lesson plans in advance and working around them, both the audiologist and the teacher will achieve their own objectives, with the child receiving a continuity of service appropriate to his or her needs.

The method of providing services will vary with the educational setting. In the regular school the audiologist may begin the year with a demonstration of the function of hearing aids, charts of the ear, and simple explanations of hearing impairment. By using the child's own hearing aid as an example, the audiologist can check its performance. Subsequent monitoring can be more direct and probably more acceptable to the child, the rest of the class, and the teacher. In the integrated class and at special schools, a period of time scheduled for checking both personal hearing aids and classroom units is beneficial so that the learning process is not disrupted.

The above discussion presupposes that the audiologic work load will allow for such individualized attention. It is most unlikely, however, that the audiologist can afford this much time, especially if four or five schools must be served. If aides are available, the audiologist can train an aide to perform such tasks as checking the battery, earmolds, tubes, and cord continuity.

In other settings, audiologists have arranged in-service sessions for the teacher. This technique, however, produces varying levels of success. Many teachers, knowing that an audiologist has been assigned to the school, prefer to assume that the monitoring task will be performed by the audiologist and are inclined to "forget" or pass over the responsibility. Prejudices against mechanical devices must also be recognized, and a charitable approach should be used with teachers who show this attitude.

After the school audiologist has had a chance to visit the pupils in their classroom and observe their performance, he or she may notice that, although the hearing-aid model and type are apparently satisfactory for the type of loss, the child is not attentive and may actually be failing in the classroom. Other resource specialists may have no other constructive information bearing on achievement, health, or learning. It has been demonstrated that the hearing aid itself may be the crucial factor. The Bess (1971) and Chial (1977) studies have shown that up to 30% of hearing aids tested in the schools are not performing up to the manufacturer's specifications and that some 50% of the hearing aids are malfunctioning. These studies suggest an urgent need for the coordinating role of the school audiologist and the necessity for hearing-aid test equipment in the schools, including real-ear test measurements (the hearing aid *in situ*).

*Classroom Training Units.* Auditory training units (ATUs) over the years have evolved into fairly sophisticated electronic systems. Although some districts may still prefer the portable desk units, the general trend in the past 15 to 20 years has been toward high-powered frequency-modulated radio-frequency (FM-RF) body units. These units operate as a one-way wireless system on radio frequency bands approved by the Federal Communications Commission. The pupil wears the receiver unit and the teacher a microphone transmitter antenna unit. These devices appear either as combined units (regular body-type aid with a snap-on FM unit), closed-loop FM units, or the open RF unit that may be switched either to a conventional hearing-aid circuit or to the RF circuit. Multiple or individual charger units are available as most ATUs employ rechargeable batteries. Obviously both the teacher's microphone and the student's receiver must be compatible for frequency. Adjacent classrooms, of course, must be on different frequency bands.

The school district will be well advised to secure audiologic consultation during the purchasing or leasing negotiations for this type of equipment. The district must also know the warranty terms and maintenance contract conditions in advance of the purchase. The school purchasing agent must be adequately familiar with the philosophy of the program so that the contract will specify suitable amplification without interruption during the school year. These facts must be known, as local hearing-aid repair depots will usually not handle this type of equipment. Audiologists should closely examine the contracts to avoid future problems related to repair time, loaner ATUs, and exchange of frequency modules. As motivation for sales often exceeds facilities for maintenance and repair, the audiologist must coach the school staff to see that units are repaired on schedule and that the pickups are made at times suitable to the school. School districts should be encouraged to purchase or lease extra units and modules for emergencies. It is a matter of great importance that the audiologist meet with the repair technician to learn basic circuitry, simple troubleshooting procedures, and adjustment of internal controls (particularly for low-frequency and maximum-power modification). It is advisable to set the output at 130 dB SPL as a safety precaution. This setting should be verified, however, with a hearing-aid analyzer. Performance characteristics are sometimes not supplied with the ATU nor is it always possible to secure them from the factory. There are as yet no standards for these units.

Parents should be informed by letter that the children will be provided with units for classroom use and that earmolds must be made. Although the cost of impressions and the mold may be carried by the school, parental approval must be granted. Some school systems also provide the ATUs for home use in agreement with a state or private funding source.

Encouraging the use of units in programs whose philosophy is based on total communication can be an exhausting and sometimes futile task, especially if the classroom teacher's orientation is more manual than oral-aural. If the school policy is avowedly dedicated to total communication, the audiologist has no recourse other than to dig in and ferret out those children who can profit by amplification, explain its benefits to the teacher, and demand its consistent usage—a formidable task!

*Hearing Aids versus Classroom Units.* The discussion of classroom units is not complete without mention of their value in comparison with personal hearing aids. The audiologist must make decisions regarding the relative merits of ATUs with earphones or earmolds. If the latter coupling is preferred, the problem is diminished. However, if the child has standard body-type molds for his or her personal hearing aid, the internal ATU volume control will have to be adjusted to avoid blasting.

The matter of hearing aids versus trainers arises chiefly in cases where children have severe losses. Shall the child with a personal aid or aids wear the classroom unit only during school hours? Only during special speech classes? Not at all? Regardless of size, bulk, and the placement of the unit, the child's ears are only 6 to 8 inches from the teacher's mouth when RF units are employed. This intimacy or ''presence'' is not available to the child wearing personal hearing aids. Despite this advantage, pupils at the upper elementary, junior high, and senior high levels resent the conspicuousness of most training units—a body-type aid. A practical solution, and a compromise acceptable to the teen-ager, may be to restrict the use of this equipment to speech and language classes and to allow use of a personal aid during the remaining hours of the school day.

These arguments have been complicated by more extensive use of ear-level and even in-the-ear aids for severe losses. Undoubtedly the microphone is far more effective at ear level than at chest level. The rationale for each type is defensible, but the human variable has yet to be satisfactorily explained. The task, then, for the audiologist is clearly defined: types must be investigated against the criteria of wearability, communication skill, and educational achievement. Unfortunately, the problem cannot be solved in a single sentence; its solution still rests on the shoulders of the school audiologist. It is the audiologist who must spearhead a team approach consisting of the otologist, audiologist, hearing-aid dispenser, parents, child, educational resource personnel members, and often public agencies providing hearing aids.

Experience with this matter leads one to believe that the question of body versus ear-level aids for the child with severe sensorineural hearing loss is still one of the most crucial issues confronting the pediatric audiologist today. The audiologist must exert considerable caution when confronted by irate parents who have been subjected to a sales pitch on ear-level aids by teachers and hearing-aid dispensers. Fortunately (perhaps) for all of us, new advances in powerful ear-level aids have led to the near extinction of body aids. The past 10 years have also been marked by the emergence and popularity of in-the-ear and canal aids.

It is logical to assume that the best amplification will provide the best educational results. Undoubtedly, children with mild to moderate losses, when subjected to tests of educational and communication skills, can show success with ear-level instruments. However, such definitive results for children with only low-frequency residual hearing are hard to come by. At the present, we have only a vague idea of what the severely impaired child must hear. We have yet to develop an electronic filter that can simulate the severe loss. Currently, audiologists have tended to maximize the results of tests of performance, frequency response, maximum power output, and harmonic analysis as a positive indicator of wearability. Such nonsense will continue as long as ignorance regarding true parameters of human hearing loss prevails. As a check on manufacturers' quality control, performance analyzers yield results that may provide useful data. How many of these analyzers, though, utilize new coupler designs? What happens to the ear when signals come through the human system at 130 dB SPL? Such questions may be answered in the future, to be sure, but our strategy for the present must consist of elements of time, patience, and creative observation that are often avoided due to the exigencies of the occasion.

## Auditory Training

It is truly unfortunate that audiologists have been associated more with hardware than with the rehabilitative-educative process. Perhaps some find it more rewarding to deal with electronic gadgets than with people. Whatever the reason, the fact remains that the majority of audiologists prefer to work as diagnosticians; they are somewhat reluctant to take on the role of rehabilitators. The diagnostic process is neat and relatively quick.

In the short history of the study of human communicative disorders, the therapeutic aspects of the field have historically been the domain of the speech pathologist because audiology, as a separate discipline, is new and its rehabilitative aspects generally untried. When cornered, audiologists protest (mightily) that the hearing-aid evaluation is rehabilitative and thus not their responsibility.

School audiologists resist their role as rehabilitators and generally explain that their other duties are so great that they have no time left for this activity. Even if there were one audiologist for every 75 to 100 hearing-impaired children, aural rehabilitation would still play a minor role, since this function is stated as one of the responsibilities of the teacher of the hearing-impaired. These teachers are doing a tremendous job, and many incorporate communication skills in every subject area, particularly in oral-aural schools for deaf children.

Although the new audiologist may have received only 300 to 500 hours of practice in clinical audiology as a student, some of the training should have engendered a feeling for basic principles of the rehabilitative process. Having already tested the child and investigated the efficiency of the amplification utilized, the audiologist is in the unique position of advising the teacher of the child's potential to apprehend certain sounds and suggest techniques for incorporating them into speech. A simple template or overlay showing energy levels of speech sounds as a function of frequency on the audiogram may illustrate this point. Sound-level data collected during classroom activity may modify the teacher's approach to speech, language, and environmental sounds. Although the audiologist may regard this role as assistive, it may prove to be one of dominance.

The fact remains that after the otolaryngologist, the audiologist, and the hearing-aid dispenser have completed their evaluative examinations and fittings, it may be from 6 months to a year before a child is again evaluated, and then the results are measured only in terms of a few hours of observation. Such relatively infrequent visits do not provide the continuous evaluation required for growing children. This situation is an interesting commentary on our philosophy of child care in a culture that specifies a brief evaluative period on the one hand but expects continuity of academic education on the other. Intimately related to this problem are supplementary rehabilitative programs offered to selected children by community and hospital clinics. The selection is primarily based on economic considerations, since current federal subsidies may not be applied to children of the poor. The basis for this determination is that it is the mandate of the public schools to provide such services to children from 3 to 21 years of age. For those who can afford extra training, it is effective only if communication is open and continuous between the public school and the clinic. This communication must not occur just at the specialist level but at the administrative level as well. Audiologists must understand that the legal responsibility for a child enrolled in the public schools rests with the schools. Aural rehabilitation is a technique for facilitating the learning process, wherever it takes place.

## Reports and Forms

The school audiologist, like other public servants, is caught up in a paper-work explosion that inevitably consumes time that could more valuably be spent with children. Audiologists should accept this fact only with great reluctance. A partial solution may rest with the now ubiquitous technique of assigning priorities. The chief priority relates to the child and should always take precedence over other matters of importance to the system. To save time, report forms should be designed so that with a minimum of time a maximum amount of pertinent information can be stated. Computerized programs can be a time-reducing solution in the future, but much thought should precede their use. Software is the problem.

*Evaluation Report.*   The evaluation report should clearly state the findings of the audiologic evaluation. The results of the evaluation should appear on a printed form.

By exercising some ingenuity, most items may be reduced to numbers, check marks, or very brief one-line comments. This report is most important for future reference and as support for a recommendation. The crucial elements are the impressions, observations, and recommendations. In these sections the audiologist specifies operationally the child's behavior, procedures to be followed, the personnel to be informed. The findings are then sent to the principal of the child's school. It is then their joint responsibility to inform both internal and external school personnel of the findings and request subsequent action. A variety of individuals and agencies may be required to fulfill these requests: physicians, school nurses, counselors, teachers, and other resource personnel.

Of equal importance may be the necessity for further testing at some specified date. The form should bear the signature of the audiologist and the supervisor who is legally responsible for the audiology program.

The original copy of the report should stay in the audiology office. Legible copies should be sent to principals and other administrators as necessary. This seemingly minor detail can prove to be of major importance for future retrieval.

Along with this form an audiometric worksheet can be helpful by including a graphic display on a standard audiometric form. Often this kind of display can help explain test results to untrained personnel. According to current regulations in many states, the form must be shown to the parent, if requested. If such is the case, only the audiologist is capable of reviewing test results with the parent, and then only at the school site. The audiogram may be posted on a class bulletin board, but then only with parental approval.

*Referral-for-Service Form.* The purpose of this form, addressed to the audiologist to request evaluation, is to give signing authority to the referring school principal, who validates the form with a signature and date. The procedure holds true even if the actual referral is requested by a classroom teacher, counselor, or other resource personnel at the school. The form should be relatively simple, consisting of identifying data, reason for referral, amplification status, a brief description of classroom behavior, and pertinent physical information.

*Classroom ATU Monitor Form.* With few exceptions, classroom auditory training units are either purchased or leased by the district and therefore subject to some form of audit. Responsibility can rest either with a division, a department, or an individual school. The audiologist shares in this responsibility at whatever level by developing a plan to ensure that the appropriate instrument is compatible with the child's auditory status. Keeping track of the right instrument for the right child is an arduous task for the audiologist—children move on, instruments require repair and adjustment. Teachers require constant reinforcement regarding the instrument's value in the learning process. The primary reason for this form is its applicability to a problem. Monitoring forms will supply both the teacher and the audiologist with information regarding the current status of an instrument.

Teachers should have a simple but complete description of the unit, microphone, charger and receiver, and battery checker, and should be given some simple precautions regarding the maintenance of the system.

*Pupil Schedule Form.* A posted schedule allows clerical staff to inform schools of when students are to be tested, by whom, and at what schools. This control is absolutely necessary if more than one audiologist uses the same test facility. The burden may be eased by prior compromises among audiologists for their choice of test days and times. A major shortcoming is often the lack of a satisfactory solution to the problem of testing the difficult-to-test child. In certain cases two audiologists are used. A much more efficient solution to this problem would be to train aides to help with this type of child.

*Testing Log.* This type of form has proven most effective as a check on the schedule. The form should contain spaces for names, date of entry, date tested, audiologist's initials, a no-show column, and a space for comments. The form also allows for internal control of personnel as well as for a time lapse between entry and scheduling.

*Weekly Activity Report.* Probably the most controversial form that I developed, the weekly activity report is in essence a more palatable euphemism for a time and motion study of the audiologists. The form, developed in conference with our staff, was a weekly report that consisted of two main sections: direct services and indirect services to children. Indirect services accounted for approximately 70% of the clinician's time. The format used to categorize these services is as follows:

| *Direct Services* | *Other Services* |
|---|---|
| Audiologic evaluation | Parent conferences (individual and group) |
| Observation in classroom | Teacher conferences (individual and group) |
| Conferences with pupil | Conferences with other personnel (specify) |
| ATU check | School staff conference |
| Special projects (specify) | Audiology staff conference |
| Other (specify) | Conference with supervisor |
|  | In-service activities (specify) |
|  | Special projects (specify) |
|  | Audiologic reports |
|  | Travel time |
|  | Other (specify) |

Breaking down the entries into half-hour segments allows a fairly accurate accounting that can be utilized internally to compare the efficiency of audiologists. By specifying the similarities and differences in services, a supervising audiologist can explain the business of audiology. Externally the data can be used to negotiate for more space and personnel. In our program enough information was collected after a few months to justify the termination of the reports.

*Parent Forms.* Audiologists often assume that pareants are willing to cooperate with the school's requests for information. They soon learn to modify this assumption and be satisfied with a probability model. Parents are flooded with almost as many notices as are school personnel. The audiologist must enter the contest fully equipped as a personnel relations expert, ready to obtain the attention of the parents. Parents appear to be more mindful of directives sent out by the school principal than of those from other school personnel, and some principals are more skillful at this business than others. Thus, a notice should go out with the principal's signature, as well as the countersignature of the audiologist. Commonly, parents should be notified of the following:

1. Annual goals and objectives for the auditory training program

2. A malfunctioning hearing aid

3. A "forgotten" hearing aid

4. Group or individual conferences

5. Techniques for daily hearing-aid care

6. The location of testing center(s), including a map and appointment data

In districts with large non-English-speaking populations, bilingual personnel will be most beneficial. A language barrier is handicap enough, but that compounded with physical impairment is tragic. Most school districts with sizable minority groups should have translators available. Notices should be simple, clear, concise, and relevant. At the same time, they should be so contrived as to contain an amount of redundancy suitable to the importance of the notice. If the notices require a return, the principal should be requested to supply clerical help to facilitate the return of the form and eventual disposition. Although the care and responsibility for personal hearing aids rest with the parents, the audiologist should also be in communication with the hearing-aid dispenser. He or she should be responsible for putting an entry in the pupil's folder specifying the name, facility, and telephone number of the dispenser. Most dispensers are very cooperative and may provide the best entry to the home.

***Notices to Teachers.*** Although teachers of the deaf and hard-of-hearing are relatively sophisticated about the needs of these children, regular classroom teachers should receive specific information to help them serve this special population. This information can be provided as a set of guidelines* similar to the following:

---

*I am indebted to Noel D. Matkin, PhD, and Joann Sturgeon, MA, of the University of Arizona Children's Hearing Clinic for permission to reprint these guidelines.

## Guidelines for the Classroom Teacher
## Serving the Hearing-Impaired Child

1. *Classroom seating.* Hearing-impaired children should be assigned seats away from hall or street noise and not more than 10 feet from the teacher. Such seating allows the hearing-impaired child to better utilize residual hearing, the hearing aid, and visual cues (speech-reading, gestures, etc.). Flexibility in seating—movable desks and group arrangements—all better enable the hearing-impaired child to observe and actively participate in class activities.

2. *Look and listen.* Children with even a mild hearing loss function much better in the classroom if they can both look and listen.

3. *Check comprehension.* Consistently ask children with a hearing loss an occasional question related to the subject under discussion to make certain that they are following and understanding the discussion. Many hearing-impaired children smile and nod "yes" when they do not understand.

4. *Rephrase and restate.* Encourage hearing-impaired children to indicate when they do not understand what has been said. Rephrase the question or statement since certain words contain sounds that are not easily recognized by someone with defective hearing. Furthermore, most hearing-impaired children have some delay in language development and may not be familiar with key words. By substituting words, the intended meaning may be more readily conveyed.

5. *Pretutor child.* Have hearing-impaired children read ahead on a subject to be discussed in class so they are familiar with new vocabulary and concepts, and thus more easily follow and participate in classroom discussion. Such pretutoring is an important activity that the parents can undertake.

6. *Involve resource personnel.* Inform resource personnel of planned vocabulary and language topics to be covered in the classroom so that pretutoring can supplement classroom activities during individual therapy.

7. *List key vocabulary.* Before discussing new material, list key vocabulary on the blackboard. Then try to build the discussion around this key vocabulary.

8. *Visual aids.* Visual aids help hearing-impaired children by providing the association necessary for learning new things.

9. *Individual help.* The child with impaired hearing needs individual attention. When possible, provide individual help in order to fill gaps in language and understanding stemming from the child's hearing loss.

10. *Write instructions.* Hearing-impaired children may not follow verbal instructions accurately. Help them by writing assignments on the board so they can copy them in a notebook. Also use a buddy system by giving a classmate with normal hearing the responsibility for making certain the hearing-impaired child is aware of the assignments made during the day.

11. *Encourage participation.* Encourage participation in expressive activities such as reading, conversation, story telling, and creative dramatics. Reading is especially important, since information and knowledge gained through reading help compensate for what is missed because of the hearing loss. Again, parents can assist the child through participation in local library reading programs and modeling in the home.

12. *Monitor efforts.* Remember that children with impaired hearing become fatigued more readily than other children because of the continuous strain resulting from efforts to keep up with and compete in classroom activities.

13. *Inform parents.* Provide the parents of hearing-impaired children in your class with consistent input so that they understand the child's successes and difficulties.

14. *S-P-E-E-C-H.* The following mnemonic device has been found helpful by teachers and parents when communicating with hearing-impaired children.

> S = State the topic to be discussed.
>
> P = Pace your conversation at a moderate speed with occasional pauses to permit comprehension.
>
> E = Enunciate clearly, without exaggerated lip movements.
>
> E = Enthusiastically communicate, using body language and natural gestures.
>
> CH = Check comprehension before changing topics.

15. *Monitor hearing aids.* Many children with impaired hearing are wearing hearing aids that are in poor repair. The school audiologist or speech-language pathologist can give you information about how the

hearing aid works and guidance for checking its daily function. Ideally, a battery tester and a hearing-aid stethoscope will be available for the daily hearing-aid check. A small supply of fresh batteries should also be kept at school.

These guidelines are excellent for classrooms being serviced by itinerant hearing specialists. For supplementary materials the audiologist can also solicit free booklets from manufacturers of earmolds, hearing aids, and auditory training units.

## Sound Control of Classrooms

School districts have become increasingly aware of the need for more adequate control of classroom acoustics, not only for special rooms but for regular classrooms as well. Public allocation of funds for schools, however, continues to be scrutinized closely during the 1980s. The tendency has been to restore existing buildings rather than to build new structures expressly designed to include acoustic treatment. This fact poses serious problems to the audiologist, who may recommend sound treatment of classrooms for hearing-impaired children. In the first place, such improvements are quite expensive; secondly, most rooms can only be treated partially, by installing carpet on the floors and acoustically treated ceiling tile that may extend down to chair-rail height. This expense is largely negated by the amount of window space allocated for room brightness and by hard-surfaced hallways and walkways adjacent to the classroom. Administrators also question the need for quietness when the pupils have reduced hearing sensitivity. A useful technique for convincing the administration that acoustic treatment is not only desirable but necessary involves two procedures. The audiologist should take overall and band-filtered sound-level readings at peak levels of classroom activity. These results should be presented in a clear, concise form to the principal. Even more persuasive would be the playing of one of the available tapes made through a hearing aid to school personnel. A most convincing argument to teachers and administrators has been a tape made by Ross and his colleague Randolph (1976) illustrating magnificently how noise and distortion are transmitted through high-power hearing aids. They reported a relatively inexpensive evaluation system employing a cassette recorder and a crutch tip for the cavity-external microphone, with standard tubing to the hearing aid.

Caution should be exercised regarding the importance of sound-level recordings at this point. After the survey has been completed, the administration should be cautioned that much more sophisticated noise-level equipment is available and should be performed by a group qualified not only to record levels but also to advise amelioration of the noise problem. Architectural firms now employ acoustic consultants who are quite familiar with such problems. The important message here is that the audiologist should initiate the proceedings and convince the administration that sound control in classrooms is important to facilitate learning and to reduce classroom confusion and annoyance factors. The audiologist must also know the capabilities and shortcomings of instrumentation, impressing heavily upon school personnel the necessity for improving the classroom milieu.

## Relations with Community Specialists

The school audiologist also acts as a catalyzing agent and ombudsman. A close relationship with children in the schools places the audiologist in a position of authority among local agencies, physicians, clinical audiologists, hearing-aid dispensers, and the schools themselves. This unique position also poses problems that relate to prior diagnosis, medical treatment, and amplification, particularly in urban areas where a high incidence of poverty exists. Areas of poverty demand special consideration as ignorance often accompanies poverty. Some of these children receive competent medical advice and treatment, but the majority are seen by general practitioners who are not experienced with problems related to ear pathology. Children are often referred directly by the practitioner to hearing-aid dispensers, despite regulatory legislation in some states prohibiting this practice. Someone must take the lead in securing adequate diagnosis, treatment, and amplification for such children. The possibility exists, however, that this population is the one identified with almost continuous expenditure of public funds. Early attention will, in the long run, conserve significant future expense. As children grow and change between annual visits to the physician, the audiologist may, by repeated testing and hearing-aid checks, point out the need for intervention by specialists. The resolution of these problems is a long, hard, and frustrating battle, consuming hours of valuable time and requiring almost endless patience.

Public agencies must be contacted to facilitate treatment for children who have been identified as hearing-impaired but who have not been seen by specialists (or have not been seen at all) and are obviously eligible for care. These children are too often victims of understaffed bureaucratic systems whose responsibilities may be so fragmented as to defy description. These are the children who can be helped by the audiologist, who is, in the final analysis, the "court" of last resort. That this is not an impossible task has been demonstrated repeatedly by the intervention of the school audiologist. Community agencies want to help the child, but the vital link is often missing; the school audiologist can provide that missing link. The audiologist's work is follow-up work in the true sense. The rewards are great; the child is served and the community educated.

# School Relations

## Job Description

School audiologists must have a working knowledge of exactly what will be expected of them before accepting a position. Although the preceding guidelines appear obvious, the facts show that there are few precedents currently in existence on a national level. In many cases the new audiologist may be the first one ever hired in either the school district or the state. In my situation, there was no precedent, which meant I created my own job description, namely senior audiologist. In addition, it became necessary to institute positions for those audiologists who, I hoped, would implement my plans. Although I could specify responsibilities in general, I soon found out that the district had somewhat restrictive personnel policies regarding qualifications for both positions. Fortunately, I had already acquired restricted speech and hearing credentials, and subsequently, in hiring future audiologists, I specified that they possess valid credentials. This fact alone considerably reduces the number of available applicants, since most students generally take clinical courses, assuring them of employment in agencies or hospitals only requiring ASHA certification.

There are, fortunately, emergency measures being taken in many states that enable prospective employees to be hired on a temporary basis. As previously mentioned, the California State Commission on Credentials and Licensing has authorized a program certifying audiologists in the public schools.

In the meantime, the chief qualification for the position is either ASHA certification or state licensing and credentials in speech and hearing. Although state licensing in audiology is not required in the schools, it is apparent that the prestige of the audiologist is enhanced by the license.

Furthermore, if the school audiologist performs any service outside of the school system, a license is mandatory in the state of California, as is undoubtedly true with other states. A factor not to be overlooked is the numbers game; the profession must be identified, and numbers help. (Unfortunately, in some states licensure laws have been hindered by well-meaning but misinformed legislators.)

ASHA-based certification, modified to be congruent with the new guidelines specified by the Joint Committee of the American Speech and Hearing Association and the Conference of Executives of American Schools for the Deaf (1976), would be useful as a model for districts considering audiologic services. Presently, the major problem with the guidelines is an excessive amount of optimism regarding case loads and personnel requirements. The guidelines do, however, point toward an ideal that should be sought.

## Job Accountability

The audiology student who has just emerged from a university clinical program enters an environment where, by law, everyone from clerical to professionally certified personnel must be accountable to an individual in a supervisory capacity. In many states, including California, this is a formal annual or biannual requirement; an evaluation of performance and a statement of goals are contained in a written document signed by both the evaluator and the employee. In many respects this is a redundant procedure, since both the code and local district policy contain clauses relative to job accountability. However, its necessity becomes apparent when promotion or dismissal is under consideration and precise written documentation is absolutely necessary, particularly for dismissal. This procedure is extremely valuable because it forces employees to actually set down on paper their goals and objectives and requires supervisors to write out their opinions regarding the past and current performance of employees.

This procedure is of equal importance to the new teacher. Since audiology is a new specialty, the probationary period is one that can either encourage or kill a new program. Initially, the newly hired audiologist must resent being put on the spot, particularly if the evaluator is not an audiologist. However, a realization that the experience may be an educational one to both the evaluator and the district may soothe the novice's sense of pride.

To whom an audiology group should be accountable is a moot point. Traditionally, audiologists have been associated with providers of health services. In the schools, however, the power usually rests with the instructional divisions. The prospective audiologist should, therefore, take a long, hard look at the administrative structure before leaping into a division with a low budget and only intermittent contact with pupils. The temptation to be associated with the physician should be tempered by an awareness that education is the name of the game, not medicine!

## Speech and Language Specialists

By and large, audiologists are "loners" when they enter the public schools. They are often confronted with a bewildering array of specialists, all of whom have specific duties relating to the education of the exceptional child. In addition to working with teachers of the deaf and hard-of-hearing, the audiologist will be working quite closely with the speech and language specialists. The job description of these specialists generally includes working with children who have speech problems related to hearing loss and may even be called speech and hearing clinicians. Their work may often include responsibilities in special schools that encompass either the total population or special classes. This situation may create some initial confusion that may persist until the two specialists negotiate and redefine their responsibilities.

The issue of responsibility delegation with regard to the hearing-impaired child is not new. Audiologists feel that by virtue of their training, they should be the primary providers of such services. The fact remains, however, that in most systems speech and language specialists are well entrenched, simply because for years there were no audiologists available to work with these children.

Audiologists, because of their training, may prefer to restrict their activities to evaluation rather than rehabilitation and, by extension, amplification. In small school districts, the audiologist may be called on to handle an entire continuum of oral-aural training. In large districts, the load may be so great that the audiologist can act only as a consultant to both the teacher of the hearing-impaired and the speech specialist.

Schools whose specialists are currently being hired as language and speech specialists but whose credentials are in the areas of speech, language, and hearing may simply divide their personnel into two categories. By extension, the increase of responsibility regarding the hearing specialist would then include evaluation and amplification procedures. It is interesting to note that in 1975 the California State Board of Education, through one of its commissions, revised the credential structure by creating two new credentials: (1) specialization in clinical or rehabilitative services in the area of language, speech, and hearing services and (2) specialization in clinical or rehabilitative services in the area of audiology. The policy and implementation statements regarding these two specialties defy definition and leave one with the impression that some specialists with an audiologic background are better than others. The language is so stilted and so laden with terminology reminiscent of systems research that it is almost unreadable. Undoubtedly other states are burdened with this problem.

## School Psychologists

Another well-entrenched specialty in public education is school psychology. Psychologists could logically be close allies of the audiologist, as their evaluation program is important to the total evaluation of the child's psychosocial ability as a function of learning, but this is not always the case; their training appears to be negligible in the area of severe hearing loss and deafness. Psychologists are often at a loss when an evaluation must be made almost solely upon the basis of performance rather than verbal skills. If they were to accept this fact and seek guidance from the audiologist, suitable school placement could be facilitated greatly. Meetings to discuss placement of handicapped children could provide an excellent meeting ground to resolve differences in opinion, especially if time has been given to observe the child prior to the meeting. (Both parties will complain, with justification, that their other responsibilities are so great that time is rarely available for extended observation, a complaint common to all resource specialists.)

## School Physicians and Nurses

If a district is fortunate enough to employ an otolaryngologist (even part time), the audiologist will have an excellent resource for consultation, particularly about children with middle ear problems. The situation is more complicated if the physician is not an ear specialist, and action may be slower unless the audiologist builds a strong case for medical or surgical intervention. By and large, most school physicians are pediatricians; they have some knowledge of what transpires behind the eardrum, but it is usually minimal. The audiology unit of the Los Angeles schools was able to provide several lectures a year by local otologists as a component of the district's in-service program. Special invitations were sent to the school physicians and nurses. Fortunately, a large city can support a number of otologists, some of whom are really quite concerned about children and are glad to volunteer their time for such special lectures. Audiologists would be well advised to secure a reprint of the article by Bluestone et al. (1983), which is a comprehensive and thoughtful essay on common middle ear problems of children.

In the last analysis, though, the presence of school nurses is far more valuable. They are in close contact with the children on a day-to-day basis. In addition, nurses generally have the authority to refer the child to an outside physician. Again, the audiologist must come to a meeting of the minds with nurses, who, until an audiologist has been hired, may often serve as amateur audiologists.

## School Committee Functions

*Pupil Placement.*  Hard-of-hearing and deaf children are not automatically placed in special classes; they are admitted only after a school conducts formal and legal procedures that are generally functions of a committee called the Individualized Education Program (IEP) Committee, specified by PL 94-142. Audiologists, as a rule, are not specifically recognized as administrators, whereas experienced special education teachers are. Districts are wise, however, to invite an audiologist to be a member of the committee because the audiologist is the sole member knowledgeable about diagnostic findings (both medical and audiological) and amplification factors. Often the speech pathologist is an invited member of the committee. In California, the law specifies that parents must be invited to the committee meeting at which their child will be discussed, and must be notified of the meeting date well in advance.

Of primary concern to the committee is whether a child is eligible for a special program and whether the district has a program capable of meeting the child's needs. Since every state has minimal criteria for admission into a special program, the audiologist is responsible for checking the child's hearing status against the state criteria. In addition, the audiologist must be able to assure the committee that the medical statement is in general agreement with state criteria. Generally, otologists supply excellent reports, often with complete audiologic and hearing-aid data. The response from hospital clinics is another matter, and the level of their sophistication is generally a measure of the hospital audiologist's ability to secure adequate diagnostic information from a resident staff member.

Generally speaking, committee meetings are not scheduled until all diagnostic information is available. Occasionally the referring audiologist or physician will present an overzealous recommendation for a child's educational management that accomplishes little more than to infuriate the school administrators. Because the parents may be informed of the recommendation, the process can become most uncomfortable. Such recommendations tend to be made in ignorance, but with the aid of a skillful and diplomatic school audiologist, the situation could possibly be remedied.

The audiologist also contributes to the procedure with his knowledge of hearing aids. He can determine, before a child is actually enrolled in a school, whether the hearing aid is in fact functional. Although parents are requested to see that their child is wearing the aid at the committee meeting, between 25% and 50% of the children arrive without amplification. The aid has either been "forgotten" or "lost"; in many cases, it does not even work. In Los Angeles, where the Spanish-speaking population is sizable, children from families who have newly arrived from South and Central America or Mexico have never been fitted with hearing aids. This is also true of immigrant children from Southeast Asia. The recommended procedure then becomes one of trial placement until an aid is purchased or negotiated through state or federal assistance plans.

As much assistance as can be elicited from the parent, some observation of the performance by the child, and a review of the other school data can result in a decision for placement. As part of the decision-making process, the audiologist must exert experience and expertise in answering several important questions. Shall the child be admitted to a special school and, if so, to an oral or a total communication program? Would it be more beneficial to enroll the child in an integrated program within a regular school or in a regular school with itinerant tutoring services?

It is during this discussion that knowledge of the available programs is crucial. Here the audiologist must exercise caution and judgment. The audiologist is not only sending a child out into the world, but also into an educational atmosphere that must be designed to foster academic growth as well as improved communication skills. If the procedure occurs at the beginning of the school year, the decision can bring about dismissal of a teacher because of low enrollment or perhaps hiring of new personnel because of increased enrollment. The parent may have been advised by the referral source that some schools would better fit the needs of their child than others. It is the function of the referring audiologist to specify the type of treatment, not the location. Despite any number of professional opinions that may be offered, by law it is often the decision of the parent that is final.

Another function of the committee is to resolve problems in cases in which the district determines that a child is eligible for special services that are not available within the district. This is a very tense situation, since the district may have to spend a sizable sum of money to send the child to a private school. A parent, for example, might request that the child be enrolled in a private facility that allegedly supplies better individualized services than those supplied by the district. A state department of education consultant may be appointed to investigate the problem, but even so, the responsibility of the audiologist remains constant regarding admission and discharge procedures, and his or her contribution must be restricted to audiologic findings.

*Placement Review.* Frequently there is a need for change in placement of a child within the district to an integrated or a regular school setting. The school recommends that a designated school committee consider the child for a change in school placement. The usual periods for recommending change are at the end of elementary school and the end of junior high school.

In a city as large as Los Angeles, decisions must rest not only on the basis of the mainstream philosophy but also on distance from the home school. In a district of 750 square miles, transportation can pose quite a problem. In smaller districts with no alternatives, the decision is rather simple: the child moves to an area where programs are available. If the audiologist has been rendering attentive service, his or her position is generally in agreement with the teacher. However, the procedure is based primarily on educational achievement, and any information that the audiologist can offer will be seriously considered in the final decision. As the decision is based on current needs, the audiologist may also be called upon to administer further hearing tests and hearing-aid evaluations just prior to the meeting, particularly if the previous evaluation was equivocal. Following this evaluation, tests might also indicate that the child is making better use of amplification as measured by educational achievement.

## The School Principal

Coordinators and supervisors may have a high ranking in the hierarchy of a school system, but in truth the principal runs the school and ranks immediately under the superintendent in level of administration. The new audiologist should be aware of this fact. Some principals rank higher than others; the secondary-school principal is not only paid more but has a larger staff. Assuming that the majority of the audiologist's load will be composed of elementary school children, the audiologist should exert considerable effort not only in rendering services to the pupils but in trying to make the job easier for the principal. The audiologist who can understand the dilemma faced by the principal in this age of specialists is well on the way to becoming a valuable adjunct to the school team. On one hand, the principal-as-administrator would prefer audiologists to be full-time members of the school staff; but on the other hand, the principal also realizes that they are employed by a division and, therefore, must be part-time help. The work week must be planned carefully yet flexibly; schedules must be discussed with each principal. Obviously all principals are not alike, and presuppositions must be reduced accordingly. The principal is the audiologist's strongest ally, so successes as well as failures should be shared.

Principals can assist with interpretations of the administrative codes, facilitate relations with teachers, and supply important information regarding pupil status.

It might be suggested to prospective school audiologists that they obtain first-hand experience in public education by following a principal around the school for at least one full school day. In fact, it would be advisable to spend at least one day in a special school, in a school with "integrated" classes, and in a school that provides itinerant services to the hearing-impaired child.

## Education Codes and School Policies

Commonly state educational systems have, by law, a set of rules and regulations that ensure conformity by the school districts. This law is then transposed into district policy. Several small districts may join forces by consolidating or unifying services and may fall under the governance of a county, which in turn is responsible to the state. In California, for example, the state supplies partial funding according to a formula that, with local revenue, allows the district to stay in business. California also specifies certain programs to be mandatory; it then becomes the responsibility of the district to allocate necessary funding. In the case of special education programs, the school district may well be reimbursed by the state.

In many states speech, hearing, and language programs come under the heading of "physical handicaps." The area of hearing disorders is further divided into subcategories: the deaf, the severely hard-of-hearing, and the moderately hard-of-hearing. The districts are, by law, required to instruct this population between the ages of 3 and 21. Fortunately, the definitions for each are quite broad and extend by decibel level (presumably in hearing level) from over 70 dB down to 20 dB in the better ear in the "speech range." The language is somewhat quaint regarding the authority to label. As an example, note the extreme diversity in the following corrective measures. A hearing specialist and a qualified educator can recommend special placement for the deaf child; a licensed physician and surgeon can diagnose a severely hard-of-hearing child; and a licensed physician and surgeon, audiologist, or teacher holding a certificate in the area of speech and hearing handicaps can recommend remedial instruction for the moderately hard-of-hearing!

The actual reason for lack of regulations and methods of funding for audiologists is that such functions have been assumed to be accomplished outside the system. It is also presupposed that these functions can be performed, in part, by the teacher of the deaf or the speech and hearing specialist after being identified by the school audiometrist. The school audiometry identification program, incidentally, is mandated in California, and the results of pure-tone threshold tests performed by the audiometrist are considered to be one of the requirements for entrance into special programs.

The California education code also specifies that an experimental program may be petitioned by a district to the state superintendent of public instruction for deaf and severely hard-of-hearing infants, subject to an annual review for continuance. This program was not mandated, however, and despite our knowledge of optimal ages for instruction, there are few viable programs for very young children in the state. There is nothing in the code that allows for special instruction of pupils with a unilateral hearing loss unless the child has a speech or language problem; in this case, the child is then eligible for the speech program.

There may be funds available for children who are eligible for mainstreaming. As a matter of fact, there was one such clause in the California code that enabled us to hire two audiologists. This clause was interpreted by the district as authority to hire audiologists to evaluate, not identify, children with hearing losses who did not qualify for the hard-of-hearing program. Retrospectively, the acquisition of personnel by this technique may have been somewhat questionable, but the positions were obtained.

Equally important, the audiologist should systematically research current state codes and look for regulations that have even the slightest bearing on hearing handicaps. More to the point, the audiologist should enroll in either college or in-service courses relating to school finance and law. The slight amount of time spent in such continuing education efforts will pay off. One of the remarkable failings with students entering public education from our field is their apparent lack of interest in educating themselves in these vital areas of school administration.

Not all hearing-impaired pupils are found in programs for the deaf and hard-of-hearing; a sizable number are enrolled in other special programs because the primary disability is other than the hearing handicap. They may be found in the speech, developmentally delayed, autistic, aphasic, and orthopedically handicapped programs. The problem of assistance to these other handicapped pupils lies with the philosophy of the programs and the priority system developed by the audiologist. The district may want priority given to those children who are not in the hearing program, based on the assumption that these children are already being instructed by special teachers. However, the audiologist's chief responsibility rests with the severely hard-of-hearing and deaf child. If time is available, the needs of the moderately hearing-impaired come next. This ordering of priorities, however, may be a trap and can result in more intensive work with fewer children while children with moderate handicaps and higher potential are neglected.

On the other hand, there may be no options. Such was the case in the Los Angeles city schools when the program started. Enrollment in the hearing-impaired program totaled 1,000 children, and there were only four audiologists. Despite the efforts of other programs to engage our services, we had little time left over and had to take a firm stand. It was hoped at the time that as the program developed, the district would see how important it was and create positions for more audiologists. The program now has nine audiologists.

Putting our problem into perspective, we soon discovered that our priorities were quite minor when compared to those of the regular instructional program. However, PL 94-142 now includes programs for audiologists. Unless professional workers at the local and state levels do not become immediately aggressive, other special services will make their own claims. The law requires that the school file a statement through the district to the state regarding an IEP. If audiological care is not included on the IEP, funds will not be earmarked for that purpose. Great emphasis should also be placed on the importance of pushing particularly hard for required preschool services. This priority should be attractive to the district as it may secure discretionary funds for this purpose.

Audiologists need help to interpret the law, to advise on action programs, to assure front-line visibility. They stand on the threshold of one of the great areas for growth in the field. The facts should be obtained and advertised to potential lawmakers, public figures, state consultants, and school boards. Public school is where the action is!

## Aides and Assistants

There are very few professions, regardless of work setting, that do not require the use of support personnel. In public schools precedents have already been set in almost every area of instruction. The audiologist needs two types of assistants—testing and technical. The test assistants are invaluable to the audiologist, particularly with difficult-to-test children. Chiefly they act as aides in the test room, but they are also needed to assist with the details of arranging schedules and transportation. These tasks are time-consuming and relatively costly to the district when performed by the audiologist. The technical assistant can be of tremendous help in running frequency curves on hearing aids and auditory training units. In addition, the technical assistant can coordinate the details of repair and maintenance of such units. Technicians, properly trained, can also measure noise levels in classrooms.

For both types of support the chief objective is to have the assistant perform those functions that do not require the expertise of the professional. Relinquishing these functions is often threatening, but in the long run it will afford the audiologist time for the principal responsibility— the face-to-face relations with the hearing-impaired child. The addition of supportive personnel may be generally viewed with approval by the administration; providing a carefully designed proposal shows exactly how the district can conserve funds while providing more and better services to the pupil. The audiologist should take the time to get the facts and present them with clarity; the administration will listen.

## Transportation

To an audiologist in a clinical setting, transportation of patients may never become an issue. In schools that must adhere to laws governing the transportation of school children from one place to another during the school day, it certainly is an issue. If the district either owns or has access to mobile test units or satellite centers, the battle is practically won; the tests and evaluations can be performed at or near the home school site. However, in some districts, children may have to be bused to a central test site that could be miles away from their home school.

Preferably, the child should be driven by the parents to the test site. Surprisingly, few parents are available during the school day, for a variety of reasons: care for preschoolers in the family is not available, the mother does not know how to drive, or both parents work. Calls to the home, both written and verbal, may fail to elicit any response. Only a few parents can drive their children for this service. Thus, between the audiologist, the classroom teacher, and the principal a plan must be devised that will accommodate not only district transportation but also suitable scheduling dates. Some schools in large districts have assistants or aides who are bonded to perform such services, but as a rule the children must be driven only in school buses.

Procuring a special bus for such a specific purpose and for such a small group is a sizable problem of logistics. The bus may also have to be equipped with specialized accessories necessary to transport handicapped children. The buses are available only between their regular morning and afternoon runs, so the time left for testing may total only 4 hours per day. In order to make the operation minimally efficient, at least one or two children should be scheduled per day. The audiologist may not have an aide at the test site, and the home school may have to provide such personnel. This entails more paper work, telephone calls, and teacher conferences.

Audiologists become further involved in transportation when they examine noise conditions on the bus. The Los Angeles system found that the noise level at the driver's seat averaged 94 dBA. Sound-treating at high-vibration locations reduced the noise level to between 82 and 85 dBA at the cost of about $300 per bus. These facts are cited here simply to illustrate a little known area of concern that may prove to be an important one for the school audiologist and also one that should be investigated when a program is initiated.

## In-Service Training

For an individual dedicated to a career of helping others, education should never cease. Personal frustration and dissatisfaction are the hallmarks of a successful clinician. School audiologists are in a much better position to observe success in rehabilitation than fellow clinical audiologists because of almost daily contact with the children over an extended period of time. The proximity and continuity in such a working situation provide constant reminders of success and failure, which, of course, promote professional growth. Growth can be stimulated by perceptive observation, and such observations should be reported to others—not only to audiological colleagues but to other associates involved in the rehabilitative process. Individuals and the community must be served by conducting training sessions that come from such insightful experience. Just as rewarding as informing others is the process of learning how others operate.

In-service training can be divided into two categories: internal and external. Internal sessions are important to fellow audiologists in the district; external sessions benefit other resource personnel in the district as well as concerned groups in the community.

*Internal Training.*   Audiologists should know what other services within the district's system can offer in terms of information and cooperation. Directors of personnel, psychology, nursing, audiometry, speech and language, and deaf and hard-of-hearing programs are generally delighted to provide information regarding their responsibilities. Coordinators of other special education programs are also resources that should be tapped. This type of education cannot be secured from colleges and universities in the same intimate fashion that it can be obtained from fellow employees. Inevitably such sessions promote cross-fertilization of ideas that directly improve services.

In-service training provides the necessary experiences not yet generally provided by formal education. As a matter of fact, it may not even be necessary for students in training to be knowledgeable about topics that can be learned while on the job. However, what Comfort (1974) calls "the American infatuation with mandarin education" may well defeat this philosophical point of view, and the tendency for preservation may be too strong to override such a practical solution. Perhaps we lack the maturity or the opportunity to exercise our talent.

*External Training.*   The value of listening to parents and concerned professionals in the community should never be underestimated. Representatives from social and welfare agencies and hospital clinics, otologists, and hearing-aid dispensers can enable the audiologist to feel the pulse of the community. It is surprising to see how enthusiastically most speakers welcome new activities in the schools. The in-service concept can take other and equally important forms.

One in-service meeting in our district, for example, was a 2-hour afternoon session for hearing-aid dispensers in the community. The meeting was not held to inform them of ongoing activities, but rather to share the school district's pupil placement procedures in the special education division. The session apparently explained to them for the first time the school's responsibilities and restrictions concerning the handicapped child. Another meeting was held for local audiologists and otologists. Only one otologist attended, but he was the director of resident training in otolaryngology from a large county hospital. Perhaps a future generation of otolaryngologists may benefit from his knowledge.

A very successful joint conference was offered by our unit and the staff of the Hearing and Speech Clinic, Children's Hospital of Los Angeles.

The rationale developed from a community need for better communication between the public school audiology programs of the city and county and private and institutional audiologists in the greater Los Angeles area. By common agreement, the subject that required the most clarification and the most cooperation between these two forces was the general need for discussion of wearable hearing aids and auditory training units. The conference opened with presentations of a number of discussion topics. After these openers, the participants were divided into four groups consisting of 15 members each. Also included in each group were invited principals, teachers, and other related resource personnel over and above the participants. Discussion of items was followed by splendid summarizing statements from each group, and the experience generated a follow-up conference. Such in-service conferences based on the discussion concept, rather than a didactic one, are well worth the time and effort.

## School Organizations, Unions, and Professional Organizations

As an employee of a school district, the audiologist's basic loyalties and obligations are to the district. The division in which one operates may have an organization. If an interest is taken in the status of a division and how it can be improved, the most effective results can be obtained by direct involvement in the organization. The same may be said for state teachers' associations, which offer worthwhile fringe benefits that certain individuals can ill afford to neglect. Diverse backgrounds have led many people to eschew organizations. If such is the case, a review of their pros and cons should be considered, especially when contemplating membership in a teachers' union. One can be assured that the administrators are generally well organized, as are the majority of other certified and classified personnel.

These organizations have powerful lobbies in state governments. Union organization can be highly beneficial, as group representation is often the most efficient way of effecting change.

Although ties may exist to the American Speech-Language-Hearing Association by certification, its services have been designed to help and not hinder professional growth. The same logic pertains to state speech and hearing associations.

School audiology is a relatively new area, and the profession needs constant input. Another organization, the Council for Exceptional Children, through its Division for Children with Communication Disorders, welcomes contributions, as does the Academy of Rehabilitative Audiology.

It may be found, however, that a district is only interested in releasing an individual for professional meetings if that person is a contributor, which should be a stimulus for participation. The pay received may be nothing more than not being docked for released time. This indifference may stem from an anti-intellectual administration. Notice should be taken, however, of pension plans and fringe benefits, for school professionals are often the envy of their colleagues in private practice and community agencies. Besides, business-related travel, convention dues, and other professional expenses are all tax deductible.

# Summary

School audiology is an emerging specialty within the broad area of pediatric audiology. A chief difference between the clinical and the school audiologist revolves around the primacy of the diagnostic function of the former and the rehabilitative-educative role of the latter.

Although both pursue the goals of efficient amplification, the school audiologist is in the superior position of being able to monitor, almost daily, performance of both the hearing-impaired child and the hearing aid. The school audiologist is a public servant, working in an environment that is under public scrutiny and, therefore, more restrictive than other areas of audiology. However, a knowledge of school hierarchies, policies, and administrative codes may alleviate the burden considerably. The school audiologist should realize that the position offers a unique opportunity to observe and share closely the personal growth of the hearing-impaired child.

Although school audiology is apparently gaining ground, we do not have precise yearly statistics since 1975, when PL 94-142 was implemented. If the field is growing, it is probably a slow growth and may even tumble somewhat with the ebb and flow of our economy. Perhaps in the future school districts will not be able to afford full-time audiologists and may opt for contractual arrangements with a growing number of small corporate organizations. I foresee such organizations supplying a complete package offering diagnostic testing, in-service training, and the fitting and dispensing of hearing aids. I feel confident that all hearing-impaired children from infancy through secondary school will be served—regardless of the type of delivery system and the type of provider. Cost effectiveness remains the buzz phrase. All things considered, let us hope that care for these children will prosper!

# References

Berg, F. S., Blair, J. C., & Wilson-Vlotman, A. (1984). *Educational audiology directory*. Logan, UT: Department of Communicative Disorders, Utah State University.

Bess, F. H. (1977). Condition of hearing aids worn by children in a public school setting. In *The condition of hearing aids worn by children in a public school program* (pp. 13–23). HEW Publication No. 77-05002 (OE). Washington, DC: U.S. Government Printing Office.

Bluestone, C. D., Klein, J. O., Paradise, J. L., Eichenwald, H., Bess, F. H., Downs, M. P., Green, M., Berko-Gleason, J., Ventry, I. M., Gray, S. W., McWilliams, B. J., & Gates, G. A. (1983). Workshop on effects of otitis media on the child. *Pediatrics, 71* (4) 639–652.

Chial, M. R., (1977). Electroacoustic assessment of children's hearing aids. In *The condition of hearing aids worn by children in a public school program* (pp. 25–51). HEW Publication No. 77-05002 (OE). Washington, DC: U.S. Government Printing Office.

Cohen, S., Evans, G. W., Krantz, D. S., & Stokols, D. (1980). Physiological, motivational, and cognitive effects of aircraft noise on children. *American Psychologist, 35*, 231–243.

Comfort, A. (1974) The American infatuation with mandarin education. *Center Report* [Center for the Study of Democratic Institutions], *7* (5), 25–27.

Garwood, V. P. (1979). Audiology in the public schools. In L. J. Bradford & W. G. Hardy (Eds.), *Hearing and hearing impairment* (pp. 299–309). New York: Grune and Stratton.

Joint Committee of the American Speech and Hearing Association and Conference of Executives of American Schools for the Deaf. (1976). Guidelines for audiology programs in educational settings for hearing-impaired children. *Asha, 18*, 291–294.

Luterman, D. (1979). *Counseling parents of hearing-impaired children*. Boston: Little, Brown.

Miller, J. M., & Pfingst, B. E. (1984). Cochlear implants. In C. I. Berlin (Ed.), *Hearing science* (pp. 309–339). San Diego: College-Hill Press.

99th Congress produces "landmark" legislation. *Asha, 29* (1), 10.

Randolph, K. (1976). Checking hearing-aid operation using a cassette recorder. *Audiology and Hearing Education, 7* (1), 28, 40.

Ross, M. (1976). The incidence of hearing-aid malfunction: A review and some recommendations. Unpublished manuscript.

Wilson-Vlotman, A. L., & Blair, J. C. (1986). A survey of audiologists working full-time in school systems. *Asha, 28* (11), 33–38.

# Author Index

# Subject Index

**Dr. Frederick N. Martin** is the Lillie Hage Jamail Centennial Professor in Speech Communication, The University of Texas at Austin, where he won the Award for Teaching Excellence from the College of Communication. A Fellow of the American Speech-Language-Hearing Association, he is author or editor of over 100 publications in the field of audiology, including the best-selling *Introduction to Audiology* (3rd edition, Prentice-Hall, 1986), *Basic Audiometry* (PRO-ED, 1986), *Principles of Audiology* (PRO-ED, 1984), *Medical Audiology* (Prentice-Hall, 1981), *Pediatric Audiology* (Prentice-Hall, 1978), *Clinical Audiometry and Masking* (Bobbs-Merrill, 1972), and Prentice-Hall's series, *Remediation of Communication Disorders*. Additionally, Dr. Martin was coeditor of *Audiology: A Journal for Continuing Education*, has authored or coauthored more than 60 convention papers, and has written more than 75 book reviews.